Facial Volumization with Fillers

Kyle K. Seo

Facial Volumization with Fillers

Springer

Kyle K. Seo
Modelo Clinic
Seoul
Korea (Republic of)

ISBN 978-981-33-6214-7   ISBN 978-981-33-6212-3 (eBook)
https://doi.org/10.1007/978-981-33-6212-3

This Springer imprint is published by the registered company Springer Nature Singapore Pte Ltd.
The registered company address is: 152 Beach Road, #21-01/04 Gateway East, Singapore 189721, Singapore

This book is dedicated to my children, Seongwon, Hyejune, and Yejin, who give me hope and motivation in life.

Preface

Aging of the face is not merely the result of wrinkling of the skin from age-related loss of dermal elasticity but more significantly due to the loss of continuity in the facial contour caused by the sinking and sagging of the face with age. Injectable fillers are youth-restoring in this respect as they serve not only to fill etched-in grooves and creases but also to plump up facial volume depressions and thus help restore the convexity and fullness of the face seen in youth. Indeed, injectable fillers together with botulinum toxin injections represent the two most essential tools in the esthetic practitioner's armamentarium of facial rejuvenation treatments. Today, injectable fillers have evolved beyond a rejuvenation tool for recapturing youth and have become a significant beautification tool for unlocking facial beauty. Based on the multifaceted three-dimensional assessment of the face, injectable fillers serve not only to reshape the facial contour when placed in the receded chin, sunken cheeks, and areas of facial asymmetry but also to enhance and beautify individual facial features, for example, by projecting the nose and plumping the lips. While soft tissue fillers have been customarily referred to as *dermal* fillers ever since collagen fillers first made their debut back in the 1980s, it might be high time they were referred to instead as *volume* fillers in light of their increasingly larger role and versatility as volume enhancers.

In these pages, I have attempted to provide a comprehensive A to Z guide to filler injection techniques for facial volumization which have been honed and refined over my 20 years of clinical experience with soft tissue fillers. The Asian face is inherently rounder and flatter compared to the Caucasian face. Within the Asian demographic, this has created a desire for and popularity of various volumizing filler applications for adding definition and projection to the face, with augmentations of the forehead, nose, and chin being among some of the most highly requested indications. Notably, the cheeks are a common area for volumization in Korean patients, who aspire to have a baby-like face with full, chubby cheeks—a hallmark of the ideal *Korean look*, which a Caucasian patient may happen to find less appealing.

On top of this robust demand for facial volumization with soft tissue fillers, the Korean market for HA fillers is capable of supplying HA fillers at prices more affordable than anywhere else in the world due to the fierce competition among different brands. It is thus reasonable to conclude that this interplay between the supply- and demand-side factors puts Asia ahead of Western countries in terms of the sheer number of facial volumization treatments performed. As a testament to this buoyant trend, I have had the pleasure of being recognized as "Asia's Top Belotero® Injector" by Merz, Germany, for three consecutive years from 2018 to 2020. In 2019 alone, as it turns out, I used over 7000ml of Belotero® HA fillers in my practice. Besides Belotero, I also regularly use Restylane® and other local HA filler brands for treating between 20 and 30 patients per day, which translates into more than 5000 cases performed annually. The ten thousand hour rule popularized by Malcolm Gladwell famously dictates that it takes four hours of practice per day for ten years to achieve mastery in a given field. By this standard, I suppose I qualify as a master injector, considering I have been practicing injectable filler procedures for over 20 years, the recent ten years of which I have dedicated exclusively to botulinum toxin and filler treatments,

However, to reach this stage in my career, I admit numerous trials and errors have been made along the way. Several episodes come to mind. Back in 2000 when I had first started injecting fillers, fillers had yet to be used for facial volume replacement. Thus, when an elderly patient in her 70s presented for treatment of her severe nasojugal grooves, I applied the same approach I had typically used for treating the glabella frown lines, injecting only minimal amounts of HA filler superficially in the dermis and sub-dermis of the anterior malar, and was left to wonder why nothing was happening. Indeed I had my moments of highs and lows and everything in between during my years of practice with filler treatments. I recall how I almost leaped with elation upon learning hyaluronidase could be used to melt away irregularities from HA fillers and, conversely, how I agonized over the unexpected allergic reactions suffered by a patient after her hyaluronidase injections. There were also times when, for lack of knowledge, I resorted to antibiotics for treating a delayed-type hypersensitivity reaction related to BDDE or HA impurities, misunderstanding it to be an infection-related inflammation. Of course, as a practitioner I have also had my fair share of vascular complications from inadvertent intravascular injections of HA filler, though fortunately, none of these events ever escalated to disastrous skin necrosis. In fact, most of the HA filler- related complications described in this book are based on my own clinical experience. It is against this backdrop that this book was written, in the hope of providing fellow practitioners who are either just starting out on their practice with injectable fillers or who still lack the confidence in performing this procedure with the equivalent of a Drivers Manual, and lay out the safe and effective treatment practices drawing on the trials and errors I confess to have committed in my practice while learning things from scratch.

The three key factors physicians typically consider when selecting a filler product are safety, longevity, and price. Among those, safety takes first priority as injectable fillers represent an extraneous substance introduced into the human body. While collagen stimulators or semipermanent fillers provide a better, more prolonged duration of effect, HA outperforms all other types of soft tissue fillers currently on the market in terms of its excellent safety profile. Not only does HA consist of the same substance naturally occurring in the human body, but it represents the only type of injectable filler reversible with the injection of hyaluronidase should problems occur. It is for this reason that I almost exclusively use HA fillers in my practice and why this book also primarily describes the use of HA fillers.

Meanwhile, Asians and Caucasians differ both in their structural facial anatomy and the respective facial beauty standards they pursue, which should be appreciated when undertaking filler treatments. For example, the Asian face is wider and flatter compared with the more dimensional and narrower Caucasian face. This explains why a prominent zygoma and well-defined jaws are regarded as desirable beauty traits within the Western culture, while square jaw reduction with botulinum toxin are so popular among Asians who wish to slim down their broad faces. In the same context, while a midface augmentation in a Caucasian patient typically consists of increasing the lateral cheek projection to accentuate the coveted Ogee curve, such an approach is rarely practiced in Koreans as they tend to disfavor having a prominent zygoma. Conversely, whereas Koreans generally aspire to have a baby face with full plump cheeks, Caucasians tend to find such soft rounded features less appealing.

Such differences in ethnic esthetic standards are a constant theme running through many of the discussions contained in this book. I do accept, however, that a relatively larger portion of the book has been dedicated to strategies relevant to Asian patients, for which I seek the reader's kind understanding. That said, given that most of the available literature or publications dealing with the use of injectable fillers are written solely with the Caucasian patient in mind, this book may perhaps offer more balanced guidance, reflecting the facial aesthetic standards of both Asian and Caucasians and allowing practitioners to deliver adequately customized treatments tailored to the aesthetic needs of different ethnic patients. Driven by the strong influence of the Korean wave throughout many parts of the world via K-pop and K-drama, the Korean look has been established as a distinct and dominant feature of the Asian aesthetic standard. In some respects, therefore, the strategies laid out in the book may generally resonate with the broader Asian demographic who also favor the prevailing Korean beauty standard.

The injection techniques prescribed in this book are based not on the Consensus Data but instead on the specific approaches I actually employ in my own practice. In fairness, different doctors may hold different views on some of the points I cover. That notwithstanding, the effectiveness of the injection techniques presented in this book has been established based upon the extensive patient cases I have performed over the past 20 years and will be of relevance for those seeking some practical pointers in performing facial volumization with fillers. To the extent no single method can be upheld as absolute, however, I am more than happy to entertain any further input and constructive critique from respected colleagues reading this book,

While my primary motivation for writing this book was to put together an equivalent of *a Drivers Manual* to help other physicians navigate a safer and more pleasant journey through the complexities of volumizing filler treatments, part of the reason was also to give myself an opportunity to look back and take stock of the past 20 years of my career built mostly around injectable filler treatments. If my previous book "*Botulinum Toxin for Asians (Springer, 2017)*" published four years ago represented my first child, this work represents the second child I bring into this world, for which I have both high expectations and corresponding concerns. Finally, it is my sincere hope that "Facial Volumization with Fillers" and, hopefully, its future 2nd and 3rd editions with updated and expanded information will continue to serve as a valuable and relevant source of current knowledge and insight on filler injection procedures for interested readers all over the world.

Kyle K. Seo
March, 2021 Seoul, Korea

Acknowledgment

There are plenty of people who helped in bringing this book to fruition, whom I wish to recognize and acknowledge.

Words *cannot* express my feelings of gratitude for Ms. Sanhyo Kim, who was responsible for translating this book into the English language. As a conference interpreter, Ms. Kim has worked closely with me during the past 10 years as my English teacher, based on which she was able to accurately convey the subtlest of nuances in my original manuscript with exceptional flair. It was also her occasional prodding that helped keep my progress on schedule. I especially appreciate how she put this work before all her other commitments during the final weeks to allow timely completion of this book.

As always, I am eternally grateful to my dear friend professor Hee-Jin Kim of Yonsei University for lending his rich and invaluable insight into the discipline of facial anatomy for this work and for graciously providing me with the brilliant selection of photographic images. Without his experiences and support, this book would not have the robust and rigorous anatomical foundation upon which it stands

A very special thanks indeed to Ms. Hye Won Hur, one of the greatest illustrators I could ever imagine working with, who truly took this book to the next level by enriching it with her beautiful and super accurate anatomic illustrations. Ms. Hur is a student of Prof. Kwan-Hyun Yoon of Incheon University and Representative of Mediart, who had been responsible for providing the illustrations contained in *Botulinum toxin for Asians (Springer, 2017)*. Having obtained her degree as a Bachelor of Fine Arts, she is currently studying anatomy as a Ph.D. student at the Department of Orthodontics, Yonsei University. Judging from the phenomenal energy and brilliant ingenuity she demonstrated throughout the course of this project, I have no doubt in my mind that she is indeed a master in the making in the field of medical art illustration. *The student has become the master*, as the saying goes.

I would also like to express my sincere gratitude to Dr. Per Winlof of Galderma and Mr. Sin-Gu Lee (head of R&D center, JETEMA) for their invaluable insight and advice regarding HA filler manufacturing and filler rheology, topics on which the author cannot claim to be an expert. Their experience and support has been indispensable to preparing Chap. 2 Volumizing Fillers of this book, and any credit for the level of detail and perfection embodied in the said chapter should go to them.

Finally, I wish to give a big shout out to my amazing staff for their hard work in compiling the copious amounts of material and images accompanying the manuscript as well as contributing their photographs for inclusion in the book. I am forever in their debt.

My heartfelt appreciation also goes to Galderma and Merz for their generosity in providing me with the numerous invaluable photos that significantly helped to enrich the content of this book.

March, 2021 Kyle K. Seo

Contents

About the Author

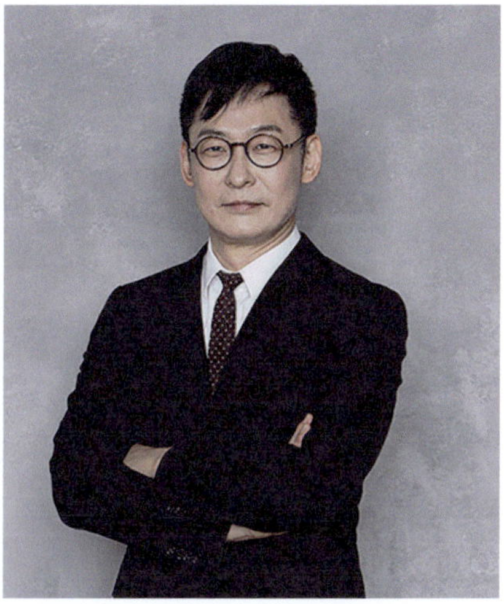

Kyle K. Seo is a dermatologist based in Seoul. He received his M.D. and Ph.D. from Seoul National University College of Medicine, Seoul, South Korea. He became a Clinical Professor in the Department of Dermatology of Seoul National University College of Medicine as a chief of the Botox Clinic. Presently, he is also the Director of Modelo Clinic in Seoul, South Korea. He also leads the Korean Dermatology Society as a President of the Korean Society for Dermatologic Surgery.

He has worldwide reputation as an authority in the field of botulinum toxin and fillers. He was the first doctor in Korea to have launched a hands-on training course on botulinum toxin and fillers, namely the "Modelo Academy," open since 2002. He has also published extensively on the areas of botulinum toxin and filler treatments including "Botulinum Toxin for Asians (Springer 2017)" and "Clinical Anatomy of Face for Botulinum Toxin and Filler Injection (Springer, 2016)." His extensive experience provided him many opportunities to lecture internationally on the subject of botulinum toxin and filler. In recognition of his exceptional dedication and prominent academic achievements, he was ultimately selected as the sole keynote speaker to represent the entire global cosmetic field at the plenary session of the 23rd World Congress of Dermatology (Vancouver 2015) and also chaired the botulinum toxin and filler session of the 24th World Congress of Dermatology (Milan 2019).

He also dedicated himself to promoting global academic activity in the dermatology society as the Vice President of the local organizing committee for the 22nd World Congress of Dermatology (WCD) (Seoul, 2011) and the Secretary-General of the local organizing committee for the 36th annual meeting of the International Society for Dermatologic Surgery (ISDS) (Seoul, 2015).

1 Pretreatment Assessment

1.1 Introduction

As with all other aesthetic procedures, the value of an individual approach cannot be emphasized enough in facial filler procedures. Delivering elaborately tailored treatment outcomes starts with a detailed assessment of the individual face, based on which a customized treatment strategy catering to the unique needs of each patient should be established. Factors to be considered during this assessment consist largely of subjective and objective appraisal of the face. Other relevant aspects including the sociocultural environment of the patient, ethnic aesthetic preferences, and gender-specific characteristics should also be broadly taken into consideration. This chapter outlines the approaches for identifying the patient's subjective aesthetic desires and expectations and covers the steps for undertaking an objective evaluation of a patient's face, including the assessment of facial shape, aging-related changes, facial symmetry, overall balance of proportions, profile view of the face, and dynamic expressions during facial animation. On this basis, the following pages explain how to formulate an individualized treatment plan which also comprehensively considers such other relevant factors as past medical history of cosmetic interventions, socioeconomic conditions, ethnic aesthetic ideals, gender-based differences, and budgetary considerations of the patient.

1.2 Individualized Assessment

During pretreatment consultations, it is important to establish the relevant patient factors that may potentially affect treatment outcomes. These include subjective, objective, sociocultural, and financial conditions as well as past medical history of aesthetic procedures. *Individualized treatment* in the truest sense can be delivered only by a treatment strategy that caters to the unique needs of the individual patient across each of these aspects.

1.2.1 Subjective Factors

Given the subjective nature of beauty, it is vital first and foremost to establish precisely what the individual patient perceives as a key aesthetic concern in his or her face. In order words, it is necessary to clarify the patient's main treatment goal and to make sure both the patient and practitioner are on the same page regarding this aesthetic goal. While some patients may be more concrete in articulating their exact aesthetic concerns down to the specific type of wrinkle they wish to have addressed, others may be more vague in their request and ask simply to have, for example, *a more youthful look* or *a softer appearance*. In this case, the practitioner is advised to dig deeper into the question and encourage the patient to specify their treatment priorities in more precise terms. This is because patients will not be pleased with the treatment outcome at the end of the day unless their initial presenting com-

K. K. Seo, *Facial Volumization with Fillers*, https://doi.org/10.1007/978-981-33-6212-3_1

plaints have been satisfactorily resolved even if positive improvements have been made in other respects. To this end, in my practice, I usually hold a mirror to the patient and ask them to pinpoint what it is exactly that bothers them about their faces (Fig. 1.1a). Such "mirror consultation" has the advantage not only of allowing the perceived defect(s) to be appreciated and expressed in richer detail but also of allowing the patient to realize any other issues that they may have previously failed or neglected to notice and inspire them to seek solutions for those as well. Moreover, applying the spreading test or the compression test at this stage can further help the patient visualize the expected outcome post-treatment (Fig. 1.1b).

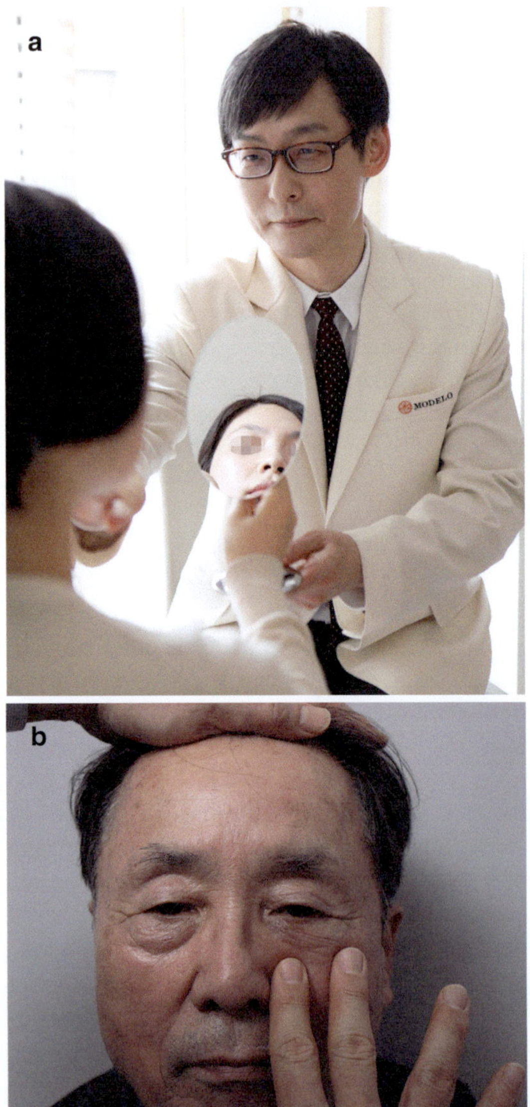

Fig. 1.1 (**a**) Mirror consultation, (**b**) An 72-year-old subject with bulging eyebags and tear trough is shown the simulated result after filler injection through mirror consultation

Having nailed down the treatment priorities, the next step is to manage patient expectations regarding the treatment outcomes. This is crucial to optimum patient outcome as patients who have unrealistic expectations or the strictest standards are most likely to be dissatisfied with the result no matter how good it may in fact turn out to be. Indeed, 'expectation management' is an established field of study within the discipline of business administration, according to which the customer's satisfaction with a product or service is said to be inversely proportionate to their level of expectation. This implies, assuming the goods or services concerned meet required quality standards, it becomes impractical to satisfy a customer whose expectation level is set too high. In aesthetic procedures such as injectable filler treatments, accurate communication of expected outcomes is absolutely key to managing patients' expectations at levels achievable by the practitioner. In this regard, it is essential first and foremost, to lay down what the practitioner may or may not reasonably be expected to achieve with injectable fillers, so patients with unrealistic expectations may be guided in the right direction. For example, patients should be counseled beforehand that filling the tear troughs may not be of much benefit in case puffy eye bags are also present above the tear troughs. In this respect, visual representation is by far the most effective method for managing patient expectations. While sophisticated 3D imaging devices such as Vectra can be used to help patients visualize what they might look like *after* their treatment, in its absence, a mirror can be used as a simple method for simulating the postoperative results. A few useful tests or manoeuvers can be done during the mirror consultation to help patients foresee the results, such as the "spreading test" for deep glabella grooves or by pushing up the anterior malar fat to see if it corrects the tear troughs.

Episode: The Light in Your Eyes

If you assumed botox and fillers were simply the preserve of old people, given how they are used as near synonyms of "wrinkle treatment" you'd be surprised to learn how over the years, there has been a steady and notable growth of young people in their 20s and 30s opting for these treatments. Originally developed as anti-wrinkle treatments, botox and fillers have now evolved beyond their initial indication and have emerged as viable tools for purposes of facial beautification. Typical examples include masseter reduction with botox for facial slimming and the use of fillers for reshaping and recontouring the nose, lips, and chin. Rather than aimed at counteracting signs of aging, these treatments are focused on aesthetically enhancing and optimizing the congenital structural deficits of the face and body, for which, I suppose, there exists a ready market across demographics of all ages.

Obviously, the fact that the threshold age at which wrinkle-prevention starts has been lowered to the late 20s or early 30s also explains why the market for botox and filler is getting increasingly younger. As regards botox injections, they serve not merely as a quick fix for expression lines but upon repeat use offer the long-term benefit of keeping the face less wrinkle prone, as was already established worldwide some 10 years ago. As a matter of fact, when it comes to botox treatments, the younger you start, the better. Since young skin is naturally high in elasticity, wrinkles on a young face can be successfully tackled with botox alone. By the time you get to your 60s and 70s however, expression lines left neglected end up becoming deep static wrinkles permanently etched on the face like scars; the aging face also undergoes volume depletion and soft tissue ptosis, none of which can be satisfactorily addressed with the use of botox alone. Nonetheless, every now and then, I meet patients in their 40s and 50s who come in for anti-wrinkle consultations and even after hearing out my explanation in full, decline to get botox until much later in life.

Understandably, undergoing an aesthetic procedure can be unnerving the first time around. After all, the image of having toxin, that is, botox, or a foreign material, that is, fillers, shot in the face is perhaps not the most comforting thought one can imagine. Some might feel uneasy about the prospect of having to rely on botox and fillers for the rest of their lives, given the temporary nature of these injectables and fret whether they might not be starting too early on. However, for those who refuse botox for reasons falling outside these vague concerns if not for financial considerations, I simply smile benignly and advise them to "Get started while you're still young and pretty. Why hold out until you've become a granny?"

Personally speaking, I am at that stage in my life where I'm not getting any younger or fitter. If I'm getting any wiser though, I've come to realize the value of living for today. As the old Korean adage goes, *the reddest flower cannot last beyond 10 days* and *even a grasshopper has its own season.* It is a simple fact of life, just as the moon waxes and wanes and flowers bloom and wilt that nothing lasts forever including our transient youth and beauty. For all the euphemism about wrinkles being "the medals of our passage of life," let's face it; it is a basic human desire to stay forever young and beautiful if possible. Though we may never regain the vitality of fresh green spring leaves we once embodied as teens or recover the lusciousness of a blooming flower we radiated in our twenties, advances in modern medicine however have brought us the next best thing; the ability to continue looking our best and remaining elegantly beautiful even in our 40s and 50s, with proper maintenance and upkeep.

This year's Baeksang Arts Awards for Best Korean TV Drama was awarded to Kim Hye Ja in honor of her overwhelming and transformative performance in the drama series *The Light in Your Eyes* in which she played the role of a young woman in her 20s who suddenly finds herself bumped up to old age. Kim's exceptional performance which transcends generation to capture both the sweet innocence of a 20 something and the calm poise of an elderly woman, combined with a brilliant screenplay carrying a massive surprise ending, led the series to become a smashing hit with a peak rating of 9.7%. The series purports to be a fantasy drama about a young woman who is suddenly transformed into an elder due to some inexplicable circumstances which rob her of all her time; but it turns out—*spoiler alert!*—that the whole narrative all along had been one told by the old woman who in fact was suffering Alzheimer's disease.

The drama shed light on the preciousness of time and life, and a line from the final episode resonated in particular with many; "Don't let the regrets of yesterday or uncertainties tomorrow spoil your present. Live for today. Let the light into your eyes. This is your moment to shine. You deserve nothing less" And that is exactly what I remind myself at this very moment. May those dazzling words of wisdom guide us both in our lives and in removing our wrinkles. *Carpe diem (May, 2019).*

1.2.2 Objective Factors

An objective evaluation of a patient's face consists of a comprehensive assessment of the patient's biological factors such as gender and age, as well as the extent of facial aging as manifested by the lack of continuity in facial contour, characteristic of facial lines and wrinkles, visibility of pores, facial volume depression and sagging, and skin thickness and elasticity, among others. As with all other medical treatments, it is essential to define the problem correctly before finding the right solution, as an accurate diagnosis is the first step toward achieving a successful postoperative aesthetic result.

As such, prior to an injectable filler procedure, each face should be assessed individually to identify the characteristics and aging changes specific to the patient's face. On this basis, it should be determined whether the patient is the right candidate for the filler treatment, whether the procedure may not disrupt balance with the rest of the face, and whether combination with other treatment modalities should be considered. For example, deep glabella furrows cannot be satisfactorily erased with HA fillers alone but instead requires the adjunctive use of BoNT-A. Likewise, the sunken cheeks lateral to the nasolabial fold need to be filled concurrently during a nasolabial fold correction in patients with severely sunken cheeks, to create a confluent transition between these adjacent anatomical units.

1.2.3 Facial Assessment Flow Chart

As illustrated, a thorough and accurate assessment of the patient's face guides the artistry of injectable filler injections and represents the starting point for delivering elaborately tailored treatment outcomes. To this end, a step-by-step guide for analyzing the face can help ensure that all necessary objective factors are considered in a sequential manner. The flow chart in Fig. 1.2 has been drawn up to provide a visual illustration of the relevant steps to be performed. The first step of a customized facial assessment consists of facial shape analysis. With the oval facial shape defined as the aesthetic ideal, the other facial shapes are stylized into seven categories, including round, oval, square, pentagon, oblong, rectangular (or slender), and inverted triangle shapes (Fig. 1.3). After placing the face into the relevant category, the next step is to formulate the aesthetic strategy for bringing the face closer to the ideal oval shape. In square, pentagonal, rectangular, and round faces where the prominence of the masseter m. or temporalis m. is the underlying cause, combination treatment with BoNT-A is recommended for reducing the facial width. Meanwhile, in faces featuring a pronounced

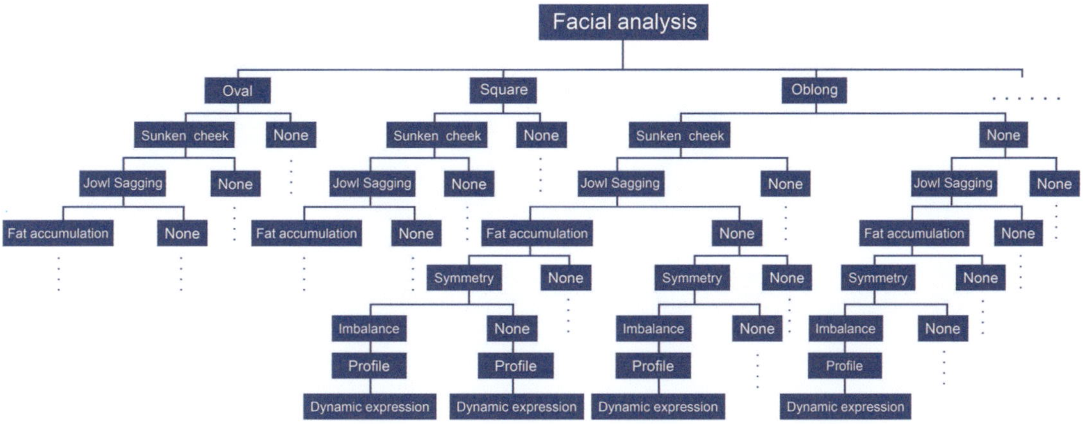

Fig. 1.2 Facial analysis flow chart

zygoma, while the bony zygoma itself cannot be reduced via injectable fillers, volume restoration simultaneously in the temporal and lateral cheek hollows can visually diminish the zygomatic emphasis by blending its superior and inferior borders with the lateral facial contour (Fig. 1.4). Volumizing the zygomatic arch and sunken cheeks in slender or inverted triangle faces not only helps to ovalize the face but also creates the illusion of a shorter facial length by adding facial width. Conversely, chin augmentation in round or square faces has the effect of slimming the face and bringing it closer to the ideal oval shape by adding the facial length (Fig. 1.5). While assessing the facial shape, it is also essential to consider the size of the face. It bears reminding in this regard that patients with a naturally large, voluminous face should be injected with conservative amounts only as injectable filler procedures serve primarily to add volume to the face.

The second step involves assessment of the aging changes present in the patient's face, including the appearance and extent of facial wrinkling, sagging, and depression, and clumping of facial fat (Fig. 1.6). Depending on the severity of such symptoms, combination with other adjunct procedures may be explored. For example, in patients presenting with pronounced jowl fat and jowl descent, volume correction of the sunken cheeks alone may exacerbate the heaviness of the jowls. In this case, the adjunct use of thread lifts or energy devices such as high-intensity focused ultrasound (HIFU) or fat-reducing injections should be considered for lifting and tightening the sagging face (Table 1.1). By the same token, patients with under-eye bags presenting for tear trough correction should be advised to also seek surgical removal of the herniated infraorbital fat for optimum results.

In the third step, facial symmetry should be considered. Slight asymmetry is common in most people and may even contribute to a more natural-looking facial appearance. That said, those with more pronounced forms of facial asymmetry require adequate medical treatment, as such discrepancy can be aesthetically displeasing. While a definitive correction requires an orthodontic or even surgical interventions including upper and lower jaw surgery in severe cases, patients can also benefit from moderate cosmetic improvements with injectable fillers. Here, injectable fillers can be placed strategically to augment the weaker side of the face and to realign the canted maxilla/mandible to lie closer to the facial midline (Fig. 1.7).

The fourth step concerns facial balance. When it comes to facial aesthetics, the whole is greater than the sum of its parts. A face with the most stunning and prominent eyes, nose, and mouth may detract from beauty if each feature is not congruent with each other. It is for this reason that assessments should be performed regarding the relative size and position of individual facial features and the proportionality of the facial contour to determine the overall balance and propor-

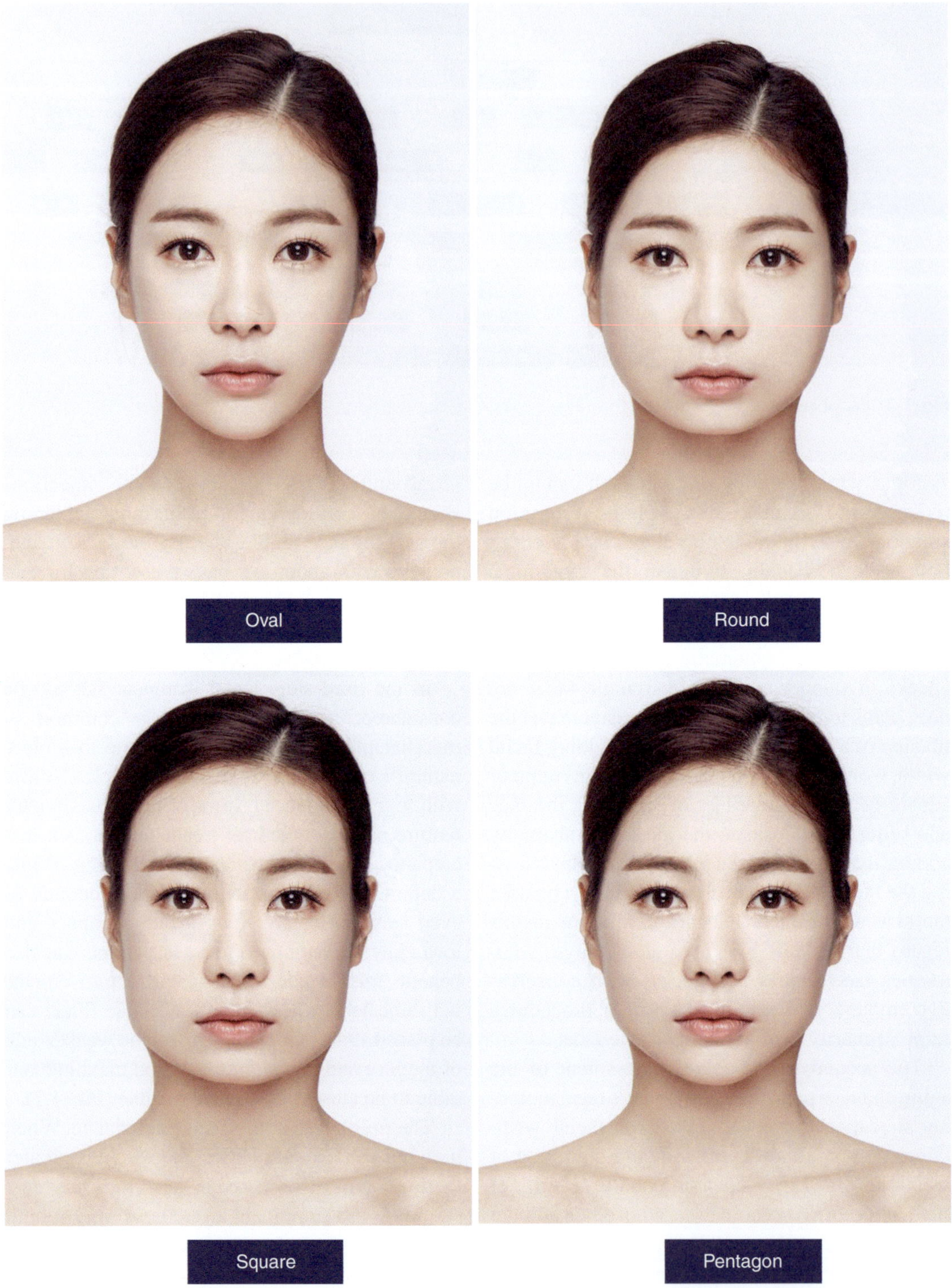

Fig. 1.3 The facial shape analysis. Oval, round, square, pentagon, oblong, rectangular, and inverted triangle shapes

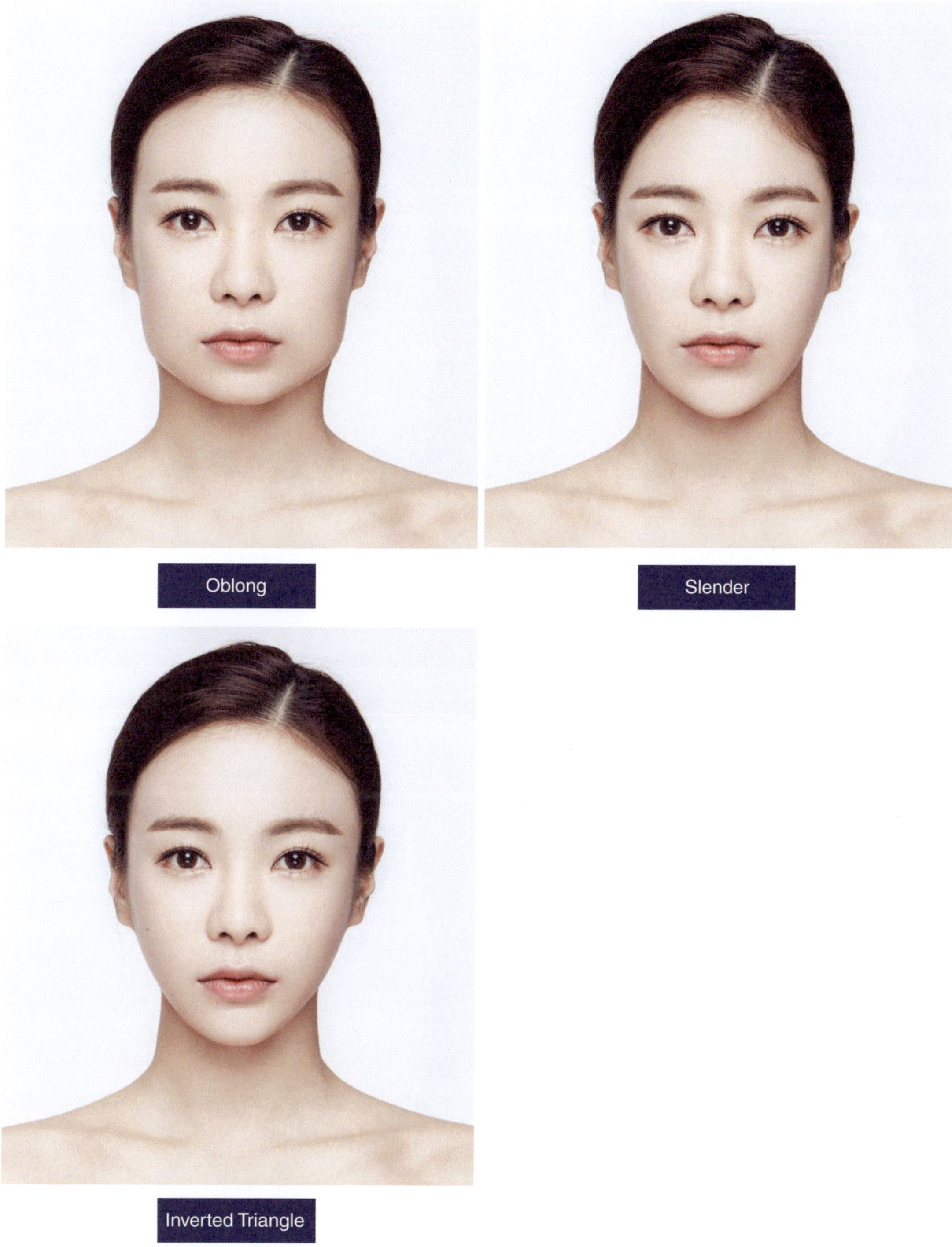

Fig. 1.3 (continued)

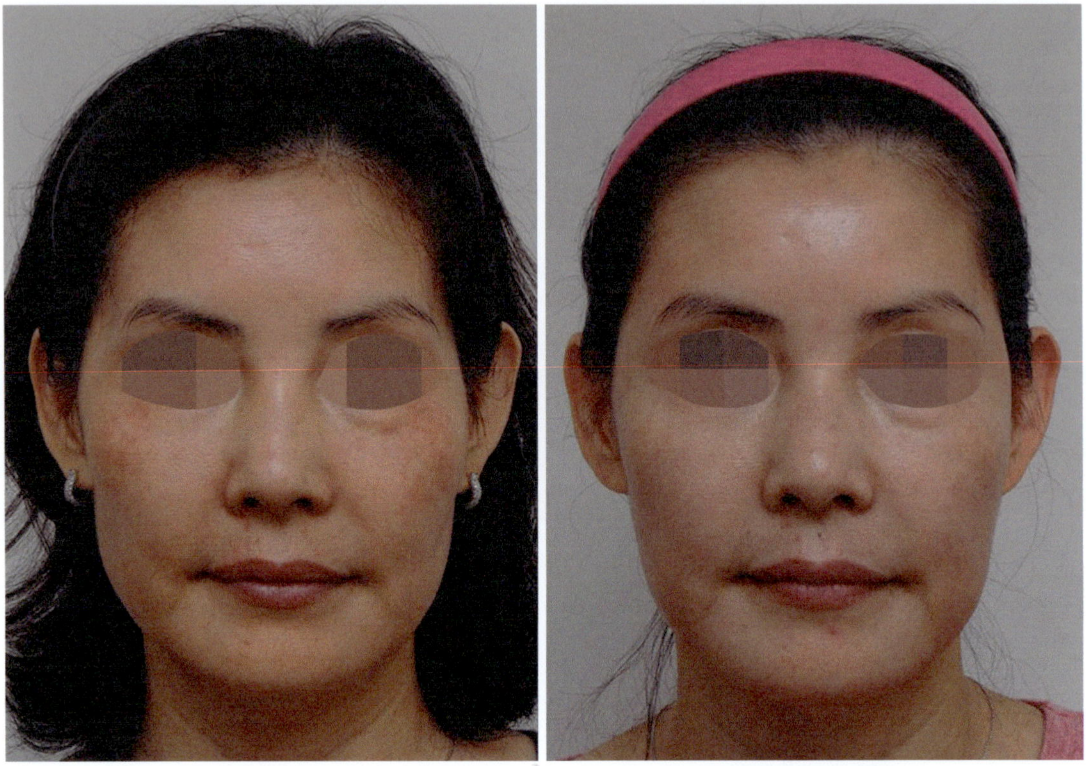

Fig. 1.4 A pronounced zygoma can be camouflaged by volume restoration simultaneously in the temporal and lateral cheek hollows leveraging optical illusion

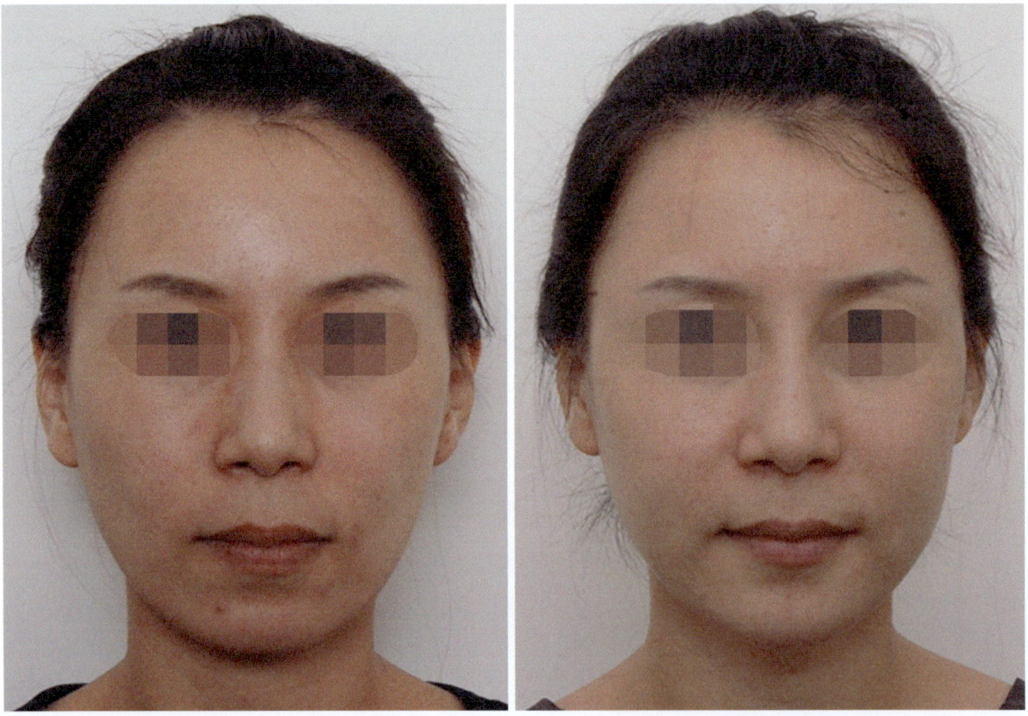

Fig. 1.5 Chin elongation with filler injection can bring about a slimmer V line in U-shaped face

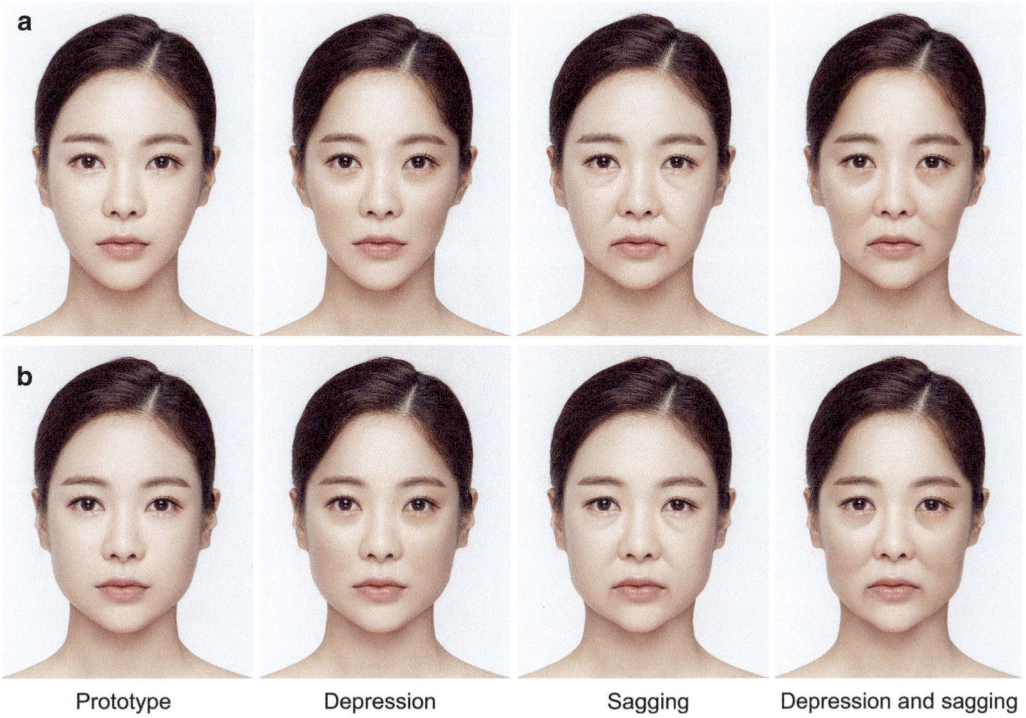

Fig. 1.6 Aging pattern (**a**) in oval shape and (**b**) in pentagon shape

Table 1.1 Treatment recommendation for square shape face depending on the aging pattern

	Depression	Sagging	Fat accumulation	Recommended treatment
Square	None	None	None	FC_BoNT_A
Square	None	None	Yes	FC_BoNT_A, FRI or liposuction
Square	None	Yes	None	FC_BoNT_A, HIFU or thread lifting
Square	None	Yes	Yes	FC_BoNT_A, FRI, HIFU or thread lifting
Square	Yes	None	None	FC_BoNT_A, filler
Square	Yes	None	Yes	FC_BoNT_A, filler, FRI, (HIFU or thread lifting)
Square	Yes	Yes	None	FC_BoNT_A, filler, HIFU or thread lifting
Square	Yes	Yes	Yes	FC_BoNT_A, filler, FRI, HIFU, thread lifting

FC_BoNT_A facial contouring using botulinum toxin, *FRI* fat reduction injection, *HIFU* high-intensity focused ultrasound

tion of the face. For example, a face that has a disproportionately small mouth, as shown in the composite image, tends to looks odd and out of balance (Fig. 1.8). Further, even where the size and shape of individual features remain attractively adequate, if one were to tip the balance of their relative positions by, for instance, narrowing the distance between the eyes or elongating the length of the philtrum, this can also diminish facial attractiveness (Fig. 1.9). Balance of proportions is also important in assessing the facial contour. Altering the proportions of the facial contour by narrowing the width of the forehead or chin, or widening the facial width can distort the face and cause it to lose its proportional quality, even where the size and location of individual features remain intact (Fig. 1.10).

In the fifth step, the face must be assessed from the profile view. A side view of the face is particularly important prior to the augmentation

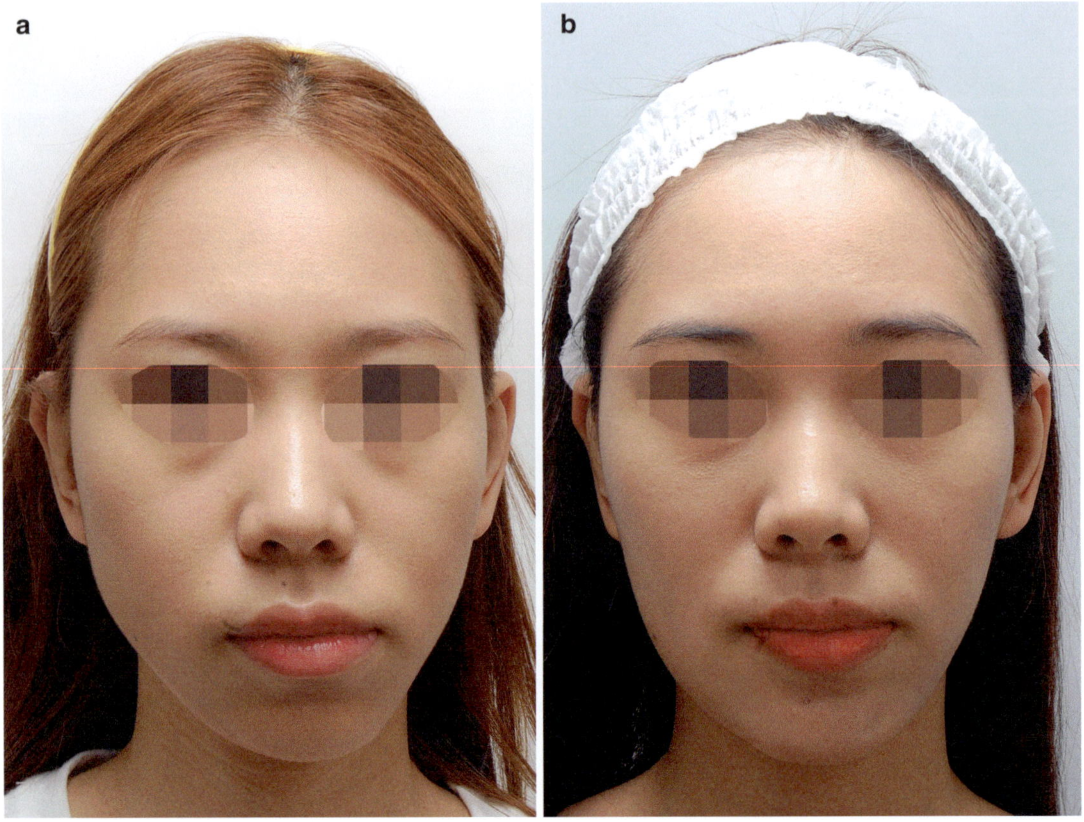

Fig. 1.7 Facial asymmetry can benefit from cosmetic improvements using injectable fillers. (**a**) Before and (**b**) after filler volumization

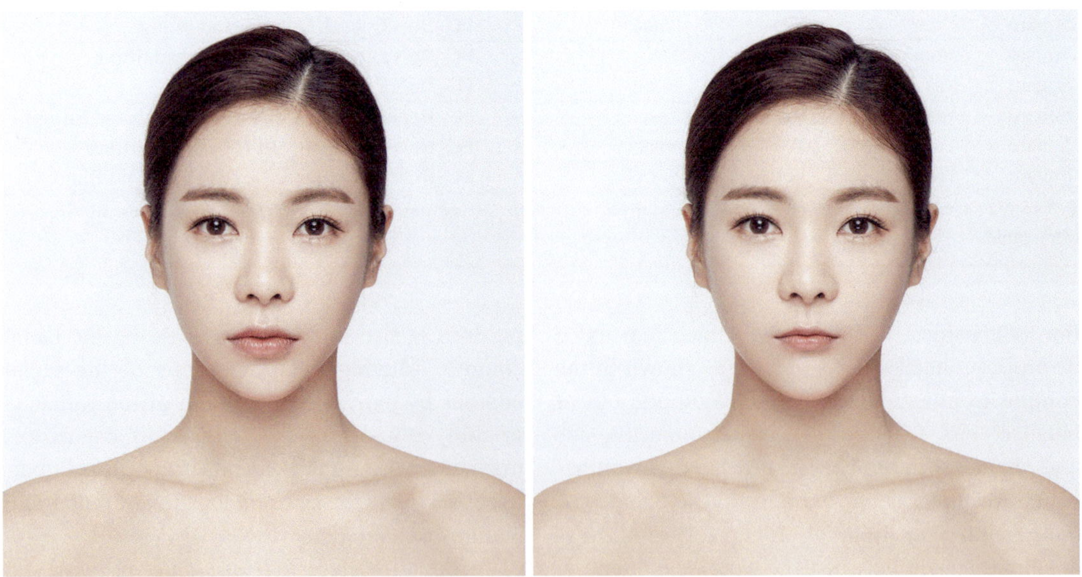

Fig. 1.8 A face that has a disproportionately small mouth, as shown in the composite image, tends to looks odd and out of balance

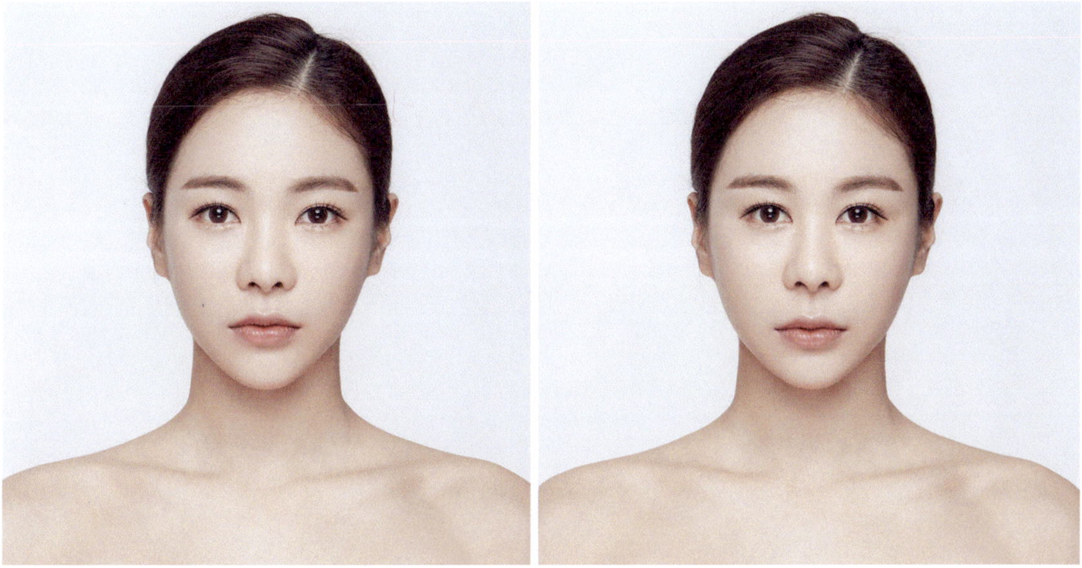

Fig. 1.9 Imbalance of relative positions between individual facial features can diminish facial attractiveness

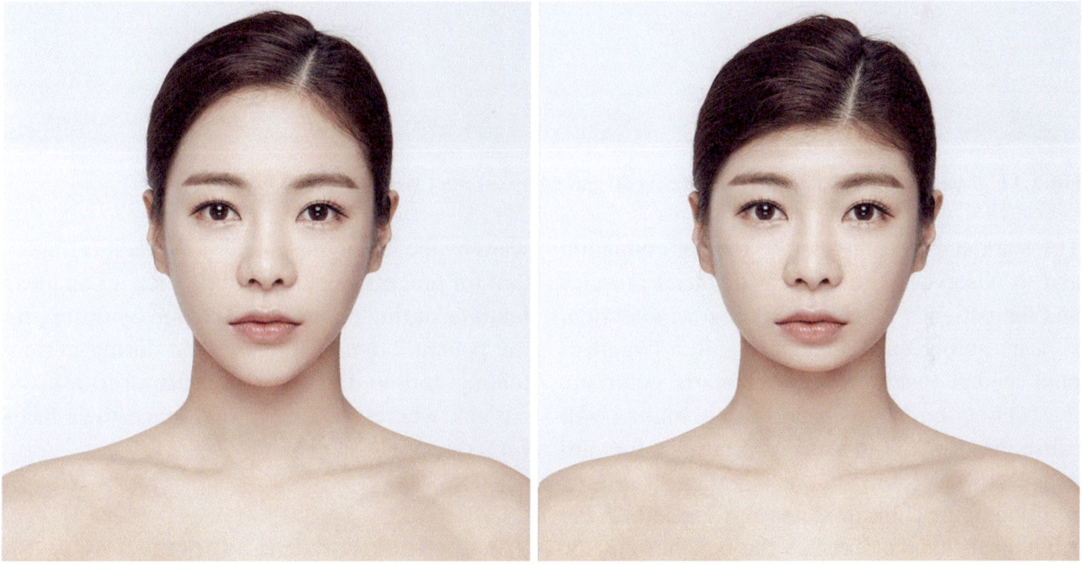

Fig. 1.10 Balance of proportions is also important in the facial contour. Altering the proportions of the facial contour by narrowing the width of the forehead or chin, or widening the bizygomatic distance, can distort the face and cause it to lose its proportional quality, even where the size and location of individual features remain intact

of the forehead, nose, lips, and chin, as it gives the best view of the incline of the sloping forehead, presence of a nasal hump, protruded lips, receded chin, or protruded jaw, none of which may be immediately apparent on the frontal view (Fig. 1.11). This assessment should form part of the decision-making process and inform, for example, that a chin filler is not indicated in a patient with a prognathia (protruding lower jaws).

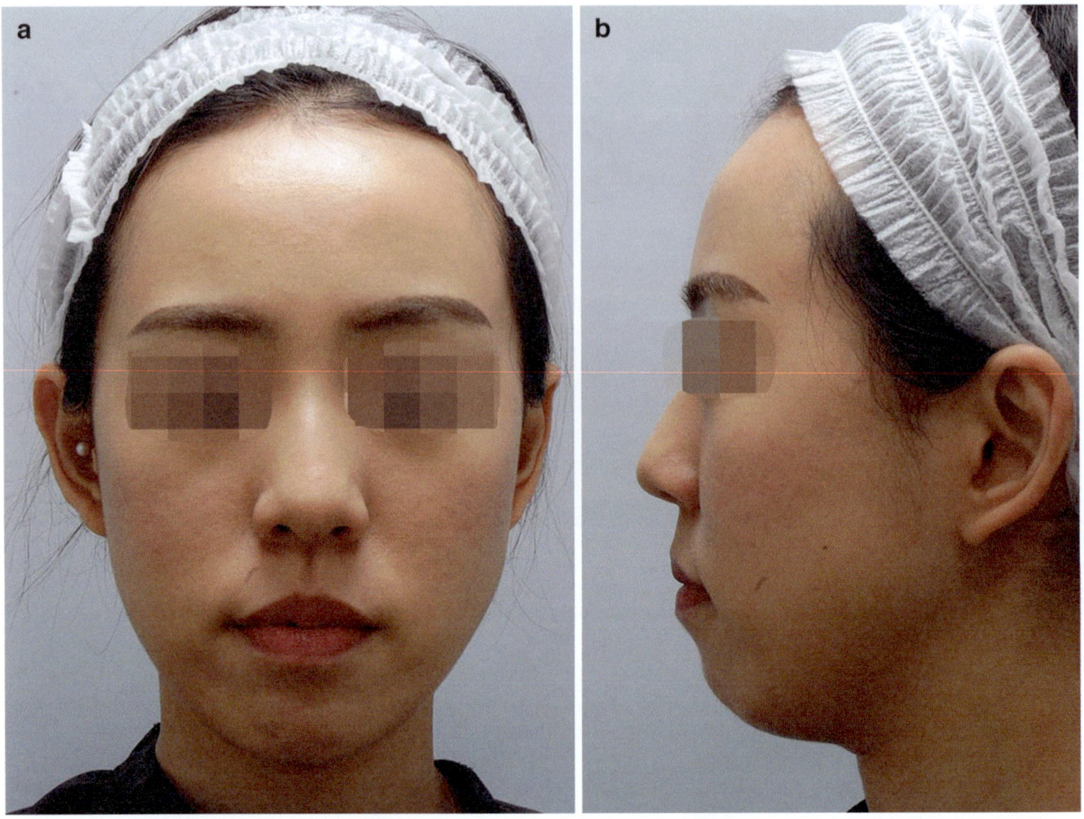

Fig. 1.11 Recessed chin can be more accurately diagnosed by (**a**) front view and (**b**) profile view

The sixth step is to assess the face in animation and to observe the movement of facial muscles and the patient's dynamic expressions in action. It bears noting that in patients with a hypertrophic medial band of the orbicularis oculi m., the contraction of this band during smiling will cause the orbicularis oculi to protrudes forward and become visible. In these patients, volume addition in the anterior malar may exacerbate the bulging of this band due to the bunching of the injected filler on muscle contraction. Such risks should be clearly communicated to the patient in advance or addressed with concurrent BoNT-A injection into the band (Fig. 1.12). Also, patients presenting with cheek dimples or whose cheeks tend to project laterally on smiling due to the partial insertion of the zygomaticus major m. into the skin (Fig. 1.13) may end up with cheeks that become puffy when they smile and stick sideways like the cartoon character Mr. Bogus (Fig. 1.14), as the injected filler is pushed outward by the facial musculature. While it is important for practitioners to tactfully pick up on these features during patient consultation by observing the patient's dynamic expression during normal talking and smiling, it is also useful to ask the patient, where necessary, to animate their faces for a direct assessment.

1.2.4 Sociocultural Aspects

It is useful to gain insight into the sociocultural aspects of the patient, including their occupation, marital status, amount of downtime they can afford to set aside for a bruise or edema to subside, nationality, ethnic aesthetic ideals, and gender-based characteristics, all of which should form part of the treatment strategy. Appreciation of such factors would guide the practitioner, for example, that lower injection volumes are appropriate for a patient whose profession com-

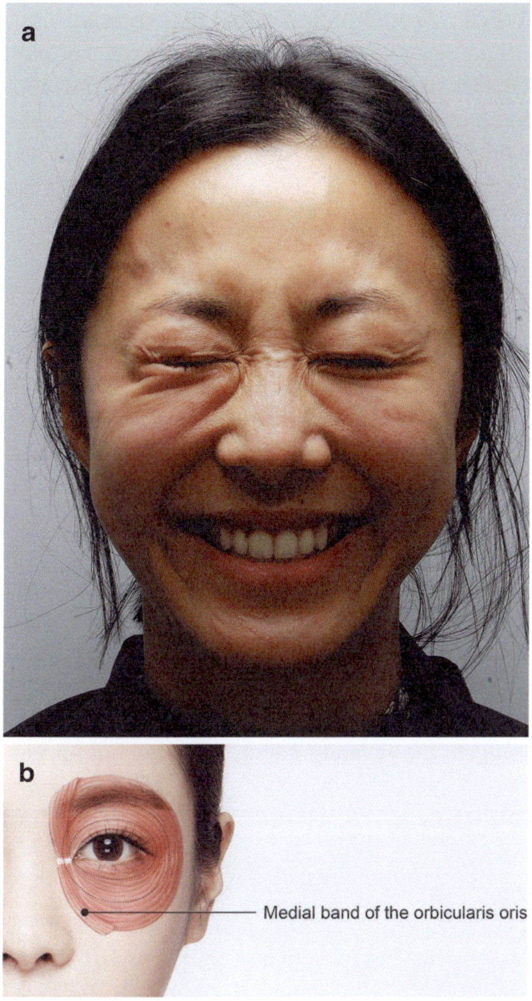

Fig. 1.12 The hypertrophic medial band of the orbicularis oris m. (**a**) Contraction of the hypertrophic medial band of the orbicularis oris m. (**b**) Anatomy of the medial band of the orbicularis oris m

pels them to stand in front of the camera, such as news anchors, celebrities, and professional models, as slightly less facial volume makes for a more photogenic appearance. When counseling a male business executive in his late 40s, the practitioner can recommend strategies for rejuvenating the face without making it look too obvious, for example, through the strategic placement of injectable fillers mostly in the glabella frown lines or infraorbital hollows.

Meanwhile, when approaching patients of different ethnicities, it is relevant to consider their

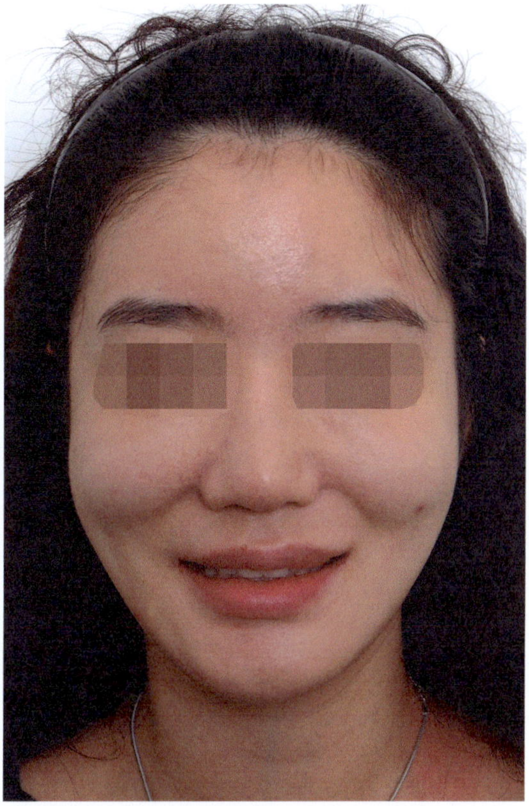

Fig. 1.13 Assessment of the face in animation

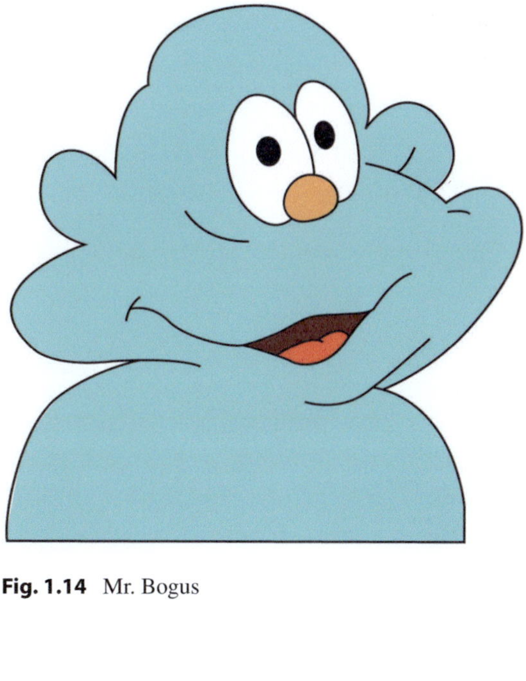

Fig. 1.14 Mr. Bogus

ethnic aesthetic differences, as the preferred facial shape and treatment goals vary widely between Caucasians and Asians (see Sect 1.3). For example, Koreans do not desire the Ogee curve coveted by Caucasians as the aesthetic ideal, as they feel it serves only to accentuate their prominent zygoma. In contrast, Caucasians are less inclined to have the characteristic baby face with full plump cheeks most Koreans find appealing. That said, the personal preference of each patient should always be enquired as well, as the patient's personal beauty standards may not always agree with that pursued by his or her ethnic group. For example, a Korean female based in Los Angeles working as a professional model or married to a Caucasian spouse may elect to espouse the Caucasian standard of beauty that prevails in her profession or her circle of relationship. As an aside, it is worthwhile to note that when treating temporal recessions in a Chinese female patient, larger doses are preferred, as full, rounded temples are considered an auspicious trait that may potentially bring a woman a perfect husband in the Chinese culture.

1.2.5 Gender-Specific Differences

Gender-specific differences must also be incorporated into the treatment plan. As portrayed in the Composite Image of Attractive Korean Male and Female Faces made from 10 input faces of Korean celebrities (Fig. 1.15), men ideally have smaller eyes and a larger nose compared to women. Also, the zygomatic bone is ideally more prominent and cheeks more flatter, if not slightly depressed, on a man. The male chin is more extended and broader than that of a female, which is smaller and pointier in shape [1]. Concerning the ideal facial shape, whereas a smooth oval face is desirable for females, a strong, angular contour built on a well-defined mandibular angle and robust masseter m. is considered more manly and charismatic in men. It is thus vital to respect these sexual dimorphic traits and vary the approach for male and female patients accordingly. For example, when treating the infraorbital hollowness or sunken cheeks, injection of discreet amounts is advised in men—just enough to mitigate the severely gaunt, hollowed-out appear-

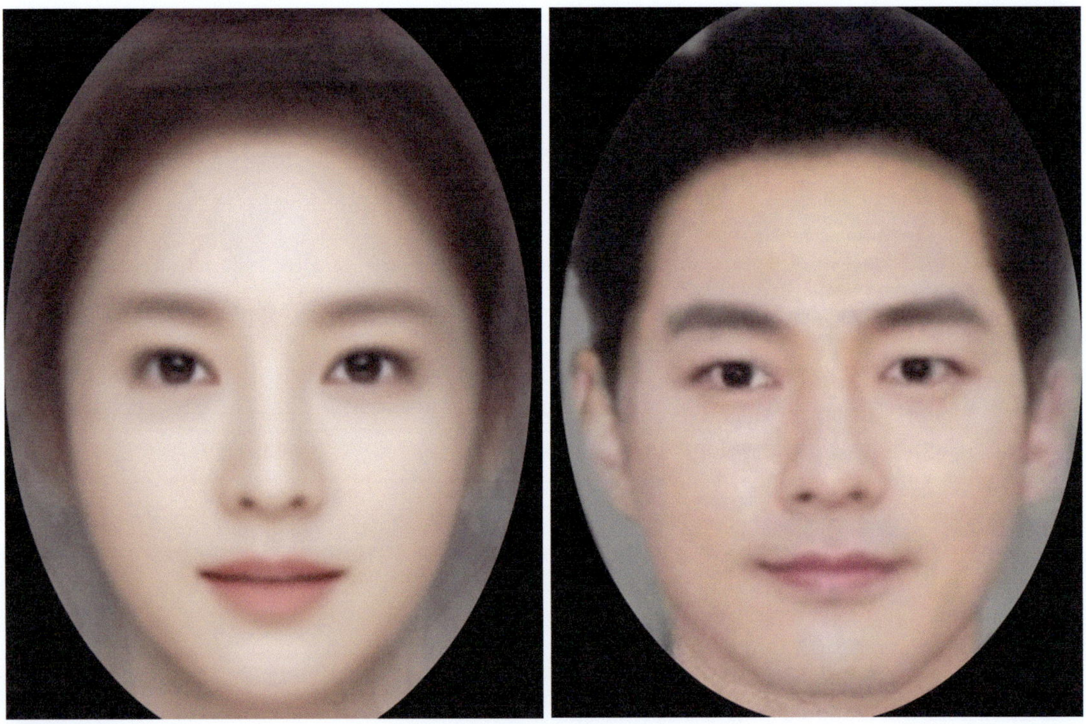

Fig. 1.15 Attractive composite faces of Korean males and females made from 10 input faces of Korean celebrities

ance, whereas larger volumes to create a fuller, a more voluminous contour is acceptable in females. Too much volume in the male cheeks serves to feminize a male face by taking the edge off the desirably chiseled masculine contour. Regardless, it is always appropriate to confirm with each patient regarding his specific aesthetic preferences, as more men in recent times opt to favor an androgynous or effeminate appearance than before.

1.2.6 Past Medical History of Aesthetic Procedures

While some patients would be undergoing the injectable filler treatment for the very first time, many have experiences with various different cosmetic treatments ranging from BoNT-A injections, injectable fillers, liposculpture, and thread lifts to surgical facelifts. In patients with a history of past filler treatments, it is relevant to ask when they had the procedure done and where, using which product. Also, it is useful to review their level of satisfaction from those procedures and the occurrence of complications, if any.

While the results of these previous procedures may appear to be favorable on the surface, they typically leave tissue adhesions and scars in the underlying subcutaneous tissue due to neocollagenesis, which can be very hard and painful to penetrate with a cannula during a subsequent HA filler procedure. Further, the blood vessels trapped within the substance of the scar tissue present a greater risk of inadvertent intravascular injection of HA filler and extensive bruising due to vessel rupture. Where tissue adhesions are present, injecting HA fillers under the tissue can be a challenge, as the tightly bound scar tissues prevent the even deposition of HA filler and cause surface irregularities. This can be particularly problematic when treating the forehead, where only limited space is available for filler placement. Here, tissue adhesions dotted across multiple areas of the forehead may conspire to restrict the creation of a smooth, even surface contour. The situation is worse for patients presenting with lumps and bumps in the forehead left from an inadequately performed previous procedure, be it implantation of injectable fillers, autologous fat, or thread lift sutures. In the case the previously implanted material consists of HA, hyaluronidase injections can be administered to remove existing irregularities before the procedure; however, in the case of collagen stimulators such as Sculptra® or El Ellansé™ or autologous fat, irregularities are harder to treat since they are the result of scar tissue adhesions created by neocollagenesis. In such cases, it is necessary to bring this to the patient's attention prior to any treatment, to prevent the patient from wrongly attributing the less favorable outcome to the present HA filler procedure.

To some extent, the patient's past medical history of cosmetic interventions can lend precious insight into their attitude toward the filler treatment. First-time filler patients with no prior experience of aesthetic procedures naturally tend to be more concerned about the treatment and the associated social downtime from bruising and swelling. On the other hand, a *few pokes of a needle* is hardly an issue for a patient who has previously undergone more invasive procedures such as mandibular angle resection or a surgical facelift. This is particularly the case for patients who have previously received autologous fat transfers. Note, however, that, unless asked directly, aesthetic patients would rarely volunteer information regarding their past cosmetic interventions. This is particularly true of patients who received facial bone surgeries performed intraorally, such as mandibular angle resection or malar and zygoma reduction surgery, as those surgeries would leave no apparent scars on the exterior of the face. However, it may be of value for the practitioner to ask directly if the patient had any work done if the patient happens to present an unnatural "step" below the zygomatic arch (indicative of a previous zygoma reduction surgery) or an overly linear jawline extending from the ear to the chin (undoubtedly from an aggressive mandibular angle resection) as HA filler can be used to restore the surgically removed volume in each of those cases (see Sect 4.14).

1.2.7 Financial Aspects

Costs represent an important, yet often neglected, part of the conversation with the patient. It would serve no purpose for the practitioner to extol the benefits of a procedure that the patient could not afford anyway, other than to leave the patient feeling alienated. Ideally, it would be best if the practitioner could make an educated guess of the patients' budget based on their age, profession, reaction to suggestions of available treatment options, as well as the practitioner's pure intuition. Otherwise, however, it might be a good idea to ask the patient upfront what their budget is. For patients who appear to be looking to stay within a defined budget, the practitioner and patient can work together to set priorities and determine the best fit between what the patient perceives as their biggest aesthetic concern and what, in the practitioner's professional judgment, can provide the most visible results for the money spent.

When fillers are used for facial rejuvenation as opposed to beautification of individual features such as the lips or nose, a full facial approach is commonly used to produce the optimum balance of proportions among various facial features and prevent regional disparity. However, as desirable as this approach may be, adding volume across multiple areas of the face requires the use of multiple filler syringes, which admittedly imposes a financial burden on the patient. In this case, a more preferable approach to give patients better value for money is to charge not by the number of syringes used or individual regions treated but based on a package deal where reduced prices are offered for 5–10 mL of filler used across the full face.

Episode: On Being a Dad of Miss Korea

While being an MD specializing in dermatology, I am also an aesthetic practitioner whose work involves rejuvenating or beautifying the facial appearance of clients using injectables such as botox or fillers. Helping people look younger and more beautiful can be just as enjoyable and gratifying as providing medical care to patients with illnesses. Besides, since most of the people visiting my clinic consist of good-looking people seeking to improve their already fairly good appearances, I get to enjoy the extra perk of meeting a lot of attractive faces in my daily practice.

I happened to come across one such patient a few years ago; a glamourous healthy-looking female patient in her 20s who introduced herself as the previous year's Miss Korea winner and came in to consult whether she could possibly beautify what she described as her "plain face" with the use of nonsurgical procedures. Unfortunately, I couldn't be of much assistance to her since she presented with relatively large zygoma and a wide nasal base, features which made her a bad candidate for filler volumization. Since fillers are indicated to literally fill out areas of volume deficit on the face such as grooves, creases, or sunken cheeks, if not to augment a flat nose or enhance small lips, it is not applicable to reducing a wide nose or a prominent zygoma. Perhaps, it was due to the fact that she was wearing no makeup, but I had to agree that she had more of a casual, modest girl-next-door quality to her face rather than being a case of divine beauty. The patient happened to be of similar age with my youngest daughter. Perhaps for that reason, just as the owl might think her own young fairest, I soon found myself entertaining the idea of having my own girl, who in the eyes of her doting dad was by no means less beautiful, enter the Miss Korea contest of that year, which she eventually did and won.

Sure enough, defining facial beauty remains a widely debated topic, and yet I am a strong proponent of facial proportionality which, I believe, trumps most other factors of facial attractiveness such as having fair skin, large eyes, tall nose, full lips, or a sharp jaw line. While I am no fan of any blind, across-the-board application of the golden ratio that does not respect each patient's individuality and character, without there being some sense of proportionality among individual features, the face can appear bizarrely distorted and unattractive.

To illustrate this point in my lectures and seminars, I often use multiple manipulated images of Angelina Jollie's face. Reducing the size of the eyes, nose, and mouth on Angelina Jollie's face alone does not significantly affect her facial attractiveness. However, when her facial proportions are altered by way of reducing the intercanthal distance or by elongating the philtrum, the face immediately becomes distorted and weird looking. The same happens when her eyes, nose, and mouth are left intact, but the facial shape or contour is distorted out of proportion, by narrowing the forehead, reducing the chin, or augmenting the malars. This demonstrates how balance among facial features rather than the aesthetics of individual elements play a bigger role in determining facial attractiveness. To her credit, while my youngest daughter does not exactly fit the profile of a classic beauty featuring big eyes and tall nose, she is nonetheless endowed with a small oval face with a harmonious balance between individual structures, which combine to create a sublime oriental allure. I guess this gives me some vindication when I say, in her father's trained eyes, she's worthy of the title *Korean Beauty Queen* by all means.

Beauty is not the only area where balance matters. For almost all things in life, there can be too much of a good thing, and you need to know how to strike the right balance. Korean voters have demonstrated an amazing, almost uncanny sense of balance in this regard by allowing the transition of power from the left-wing government to the right and back to the left at exactly 10-year intervals. Yet, the beauty of such harmony seems to be lost on the current government, caught up with "liquidating deep-rooted corruption" while leaving the economy to languish under the ambiguous and unproven policy of 'income-driven growth'. To borrow from the Korean movie *Friend*, "Give it a break pal. I've had enough already" (Nov 2018).

1.3 Consideration of Ethnic Differences in Filler Procedures

Attempts to define a perfectly ideal face have led some to advocate using a single universal standard such as the golden ratio or the phi mask for describing facial attractiveness. However, the qualities of a beautiful face can rarely be distilled down to a single or uniform formula. On the contrary, the standard for facial beauty constantly evolves with time and varies among different ethnic groups. While attending filler training sessions given by western practitioners many years ago as a novice injector, it was never quite clear to me how the inverted triangle drawn over Brigitte Bardot's face connecting her bilateral zygoma with the pogonion, or *the triangle of beauty* as it was called, purported to represent the gold standard for an aesthetic face. Likewise, I struggled to fathom how the prominent lateral zygoma set against the slightly concave temples and subzygomatic regions was meant to create the purported hallmark of all youthfully beautiful faces referred to as the *Ogee curve* [2]. This is because a prominent zygoma contrasted with sunken cheeks is considered an aesthetically displeasing trait by an average Korean female whose concept of facial beauty consists of an oval babyish face with full plump cheeks. As such, accentuating the triangle of beauty by augmenting the lateral cheekbones and brows would hardly translate well onto an Asian face already endowed with a congenitally wide frame and prominent cheekbones. Eventually, I came to learn how such incompatibilities arose from the differences in the underlying craniofacial anatomy between Caucasians and Asians, whereby Caucasians generally have an anteroposteriorly long and transversely narrow dolichocephalic head in contrast to the transversely wide brachycephalic facial bone structure presented by Asians. This chapter details the ethnic differences to consider when undertaking volumizing filler procedures on ethnic patients, with a focus on the treatment of Asians.

1.3.1 Definition of the Asian Population and Asian Facial Morphotypes

The Asian continent represents a vast territory spanning from the Middle East to Northeast Asia, encompassing highly diverse and heterogeneous ethnics groups who cannot be described as a uniform population. Thus, for the sake of consistency, the term Asia as it appears in this chapter is defined narrowly, referring only to the East Asians including the Chinese, Korean, and Japanese as well as the Southeast Asian populations, and does not extend to cover ethnicities from India and Arabic nations whose faces bear a closer resemblance to that of Caucasians. Even under this narrow definition, the Asian face can be categorized into three different morphotypes based on geographic regions, that is, the northern, intermediate, and southern facial types (Fig. 1.16). The northern facial type is commonly seen in the populations of Mongolia, Northern China, and Korea, while the southern facial type is typical of those from the Philippines, Thailand, and Vietnam, and the intermediate facial type is common among those from Hong Kong, Taiwan, and Southern China (Fig. 1.17) [3].

Concerning the specific morphological features, the northern facial type manifests prominent a mandible and zygoma, which conspire to produce a square facial frame; it also features narrow palpebral fissures without any supratarsal crease and a high nasal dorsum with small, narrow nasal ala (Table 1.2). The skin is usually fair, corresponding to Fitzpatrick skin types 2 or 3. The southern facial type is defined by a small oval face framed by a less prominent mandibular angle and zygoma, wide palpebral fissures with a distinct supratarsal crease, and a flat nasal dorsum with wide, round nasal ala. The skin tends to be darker and more pigmented than the northern type (Fitzpatrick skin type 4 or 5). The intermediate facial type is defined by a round face owing to a relatively small chin. The facial components of the intermediate face (eyes, nose, and mouth) represent a blend of the other two face types. Of course, this classification does not purport to be the absolute standard against which

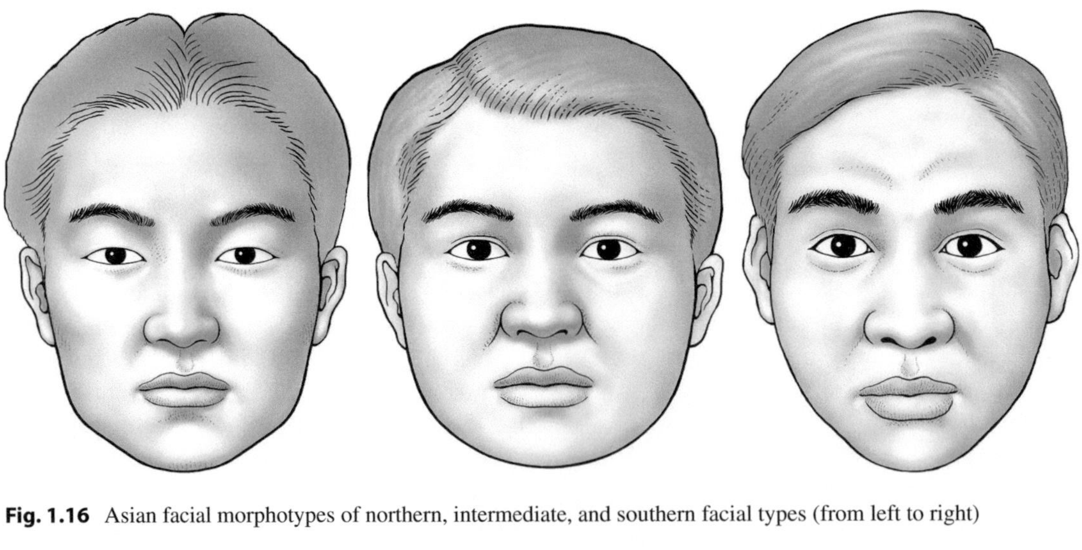

Fig. 1.16 Asian facial morphotypes of northern, intermediate, and southern facial types (from left to right)

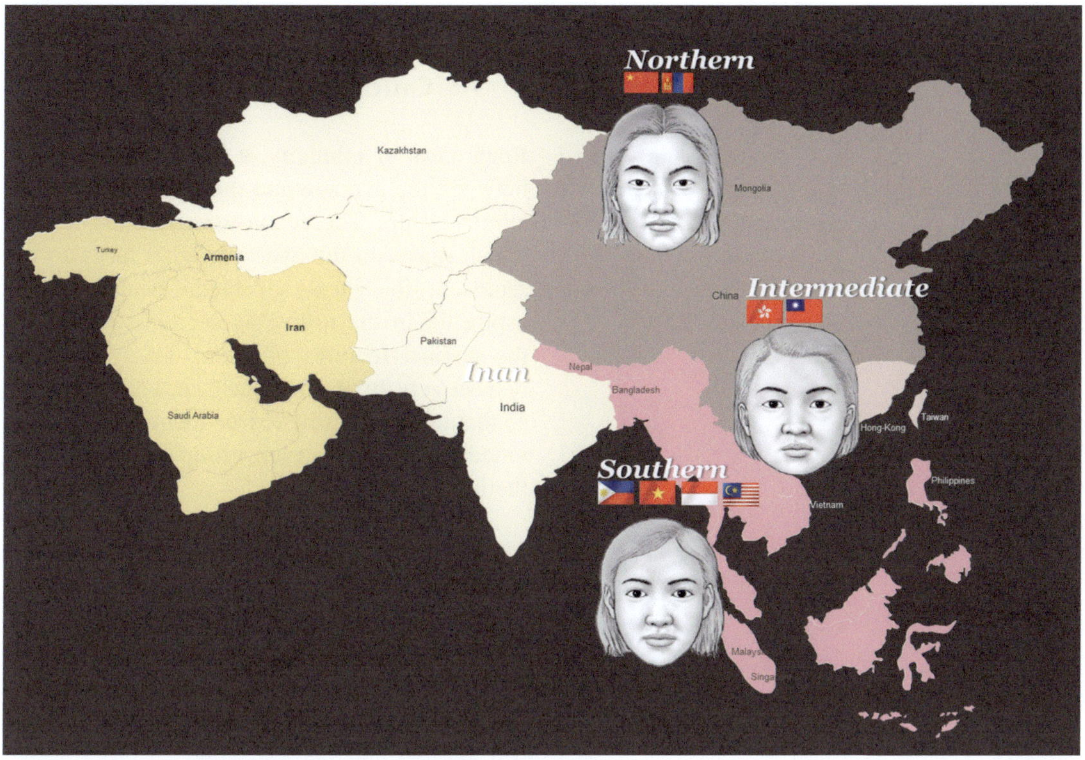

Fig. 1.17 Asian facial morphotypes based on geographic regions

Table 1.2 Characteristics of different Asian facial morphotypes

	Northern	Intermediate	Southern
Regions	Mongolia, Northern China, Korea, etc.	Hong Kong, Taiwan, Southern China	The Philippines, Thailand, Vietnam, and other Southeast Asian countries
Facial shape	Square	Round	Narrow, oval
Zygoma	Prominent	Intermediate	Not prominent
Mandibular angle	Prominent	Intermediate	Less prominent
Palpebral fissure	Narrow	Intermediate	Wide
Supratarsal crease	Absent	Intermediate	Present
Nasal dorsum	High	Intermediate	Low
Ala nasi	Small narrow	Intermediate	Wide round

to identify and discern Asian faces. Different facial morphotypes may be found within a single geographic region, while a single individual may manifest different morphotypical features across distinct parts of the face (Fig. 1.18) [4]. Nonetheless, the classification lends valuable guidance for providing individualized treatments to Asian patients of varying facial types and aesthetic desires.

1.3.2 Differences in the Skull Shape Between Caucasians and Asians

A glaring distinction between the Asian and Caucasian faces lies in their skull shape. The Asian face is characteristically wider and flatter than that of Caucasians. Whereas the dolichocephalic Caucasian head is anteroposte-

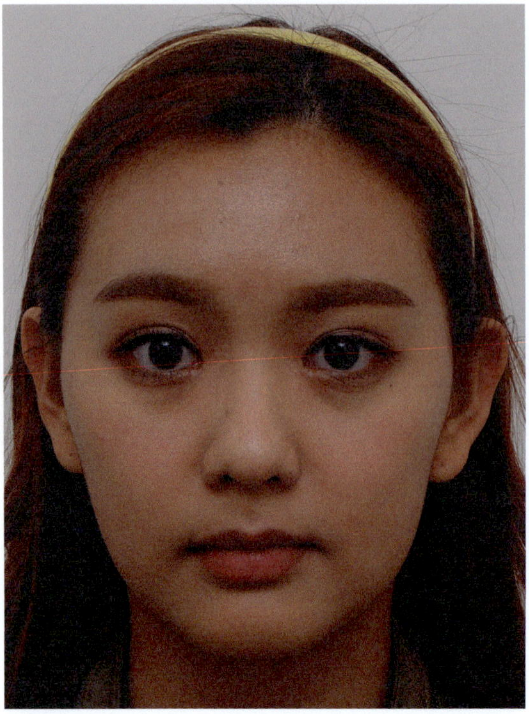

Fig. 1.18 A single individual may manifest different morphotypical features in distinct parts of the face. This beautiful Korean woman demonstrates certain southern type features such as the supratarsal crease and wide palpebral fissure but also displays distinct northern type characteristics such as the prominent zygoma, a wide face, and narrow nasal base

riorly long and transversely narrow, the brachycephalic Asian cranium is transversely wide and anteroposteriorly short (Fig. 1.19). Furthermore, the Asian head is hypsicranic, that is, with a high cranial vault, where the vertical height of the head is long relative to its anteroposterior length, while the lower face and chin tend to be relatively small [5]. Another salient feature that distinguishes the Asian face from the Caucasian is the prominence of the zygoma and mandibular angle. The relative lack of nasal dorsal projection observed in Asians further contributes to the flattened appearance of the face.

1.3.3 Differences in Facial Beauty Standards Between Caucasians and Asians

Regardless of ethnicity, a distinction is drawn between the average and the ideal faces of that ethnic group. The features mentioned earlier, which make up the average Asian face, do not represent the ideals of facial beauty Asians aspire to. In the following section, we explore the distinct features of facial beauty pursued, respectively, by the average Caucasian vs. Asian so that tailored aesthetic treatments may be provided according to each group's different aesthetic goals [6].

As illustrated in Fig. 1.20, an attractive Caucasian face tends to demonstrate the following characteristics: narrow distance between the eye and brow, deep-set eyes, and high arched brows; large, open eyes with a tall, distinct supratarsal crease; and absence of lower pretarsal fullness. The nose is tall with a sharp bridge, narrow ala nasi and sidewalls, and a well-projected pointed tip. The preferred facial features also include large, voluminous lips, a well-defined mandibular angle, and pronounced cheekbones highlighted by subtle concavities in the submalar cheek and temples. On the contrary, an attractive Asian face is characterized by the following features: straight, horizontal brows sitting relatively far above the eyes; a flat upper eyelid devoid of hollowness; small relatively large eyes without a distinct supratarsal crease; and the presence of lower pretarsal fullness. A beautiful Asian face is also correlated with a slightly rounded nasal tip and a moderately projected nasal dorsum, as well as moderately voluminous lips, all of which are framed by an oval face with full cheeks without zygomatic or mandibular prominence (Table 1.3).

Such ethnic differences in facial beauty standards have been well-established in a study whereby attractive composite faces of different ethnicities were produced for comparative

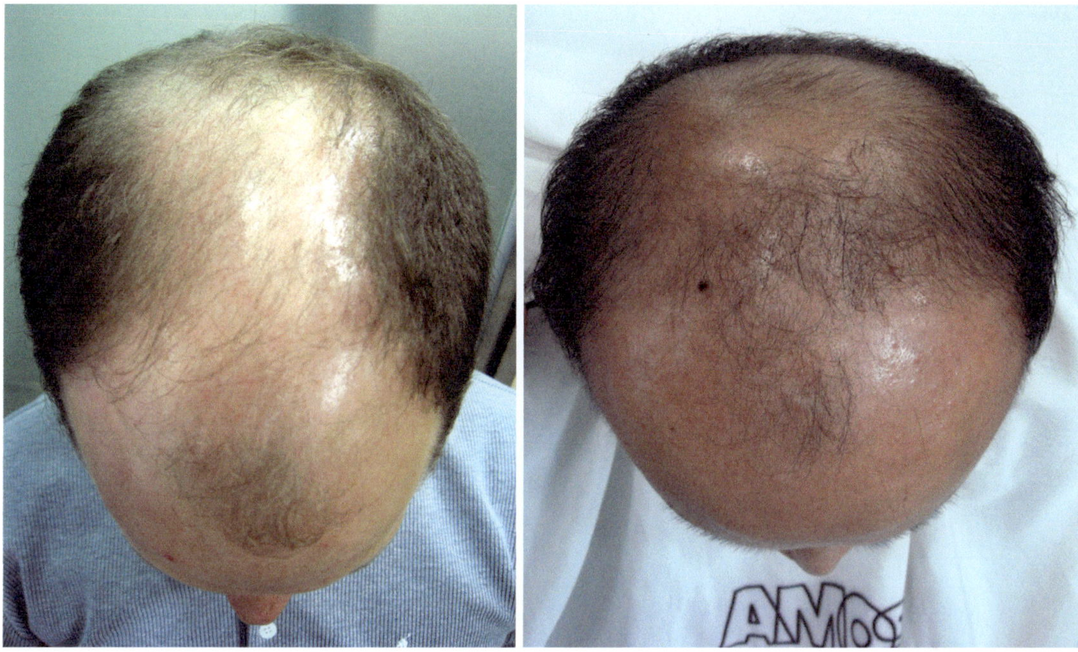

Fig. 1.19 The dolichocephalic Caucasian head (left) and the brachycephalic Asian head (right). (Photo: courtesy of Dr. Tommy S. Hwang)

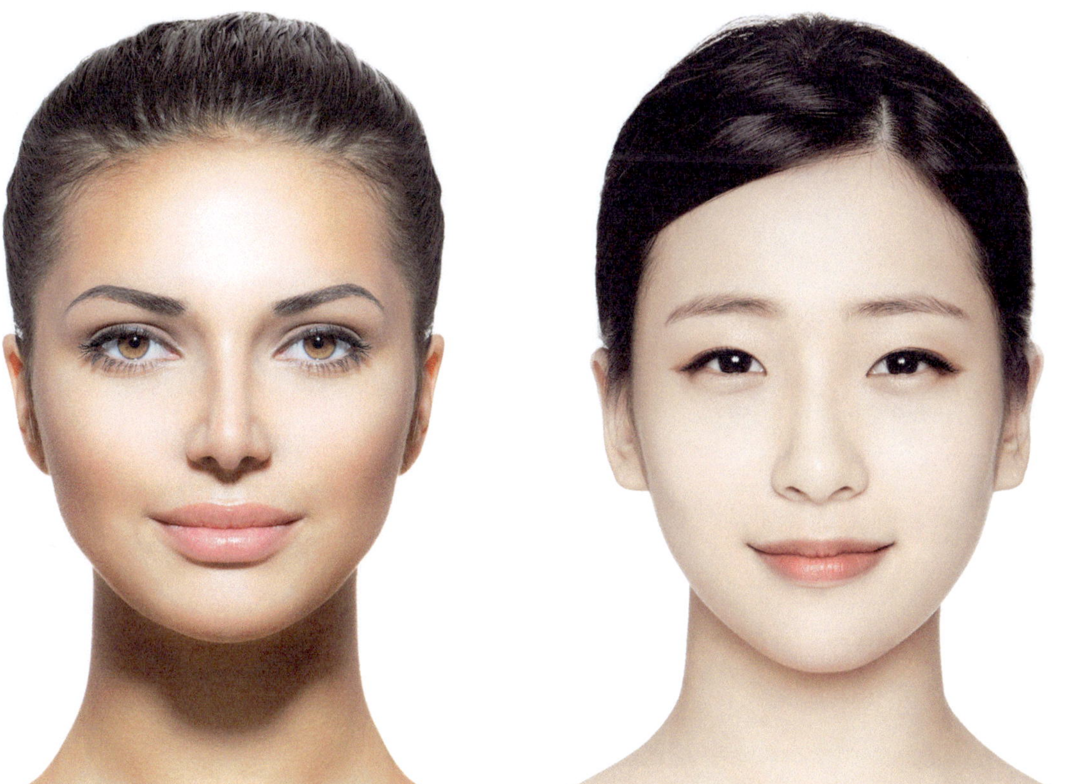

Fig. 1.20 Comparison between the attractive Caucasian vs. Asian faces (Cited from Ref. [6])

Table 1.3 Differences between Asian and Caucasian attractive faces

	Caucasian	Asian
Eyebrows	Arched	Straight
Distance between the eye and brow	Narrow with hollow upper eyelid	Wide with flat upper eyelid
Facial shape	Triangle of beauty	Oval
Zygoma	Prominent	Less prominent
Mandibular angle	Well-defined	Less prominent
Cheeks	Slightly concave	Full, chubby
Eyes	Wide	Relatively large
Supratarsal crease	Present	Absent or narrow
Lower pretarsal roll	Absent	Present
Nasal tip	Pointed	Relatively Rounded
Nasal dorsum	Tall, sharp	Moderately projected
Ala nasi	Small, narrow	Relatively wide
Lips	Full, large	Moderately voluminous

analysis based on the images of popular female celebrities representing the relevant ethnic groups [7, 8]. Specifically, if we compare the Caucasian composite face morphed from input faces of beautiful Caucasian actresses including Angelina Jolie and Hillary Duff against the Asian composite face generated using the faces of Korean celebrities including Lee Young-Ae, Kim Tae-Hee, and Song Hae-Kyo, certain salient differences can be found (Fig. 1.21). The ideal Caucasian female face tends to have a narrow palpebral height, large well-defined facial components (eyes, nose, and mouth), relatively hollow cheeks, prominent zygoma, and a more chiseled mandible, which altogether gives a more masculine appearance compared with the idealized Asian face (Fig. 1.16).

Even within the East Asian population, subtle differences exist among the attractive Chinese, Japanese, and Korean faces, with the Chinese face demonstrating the narrowest facial width and slimmest cheeks while the Japanese face dis-

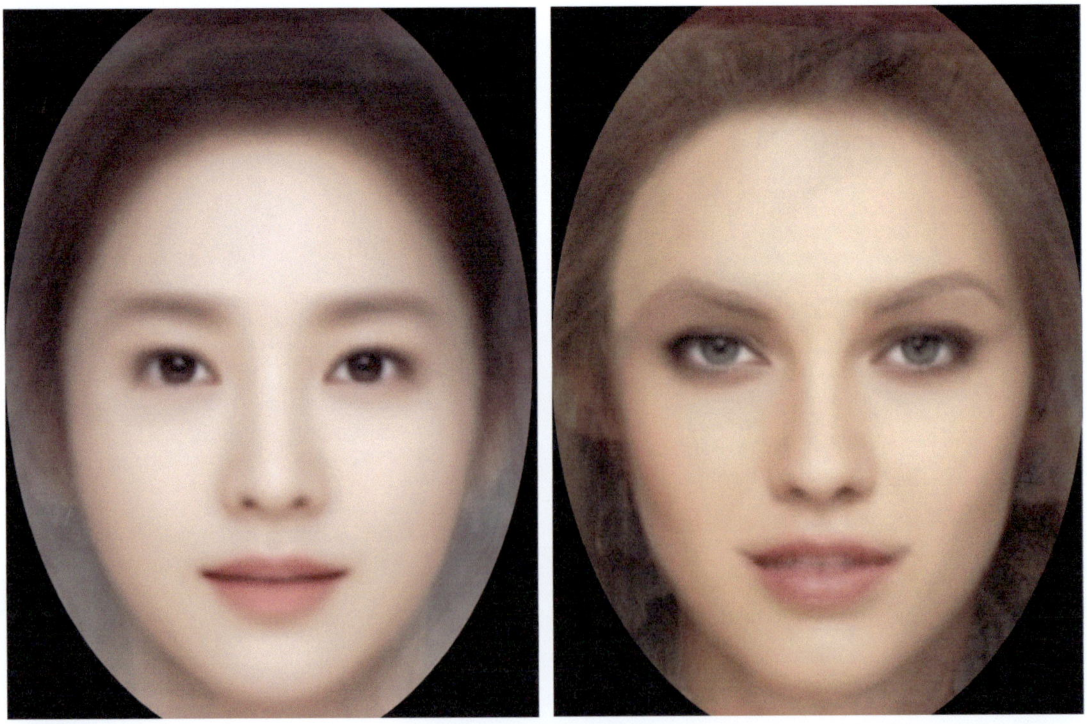

Fig. 1.21 Comparison of attractive composite faces between Caucasians vs. Asians made from 10 input faces of celebrities belonging to each ethnicity

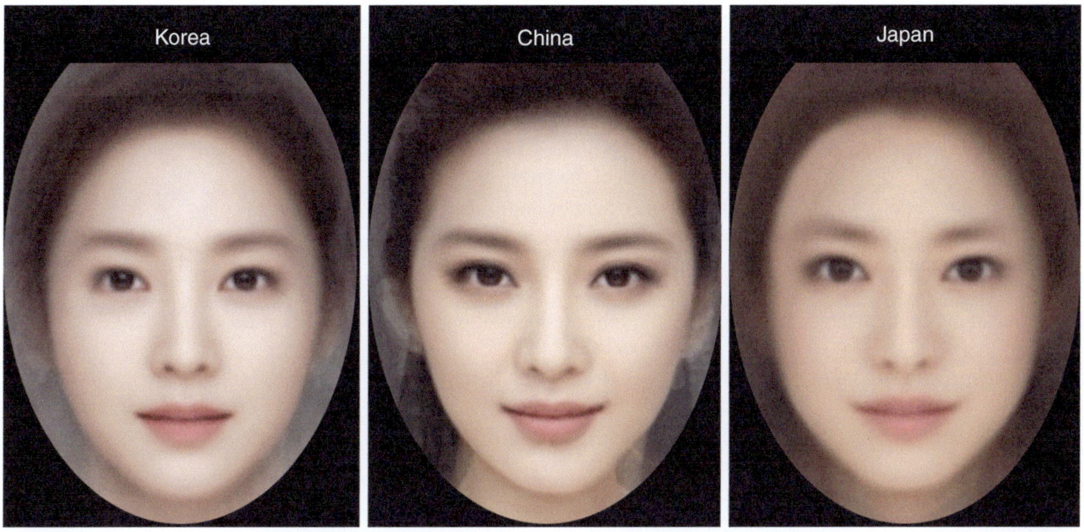

Fig. 1.22 Comparison of the attractive composite faces of Korean, Chinese, and Japanese females made from 10 input faces of celebrities belonging to each country (from left to right)

plays the most robust chin projection (Fig. 1.22) [8]. From these composite faces, we can conclude that while certain similarities may exist among the most beautiful women, the perception of facial attractiveness is never uniform across ethnicities and may not be captured solely by means of a uniform formula such as the golden ratio, but is described more as a function of the intricate interplay between various biological, cultural, and cognitive factors. Therefore, it is vitally important for practitioners to develop a keen appreciation for such distinct ethnic aesthetic preferences and provide nuanced treatment catering to the concept of beauty pursued by each ethnicity.

1.3.4 Different Filler Treatment Strategies for Caucasians and Asians

1.3.4.1 Different Strategies for Facial Contouring Based on Underlying Anatomical Differences

As mentioned earlier, due to the varying underlying structural facial anatomy between Caucasians and Asians, the ideal face shape pursued by the two groups is different, which must be respected when undertaking filler treatments. For example, since Caucasians tend to have a long, narrow dolichocephalic head, midface augmentation procedure in a Caucasian patient typically consists of volumizing the lateral zygoma to accentuate the triangle of beauty coveted by Caucasians. However, replicating this same approach, that is, horizontal midface augmentation, in a northern facial type Asian with a brachycephalic head would produce deleterious results, serving only to make their broad faces appear bigger and wider. Instead, a vertical midface augmentation which aims to project forward the midline facial features of the forehead, nose, medial malar, and chin, etc., and deemphasizing the lateral aspects is more advisable in Asians, as the anterior projection and three dimensionality added to the face serves to produce a visually slimming effect (Table 1.4; Fig. 1.23).

Likewise, while lateral brow elevation or jawline contouring with fillers (i.e., enhancing the lateral borders of the mandibular angle to give the face a squarer shape) may be suitable for accentuating and defining a narrow Caucasian face, such indications are hardly ever practiced

Table 1.4 Difference in filler indication between Caucasians and Asians by facial region

	Caucasian	Asian
Forehead augmentation	Reported mainly on forehead concavity	Popular/Adds dimension and convexity to flat Asian faces
Lateral eyebrow augmentation	Achieves brow arching via lateral enhancement of the brow	Seldom practiced
Temple augmentation	Only to the extent of improving the severity of the depression	Popular
Malar augmentation	Lateral malar enhancement	Infraorbital medial malar enhancement
Mandibular angle augmentation	Adds definition and volume support to a thin narrow face	Seldom practiced
Cheek augmentation (sunken cheek)	Only to the extent of improving the severity of the depression	Popular/creates fullness in the cheeks to resemble a baby face
Sunken eye volumization	Only to the extent of improving the severity of the hollowness	Recent gain in interest
Pretarsal roll augmentation	Rarely practiced	Popular
Nose augmentation	Confined mostly to nasal hump correction	Popular
Lip augmentation	Popular	Recently popular
Chin augmentation for receded chin/V-shaped jawline	Primarily for receded chin correction	Both indications popularly requested

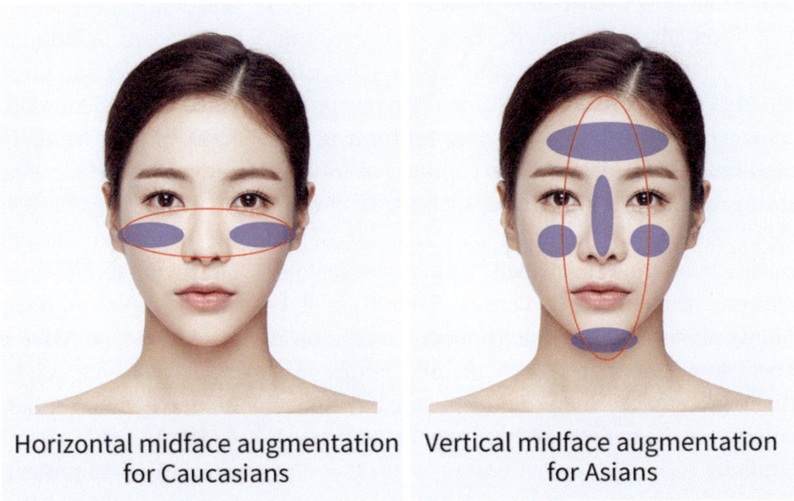

Fig. 1.23 Different strategies for midface augmentation between Caucasians vs. Asians

in Asians since laterally expanding the already broad Asian face would only serve to make the face appear wider and more rugged. On the contrary, to achieve the Asian aesthetic goal of a soft oval face, a popular indication among Asians is to volumize the sunken temples and submalar hollows to subdue the prominence of the lateral zygoma and smoothen the lateral facial contour extending from the temples toward the jawline (Fig. 1.24). However, when performing this indication in a Caucasian face, volume should be added more conservatively only to the extent of reducing the severity of the temporal and subzygomatic recesses to preserve the integrity of the Ogee curve considered aesthetically desirable by Caucasians. Chin augmentation or chin tip enhancement is also a highly requested indication among Asians to sculpt the jawline into the desired V-shape and add vertical height to the face, making it appear slimmer overall in rela-

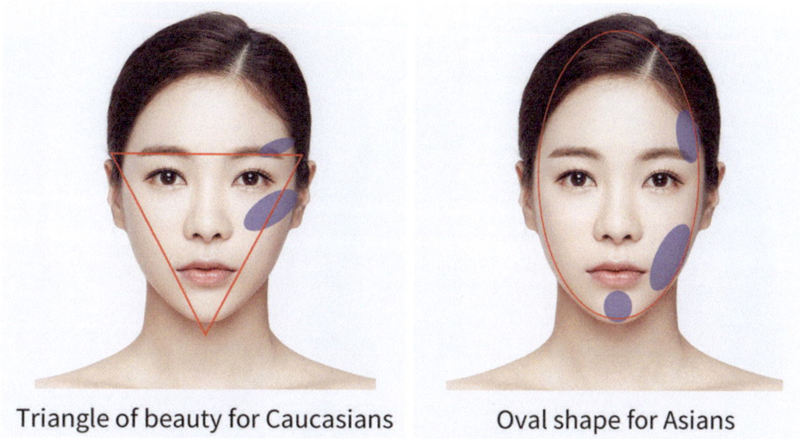

Fig. 1.24 Different strategies for achieving the ideal facial shape for Caucasians vs. Asians

Table 1.5 Filler indication for different Asian facial morphotypes by facial region

	Northern	Intermediate	Southern
Pretarsal roll augmentation	Popular	Popular	Only when favored by the patient
Malar augmentation	Confined to infraorbital medial malar enhancement	Confined to infraorbital medial malar enhancement	May optionally combine lateral malar augmentation in those with a thin narrow face
Mandibular angle augmentation	Not indicated	Not indicated	May be indicated for thin narrow face
Chin augmentation	Primarily for receded chin correction	For both V-shaped jawline and receded chin correction	Primarily for receded chin correction
Nasal dorsum augmentation	Nasal hump correction/nasal dorsum augmentation preferred	In both nasal dorsum and the subnasale	In both nasal dorsum and the subnasale

tion to the facial width. Other procedures commonly used in Asians to add dimensionality and projection include forehead augmentation, filler rhinoplasty, and receded chin augmentation (Fig. 1.18).

1.3.4.2 Different Strategies for Shaping Facial Features (Table 1.5)

Nose augmentation represents one of the most popular and well-established filler procedures among Asians who have a relatively low set nasal dorsum compared with Caucasians. This is in contrast to Caucasians for whom filler rhinoplasty is practiced more sparingly, primarily for correcting a nasal hump or bifid nose tips. Though among the Asian facial morphotypes, the northern facial type tends to feature a relatively taller nasal dorsum, nose fillers are routinely used even in this group for nasal hump correction or for the partial augmentation of the upper dorsum. This is relevant for patients with a narrow nasofrontal angle as it helps to smoothen the transition between the superciliary arch and the nasal dorsum. In southern facial type Asians who characteristically have a flat nose with a wide nasal base, filler rhinoplasty is applied not only for elevating the nasal dorsum but also for projecting and cephalically rotating the nasal tip by placing fillers in the columella and the subnasale region to open the nasolabial angle. It should be noted that Asians generally tend to have a rounded nasal tip, and therefore, direct injection in the tip is best avoided as it is likely to create a bulbous appearance. Hence, only a tiny judicious amount of filler is advised in the nasal tip just enough to provide slight accentuation.

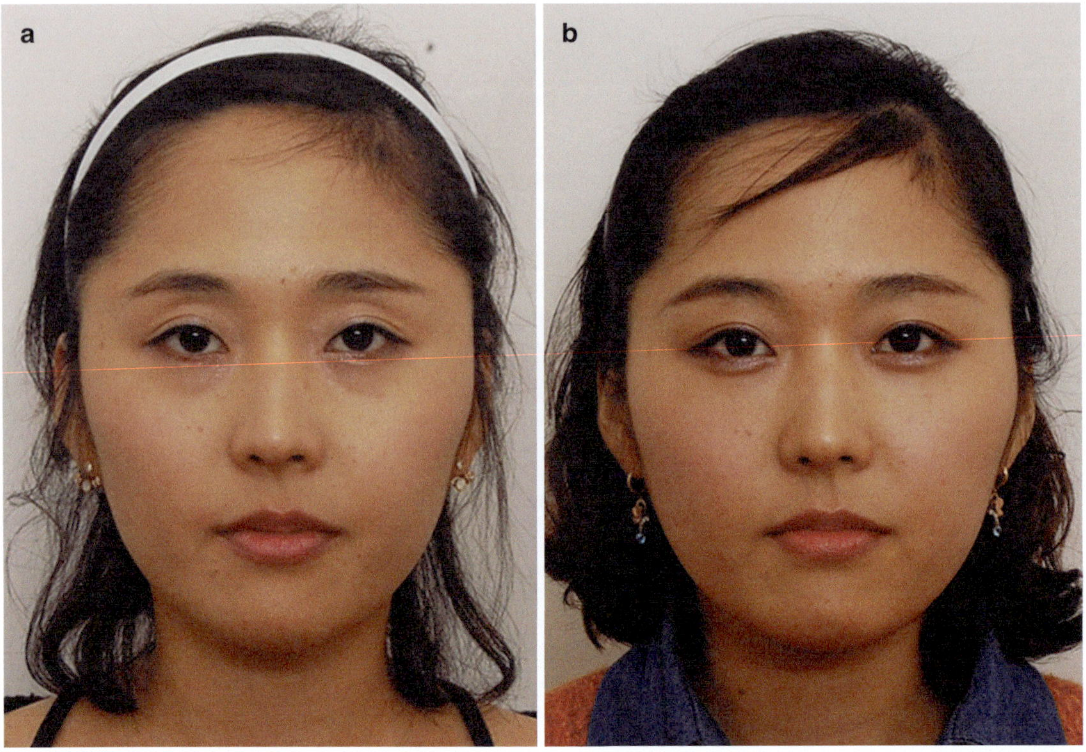

Fig. 1.25 (**a**) Before and (**b**) after pretarsal roll augmentation combined with filler volumization for sunken eyes and tear trough

Meanwhile, whereas high arched eyebrows with lateral peaks are considered a favorable feature in a Caucasian female, and thus eyebrow augmentation with fillers is commonly performed in Caucasians to gently lift the lateral brow, eyebrow arching is seldom practiced in Asians who much prefer to have straight horizontal brows. On the other hand, the use of fillers for sunken upper eyelid treatment is an indication that has recently gained popularity among Asians as it gives the eyes a more youthful and rested appearance. In Asians for whom fullness in the upper lid is the norm, the appearance of hollowness in the eyes tends to be more strongly correlated with the perception of tiredness and aging compared with Caucasians for whom deep-set eyes with narrow distance between the eye and brow is a more common facial feature.

Caucasians and Asians also differ in their aesthetic preference for lower pretarsal fullness. Pretarsal hypertrophic roll a.k.a. charming roll is a structure generated or accentuated by the contraction of the palpebral portion of the orbicularis oculi m. while smiling. For this reason, the constant presence of pretarsal fullness at rest imparts a soft, friendly smiling impression as well as framing the eye fissures in such a way to give the illusion of enlarged eyes. For this reason, they are called the 'supratarsal crease' for the lower lid. Among Koreans, augmenting the pretarsal roll with fillers is a particularly popular indication (Fig. 1.25). From the Caucasian viewpoint, however, the pretarsal roll may serve as a factor that makes the small Asian eye appear even smaller. In fact, this motivated the development of a novel BoNT-A indication for the removal of the pretarsal roll for widening the eye fissures [9].

Removing the lower pretarsal roll with this method, however, inhibits the contraction of eye fissures during a smile, which prevents the eyes from smiling along with the rest of the face, creating a rather uncanny disparity (Fig. 1.26). At rest, it results in lower white sclera show, creat-

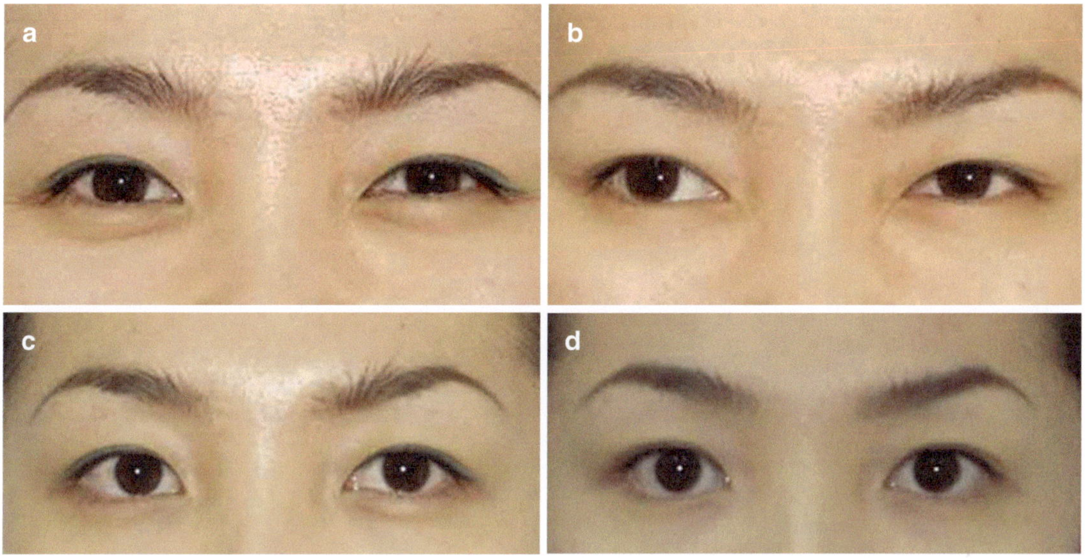

Fig. 1.26 (**a**, **c**) Before and (**b**, **d**) after removing the lower pretarsal roll with botulinum toxin injection

ing a rather negative macabre image. For this reason, this procedure is absolutely contraindicated in Koreans. Instead, most Asians, especially the northern facial types, appreciate the benefits of filler injection to their lower pretarsal roll. That said, southern facial types who tend to share the Caucasian aesthetic ideal of large, round, almond-shaped eyes may occasionally elect to have their lower pretarsal fullness removed with BoNT-A treatment. As such, the pretarsal roll treatment should be determined based on the patient's expressed preference.

Lip augmentation has traditionally been a popular aesthetic indication among Caucasians who find large, voluminous lips appealing. On the other hand, the explosion in enthusiasm for lip fillers is a relatively recent phenomenon in Asia, which has taken hold over the past few years. Attesting to this new trend, there is now even an aesthetic dermatology clinic in Seoul practicing only lip volumization procedures to the exclusion of all other aesthetic treatments. Finally, chin augmentation in Caucasians is performed primarily to restore a receded chin as opposed to defining the chin tip (a.k.a. "V-line filler") since their already long, narrow faces do not require further elongation. In contrast, a combination of receded chin correction and V-line filler is routinely used in Asians, particularly in intermediate face types, to add both volume and vertical length to the chin since the face often demonstrates not only a weak chin but also a rounded facial shape due to lack of facial length.

1.3.4.3 Summary

Knowledge of the different facial aesthetic goals between Caucasians and Asians for the ideal facial shape and facial attractiveness is the starting point for delivering the right aesthetic treatment for the right ethnic population. The same applies when undertaking volumizing filler procedures. As previously noted, the average Asian face tends to be wide and flat, presenting with enlarged zygoma and a relatively small lower facial third. For this reason, vertical midface augmentation accentuating the midline features of the forehead, nose, and chin, etc., to increase anterior projection and create the perception of a slimmer face is preferred for volumizing an Asian face and thus achieving the aesthetic ideal of an oval baby-like face. Similarly, augmenting the sunken temples and submalar hollows to obscure the appearance of the prominent zygoma is commonly used in Asians to smoothen the lateral facial contour and achieve a softer taper toward the lower face. Finally, the Asian face can be classified into three distinct morphotypes, namely, the northern, intermediate, and southern facial types, and differentiated solutions should be provided consistent with the aesthetic goals of each group.

References

1. Hu KS, Koh KS, Han SH, Shin KJ, Kim HJ. Sex determination using non-metric traits of the mandible in Koreans. J Forensic Sci. 2006;51(6):1376–82.
2. Goodman GJ. Facial attractiveness and the central role of volume. In: Carruthers J, Carruthers A, editors. Soft tissue augmentation. Philadelphia: Elsevier; 2018. p. 7–15.
3. Sundaram H, Huang PH, Hsu NJ, Huh CH, Wu W, Wu Y, Cassuto D, Kerscher MJ, Seo KI, Pan-Asian Aesthetics Toxin Consensus Group. Aesthetic applications of botulinum toxin A in Asians: an international, multidisciplinary, pan-asian consensus. Plast Reconstr Surg Glob Open. 2016;4(12):e872.
4. Seo KK. Aesthetic use of botulinum toxin in Asians. In: Benedetto AV, editor. Botulinum toxins in clinical aesthetic practice, Functional anatomy and injection techniques, vol. 2. 3rd ed. Boca Raton, FL: CRC Press/Taylor and Francis Group; 2018. p. 299–309.
5. Kim HJ, Seo KI, Lee HK, Kim JS. Clinical anatomy of face for botulinum toxin and filler injection. Berlin: Springer; 2016. p. 45–8.
6. Seo KK. Botulinum toxin for Asians. Singapore: Springer Nature Ltd.; 2017. p. 37–43.
7. Rhee SC, Lee SH. Attractive composite faces of different races. Aesthet Plast Surg. 2010;34:800–1.
8. Rhee SC. The average Korean attractive face. Aesthet Plast Surg. 2006;30(6):729–30.
9. Flynn TC, Carruthers JDA, Carruthers JA. Botulinum toxin treatment of the lower eyelid improves infraorbital rhytides and widens the eye. Dermatol Surg. 2001;27(8):703–8.

2 Volumizing Fillers

2.1 Types of Injectable Fillers

By definition, fillers refer to all materials added to provide filling efficacy in areas of volume deficit. In facial aesthetic procedures, these include materials placed in the face to lift etched-in grooves or to revolumize facial depressions. In this sense, a broader definition of the term may include autologous fat used in fat graft procedures or, for that matter, encompass even paraffin or silicon previously used widely in illicit cosmetic treatments. That said, the first injectable filler recognized as a legitimate medical device was based on collagen—a structural component of the skin matrix. In the early 1980s, bovine-derived ZYDERM® (Allergan. the US) was introduced to the market, representing the very first modern-day injectable filler to be approved by the US FDA (Fig. 2.1). However, due to their animal origin, the use of bovine collagen-based fillers was constrained by the inherent risk of *immunogenic* reactions and their short duration of effect. Accordingly, with the subsequent advent and dominance of HA fillers, bovine collagen fillers soon fell out of favor globally.

Today, injectable fillers are still commonly referred to as "dermal fillers", maybe due to the fact that the first fillers ever to be used was collagen-based. Granted, collagen does represent an essential building block of the dermal architecture, and indeed collagen fillers had originally been injected directly in the dermis to improve skin elasticity and wrinkles. However, the use of injectable fillers has since evolved significantly and today they are utilized not simply for refining lines and wrinkles but in an exciting array of new and minimally invasive cosmetic procedures that leverage the volumizing effect of injectable fillers (Fig. 2.2) [1]. Examples include enhancing a flat nose or plumping thin lips, if not reshaping the facial contour. Moreover, whereas the term "dermal filler" implies they are injected into the *dermis*, the depth of injection required for these volumization procedures is much deeper than that, that is, in the deep subcutaneous or even down onto the supraperiosteal plane. On this basis, it may be fair to suggest the term "dermal filler" has become a misnomer, and that it is high time the modifier "dermal" was duly removed.

After collagen fillers, HA came to dominate the world market for injectable fillers. The key drivers of its success were its excellent safety profile consisting of the same constituents that make up the dermis, causing minimal immunogenic responses in the body, and its unique ability to be reversible, whereby results could be dissolved away if so desired using a reversal agent. On top of its unmatched safety, HA fillers have also proven to show an excellent duration of effect. While initially HA fillers were understood to last between 6 months and 1 year in the tissue when first introduced in the early 2000s, it is now widely accepted that their longevity can last for up to several years if injected in boluses or given in repeat maintenance dosages. This is because when the HA filler is injected in the form of a

K. K. Seo, *Facial Volumization with Fillers*, https://doi.org/10.1007/978-981-33-6212-3_2

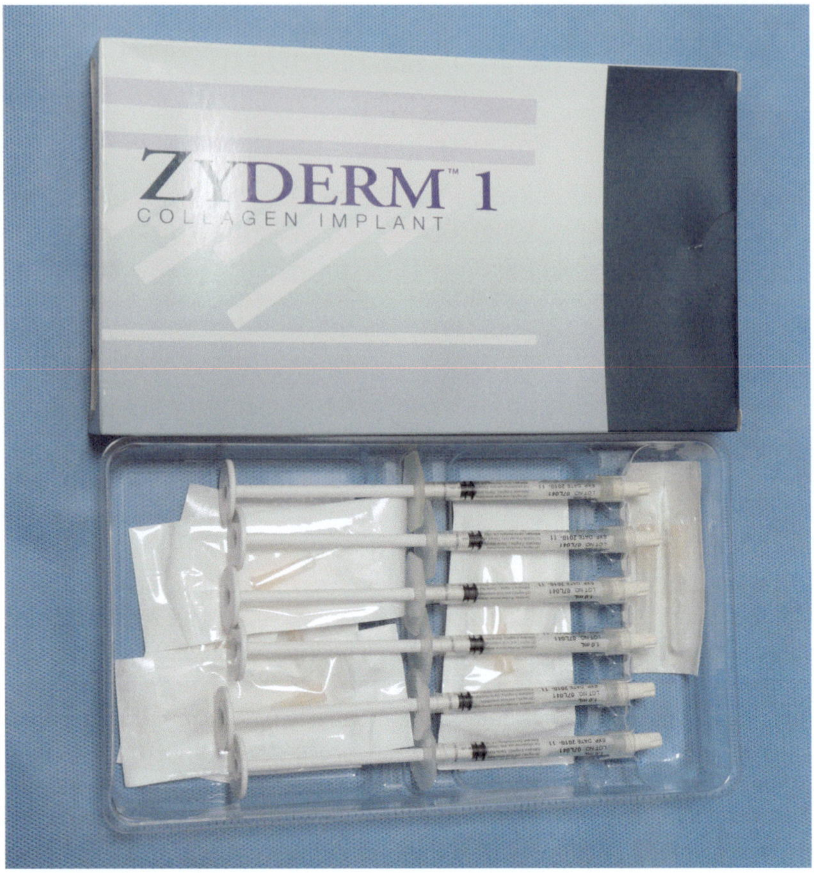

Fig. 2.1 ZYDERM®1

bolus, it limits the per unit surface area of the HA filler that comes into contact with the body's hyaluronidase, inhibiting degradation by the enzyme. Notably, HA filler placed in the forehead, nasal dorsum, and the pretarsal roll regions tends to show longevity lasting for as long as 5–10 years.

While the first HA filler to come to market was Hylaform® (Hylan B gel) (Genzyme Biosurgery) extracted from rooster combs, the product was driven out of use due to problems associated with protein impurities from avian sources and subsequently, HA fillers have been made using purified HA from bacterial sources such as streptococcus, which remain to this day to be the most dominant product on the market.

Whereas collagen-based or HA fillers are designed primarily to replace and restore lost volume ("replacement filler"), collagen-stimulating fillers, also known as biostimulating fillers, consist of biodegradable polymers that induce collagen biostimulation in the injected area while they themselves slowly degrade in the body. Prime examples of these collagen-stimulating fillers include Radiesse® for calcium hydroxylapatite (CaHA) and Sculptra® for poly-L-lactic acid (PLLA) (see the Sect. 2.4.3). In general, these collagen-stimulating fillers are known to provide better longevity compared with HA fillers. The drawback to these fillers, however, is that they do not allow customization of volume correction, as results are subject to individual variability in collagen production; and that it takes 4–12 weeks for the new collagen to build whereas the initial volume replenishment from the carrier substance, be it CMC (carboxymethylcellulose) or saline, dissipates shortly after the treatment. Moreover, the results of collagen-stimulating fillers are hard to

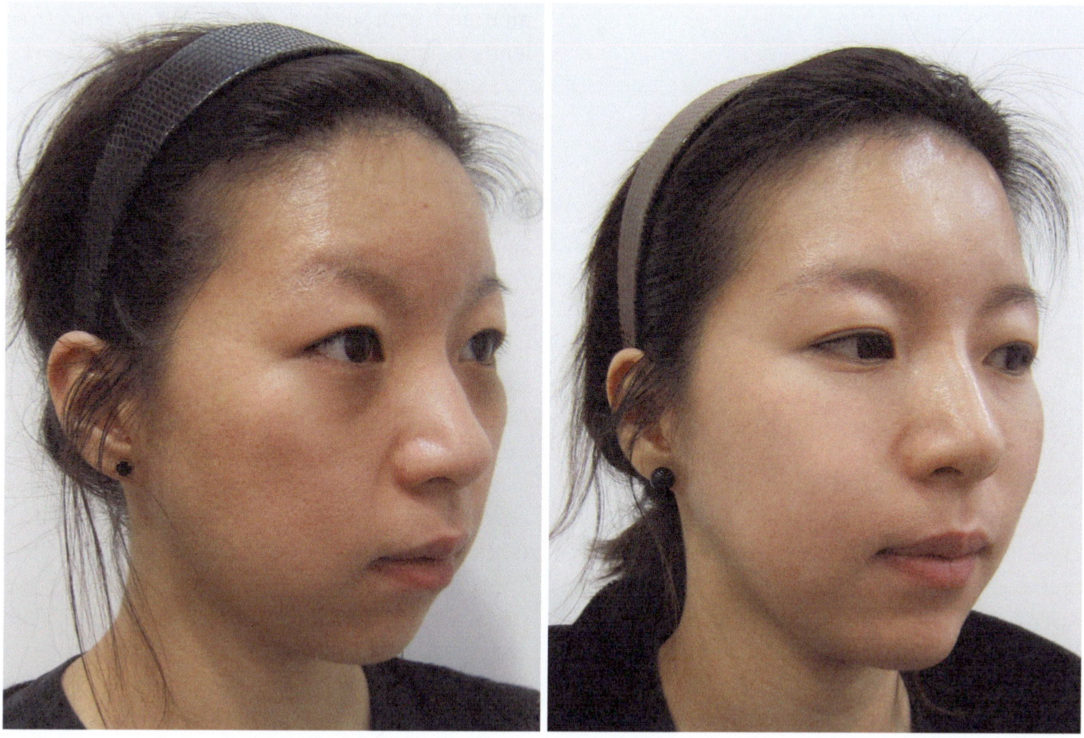

Fig. 2.2 The use of injectable fillers for three-dimensionality and volumizing effect. A 31-year-old female patient showed marked changes after receiving volumization filler injection for sunken cheeks, nose, chin, and anterior medial malar area

reverse in the event of any nodules or irregularities arising from uneven placement of the product.

Meanwhile, products such as PAAG (polyacrylamide gel)-based Aquamid® or PMMA (polymethyl methacrylate)-based Bellafill® were developed to provide prolonged longevity based on the use of permanent synthetic substances (see the Sect. 2.4.2). However, whether these permanent fillers are necessarily a good option remains open to question, considering that the underlying facial structure is not permanent. With aging, the face loses its youthful definition due to the progressive sagging and clumping of facial tissue, which continues well after these permanent fillers are placed. Consequently, this can result in a disharmonious appearance between the injected area and the rest of the aging face. Moreover, the permanency of fillers also implies that potential complications arising from such permanent or semipermanent solutions are also permanent, for which surgical removal remains the only option.

2.2 Hyaluronic Acid Fillers

Hyaluronic acid ("HA") represents the most widely used type of injectable filler in the world, with its excellent biocompatibility, low immunogenicity, and reversibility putting it far ahead of other types of injectable fillers (Fig. 2.3). While commercial HA filler products are more or less similar to each other in appearance, there exist slight distinctions in terms of their HA concentration, cross-linking technology, degree of cross-links, viscosity, gel hardness, cohesivity, etc. Differences exist even among products within the same brand of HA filler, and knowledge of such characteristics is critical for customizing the use of each product for its intended use.

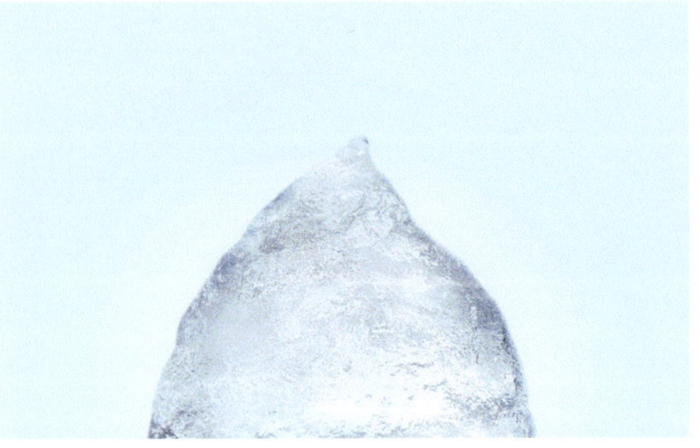

Fig. 2.3 Hyaluronic acid gel (Photo: Courtesy of Galderma)

2.2.1 Characteristics of HA

Hyaluronic acid is a high-molecular-weight polymer comprised of repeating disaccharides first discovered in 1934 by Karl Meyer and John Palmer in the vitreous body of bovine eyes [2]. Hyaluronic acid is said to derive its name from *hyaloid* (meaning vitreous) and *uronic acid*, a component of repeating dissacharide units. In the natural state, hyaluronic acid exists in the salt form, mostly as sodium hyaluronate bound to sodium (Na), a cation most widely found in the human body. In 1986, the term "hyaluronan" was adopted in accordance with the international nomenclature of polysaccharides [3]. Correspondingly, the terms hyaluronic acid, sodium hyaluronate and hyaluronan are all used interchangeably to refer to the same HA.

Hyaluronic acid constitutes a glycosaminoglycan (GAGs) molecule consisting of *polysaccharide chains* made up of alternating D-glucuronic acid and *N*-acetyl-D-glucosamine units combined together in a repetitive manner (Fig. 2.4) [2]. GAGs refer collectively to the group of long, unbranched linear polysaccharides containing amino acids that are made up of repeating disaccharide units. Representing a crucial component of the extracellular matrix, GAGs are classified into six classes based on the underlying *mono*-saccharide structures, namely, HA, chondroitin sulfate, keratin sulfate, dermatan sulfate, heparin, and heparin sulfate. Of the GAGs, HA is found most commonly in the skin [2]. However, unlike other classes of GAGs, it is not modified with sulfate groups and is not covalently bound to a protein core.

Further, it represents the only class of GAG that is present in both animal- and bacterial-sources. As a highly hydrophilic molecule, HA is also capable of retaining water up to1000 times its molecular weight [2]. In aqueous solution, the abundance of *negative charges* in HA's chemical structure generally causes the negative charges to repel each other. This allows HA to occupy a larger space, as the entire molecular network expands and is surrounded by water molecules. In addition, while HA molecules decrease in volume when subject to an increase in external pressure, they mostly recover their original volume once the external force is removed, due to the mutual repulsion between the negative charges. These characteristics allow HA to exist in a gel form when mixed with water, demonstrating the properties of both viscosity and elasticity. In a normal physiological pH environment, the carboxyl groups (–COOH) comprising the D-glucuronic acid of the HA is converted to sodium salt. HA possesses four hydroxyl groups (–OH) and one sodium salt group in each disaccharide unit [2]. The hydroxyl groups of HA form hydrogen bonds with water molecules and thus become readily soluble in water.

Each disaccharide unit of HA consisting of D-glucuronic acid and *N*-acetyl-D-glucosamine represents a monomer with a molecular weight of 400 Da, with each monomer linked together via β-1,4 glycosidic bonds to form the HA polymer. The HA polymers present in the human synovial fluid are known to consist of 20,000 monomers or a molecular mass of seven million Da. As a major component of the body's extracellular matrix, HA is responsible for absorbing moisture and keeping the tissues lubricated and hydrated while providing necessary structural support. Furthermore, it is also responsible for the modulation of cellular migration and proliferation, as well as regulating inflammation control and wound repair/regeneration. The total *HA* content in an adult weighing 70 kg is estimated to be approximately 15 g [4], with roughly half of this amount known to be located in the skin. Hyaluronic acid is also found in high concentra-

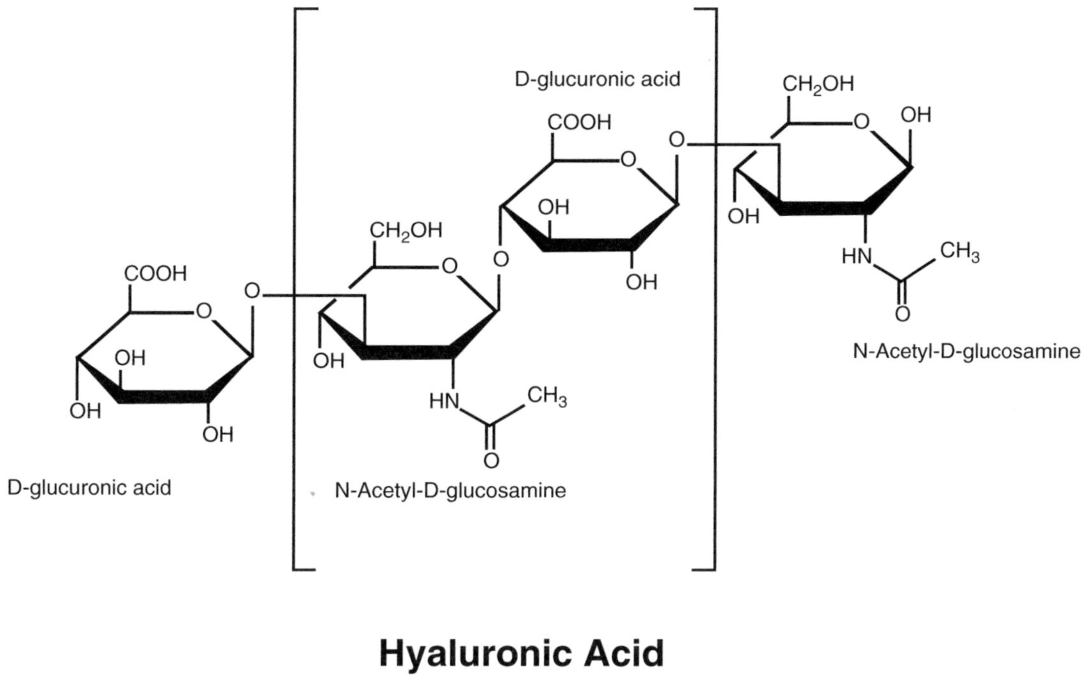

Fig. 2.4 Hyaluronic acid constitutes a glycosaminoglycan (GAGs) molecule consisting of *polysaccharide chains* made up of alternating D-glucuronic acid and *N*-acetyl-D-glucosamine units combined together in a repetitive manner

tions in the synovial fluid, cartilage, and the vitreous body of the eyes. The body is known to maintain optimum HA homeostasis, whereby *one-third* of the body's HA is turned over, that is, degraded and newly synthesized, each day [4]. While HA is continuously replenished in the human body, aging causes a gradual decrease in the natural production of HA, consequently resulting in loss of skin moisture and elasticity over time.

Unlike collagen, the molecular structure of HA remains identical across all animal species, with the only difference being the polymer length. HA polymers derived from bacterial strains are typically 4000–6000 monomers in length, shorter than the 10,000–15,000 found in animal-based HA, and thus have a lower molecular weight, 1.5–2.5 million Da [2].

2.2.2 Hyaluronic Acid Filler Manufacturing Process

In general, the HA filler manufacturing process consists of the following steps: dissolution of HA powder (raw material) in NaOH solution, addition of the cross-linking agent followed by the cross-linking reaction, cutting, cleaning, grinding, filling of the HA gel into the syringe, and sterilization (Fig. 2.5). Of these process steps, cross-linking of HA polymer chains represents the most critical stage of manufacture, as it ultimately defines the rheological properties of the HA filler while also stabilizing the HA molecules for extended longevity in vivo. Subsequent to undergoing the cross-linking reaction, the bulk HA gel is then cleaved into multiple small pieces ("cutting") to facilitate cleansing. Next, the cleaved chunks of HA are rinsed down with either purified water or saline to remove any undesired impurities. In the next step, the gels are treated to decrease the gel particle size. This is either done by crushing the gel, after which they are passed using a rotating knife or homogenizer or by passing the gel through a mesh of a defined size homogenizer. In both these cases, the gel particle size reduction allows injection of the gel into the skin through a fine gauge needle. However, as the mesh method generates particles of a controlled size, it also enables adaption of

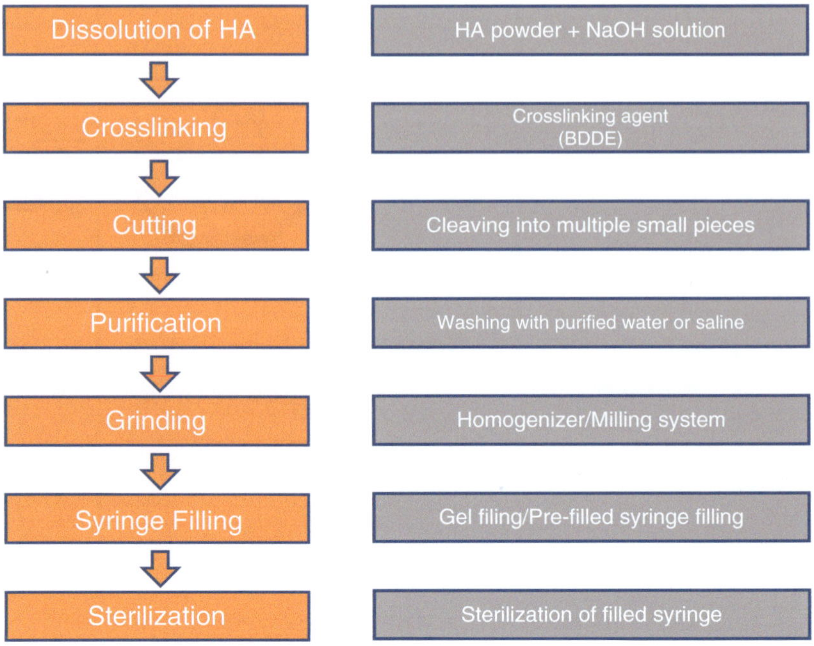

Fig. 2.5 Hyaluronic acid filler manufacturing process

the gel particles to suit the desired clinical indication. This is not the case if a homogenizer is used, as the resulting particle size is inhomogenous. After grinding, the HA gel is filled into individual syringes which are then transferred into an autoclave for sterilization [5].

A key consideration during the manufacture of HA fillers is the in-process control of undesired proteins, endotoxin, and residual crosslinking agents. Proteins are a major cause of inflammation and allergy; therefore, it is critical to ensure the HA raw material meets the requirements of the European Pharmacopoeia (EP) for protein content (<0.1% of the raw material). For most commercially available HA filler products, manufacturers endeavor to keep residual protein levels at 10μg/mL or less to minimize the risk of allergic reactions. Meanwhile, endotoxin levels are controlled at 0.5 EU/mL (endotoxin unit) or less as prescribed in the EP to avoid possible pyrogenic and/or inflammatory reactions [5]. While the BDDE levels are also regulated at below 2 ppm, in practice, BDDE is hardly ever detected in a final HA filler product.

2.2.2.1 Production of HA Raw Material

Industrial manufacturing of HA raw material (bulk HA) is based on either extraction from rooster combs or microbial fermentation using bacterial strains. During the nascent stages of HA filler development, HA biopolymer extracted from rooster combs was used for most products, as the process generated HA with naturally high molecular weight. For example, Hylaform® (Genzyme Biosurgery), approved by the US FDA in 2004, was made using HA derived from rooster combs, which had molecular weight ranging approx. 3000 kDa. However, commercial production of HA from rooster combs was time-consuming and expensive, involving numerous process steps and considerable time to complete. Furthermore, there were significant technical difficulties in eliminating possible viruses (avian) or proteins and nucleic acids potentially remaining in the animal tissue. Also, the serious incidences with Bovine Spongiform Encephalopathy showed that deadly diseases could be transfered between species (animal> human) in ways previously not known. The use of bacterially derived materials are in that aspect regarded a much lower risk than animal derived as bacteria are very different from animal cells. As a consequence of these manufacturing and safety concerns, extraction of HA from rooster combs eventually fell out of favor, and instead bacterial fermentation became the preferred method of obtaining HA [6]. Bacterial fermentation is capable of generating HA at significantly lower cost, in mass quantity, and with greater ease with which to remove residual foreign proteins and endotoxins in-process compared with extracting HA from rooster combs. Streptococcus has been the bacteria most widely used for microbial HA production, with Streptococcus zooepidemicus being the most used strain [6]. Restylane®, which represents the first HA-based injectable filler to obtain US FDA approval in 2003, is also based on HA extracted from microbial fermentation, having a molecular weight ranging approx. 1000 kDa. Driven by advances in fermentation technology, molecular weight of HA obtained from microbial HA production has progressively increased from below 2000 kDa during the early days to above 3000 kDa at present [6]. While microbial fermentation can produce HA with higher purity free of residual pathogens such as avian viruses compared with HA of avian origin, the risk of contamination with bacterial endotoxins, intracellular organelle, and undesired proteins nonetheless remains, for which complex and extensive purification is required. To this end, the bacterial cells are subjected first to centrifugation for cell separation, and subsequently to dissolution in sodium hydroxide (NaOH) solution. The resulting cell-free solution then undergoes the subsequent processes of ultrafiltration, adsorption onto activated carbon or alumina, and alcohol precipitation to remove any possible impurities or cell debris (Fig. 2.6) which may remain in the product. These purification process may differ between manufacturers. The average molecular weight of HA is controlled via e.g. fermentation conditions and the handling during the purification process.

As explained, the purity of the HA raw material is determined largely by the specific method and degree of purification applied during the manufacturing process. Key considerations in the choice of HA raw materials are bacterial endotoxins and cell-derived proteins remaining in the product, and whether their amounts fall within the required specification. The respective extent to which these impurities reside determines the biological safety of the HA, and accordingly, its clinical grade. HA raw material for industrial use is classified as food grade, cosmetic grade, or medical grade, with medical-grade HA further broken down into those for use as ophthalmic formulations (eye-drops grade) or injectable preparations (injection grade) depending on the stringency of the purification required. Eye-drops grade HA is used in the manufacture of eye drops, contact lenses preservatives, and topical preparations for oral mucosal lesions, whereas injection-grade HA is used for producing intraocular lens implants, intraarticular injections, antiadhesion agents (for preventing postsurgical tissue adhe-

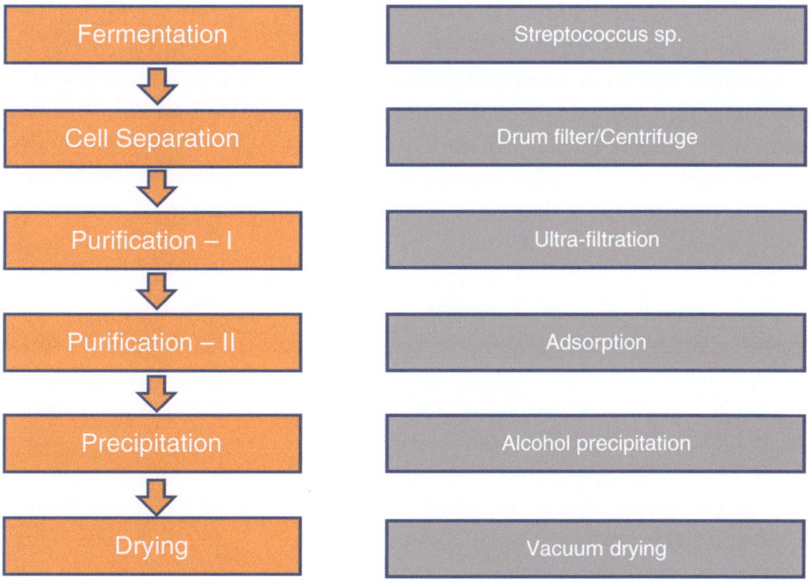

Fig. 2.6 Production of HA raw material from microbial fermentation

sion), and injectable fillers, to name a few. Injection-grade HA is generally 3–4 times more expensive than eyedrop-grade HA used for ophthalmic formulations, with HA powders for injection being of the highest purity among all formulations of HA raw material [7].

Since the safety of injectable HA filler products depends not only on the quality of additional purification steps undertaken during their manufacture but also on the underlying HA raw material itself, the quality and the purity of the source HA raw material represents a necessary, if not sufficient, component for determining the safety of the final HA filler product. At the very least, therefore, HA filler products satisfy the minimum standard for quality if they are manufactured using HA raw materials sourced from suppliers contained in the US FDA's list of Drug Master File and approved by the E*uropean* Directorate for the Quality of Medicines & Healthcare (EDQM) [7]. As of 2020, manufacturers of HA raw material contained in the FDA's list of DMF are as follows: LG Chem LTD (Korean entity); Kewpie Corp, Kikkoman Biochemifa Co, Kibun Food Chemifa Co. LTD, Kyowa Hakko Kogyo Co LTD, Seikagaku Corp, Shiseido Co LTD (Japanese entities); Bloomage Biotechnology Corp LTD, Shandong Freda Biochem Co LTD, Shandong Awa Biopharm Co LTD (Chinese entities); Bioiberica SA, Contipro AS, Fidia Farmaceutici SPA, Novozymes AS (EU entities); Dermal Research Laboratories INC, Lifecore Biomedical LLC, Maruha Nichiro Corp (US entities). In this regard, LG Chem.'s YVOIRE® is based on its own in-house HA formulation and Neuramis® by Medytox Inc. is formulated with raw HA supplied by Shiseido Co LTD (Japan) while most HA filler manufacturers do not disclose their source of HA raw material supply.

Episode: Chance and Necessity

A roofer performing repair work on a tall building inadvertently drops his hammer which hits a passing pedestrian on the head and kills him. While the roofer's dropping of the hammer was purely accidental, it inevitably led to the deterministic event of the pedestrian's death. Such is the reasoning presented in the book *Chance and Necessity* by the Nobel Prize laureate Jaques Monod to interpret the process of evolution. In essence, he postulates, it was by pure coincidence that a cell embodying the most rudimentary form of life was produced via some inexplicable and highly unlikely sequence of biochemical reactions among inorganic matter; and that today's lower or higher animals represent the necessary product of the messy and complex evolutionary process the cells subsequently underwent. Upon first reading the book back in university, I simply considered it to be a clever, if rather paradoxical, set of arguments in support of the theory of evolution. With the passage of time, however, I have come to appreciate how the ideas espoused in Chance and Necessity bore striking relevance to our own lives.

In 1998, while working as a research fellow at the Seoul National University Hospital, Department of Dermatology, I stumbled upon a fascinating study by Dr. Shelley published in the Journal of American Academy of Dermatology involving the injection of botulinum toxin on the patients' palms for the treatment of palmar hyperhidrosis. The fact that the effects were found to last for up to 5–6 months struck me as particularly intriguing. While clearly not a life-threatening condition or a contagious disease, focal hyperhidrosis, especially, palmar hyperhidrosis, can be deeply distressing to the patient himself, given how it hinders his daily activities in a host of troubling ways. Sweaty hands are subject to greater risk of frostbites in the winter; also, when writing, note taking, or completing written exams, it requires the placement of a handkerchief underneath the hand so as not to wet the paper. Wet clammy hands are neither ideal for holding or shaking and can put the person at an undue disadvantage in various social interactions. The degree of anguish felt by patients is such that according to one study, the emotional and psychological distress inflicted by hyperhydrosis was found to be greater than that of chronic rheumatoid arthritis or chronic kidney failure. Although some remedies for palmar hyperhydrosis are available, including topical agents and oral medicine, the effects are largely transient and minimal. In most cases, patients are simply referred instead to the thoracic surgery department to undergo a more invasive endoscopic sympathectomy. However, despite the permanent cure it provides, sympathectomy is not without its own share of problems, including the risk of developing compensatory hyperhidrosis. Simply put, palmar hyperhydrosis is a profoundly uninteresting business for an average dermatologist.

It so happened that during my first year of residency training at the SNUH, one of my responsibilities was measuring the amount of the sweat discharges of palmar hyperhydrosis patients as per the instructions of the professor in the Dermatology Dept. It was menial and time-consuming work; all the more so, since the precision scale used for the measurements was kept at a separate office on the twelfth floor of the building. Each trip to and from the office with the patient took up to 30 minutes. Yet nothing much materialized from those grueling daily trips and tests other than a dissertation published in the name of the professor in charge. I couldn't see what possible good it was doing for the patient when eventually they had to be whisked off to the thoracic surgery department for the actual treatment.

With that gruelling memory still vivid in my mind, it was absolutely mind-blowing to learn that a single injection was capable of providing up to months of relief for palma hyperhydrosis patients. The underlying drug was affordably priced too, at only about 60 USD per bottle of Botox®. Upon further literature review, I discovered that what scant research papers that had existed were still only in their infancy and decided right there and then that I had found my niche. Quickly, I put together a research proposal within a matter of 3 days and was set to go. The only hitch—however—was that the list price of about 60 USD in the SNUH pharmacopeia had in fact been a typo graphical error! To my dismay, it turned out a 0 in the last digit had been omitted by error, meaning the actual price was a whopping 600 USD. Two bottles for injecting both hands would cost 1,200 USD per treatment, and I had to seriously ponder whether from the patient's perspective, 5–6 months of temporary relief from sweaty hands would justify that kind of cost. In the end, however, I decided the treatment still had its appeal as a novel noninvasive treatment involving the use of injections and pushed ahead with the plan. That's how I first got started on my practice with botulinum toxin. The rest I suppose is history.

Sure enough, life works in mysterious ways. Had it not been for the drudgery of those sweat measurements, or that chance perusal of the JAAD paper on palmar hyperhidrosis, *or* the incorrectly listed Botox® price in the SNUH pharmacopeia, I wonder whether I would have ended up performing botox procedures at all. We are the ultimate product of the countless coincidental events that have occurred in our past. The only distinction between our lives and the evolutionary process is that human life does not stretch out for billions of years, and hence requires some form of exertion on our part to bridge the gap between chance and the necessary outcome that we desire. Similar to how we inevitably discovered our life partners out of the many random encounters in life, it is the passion, devotion, and sweat, I suppose, that ultimately turn mere accidents of yesterday into the well-earned fruits of tomorrow (June 2019).

2.2.2.2 Incorporation of Cross-Linking Agent/Cross-Linking Reaction

Dissolved in water, HA powder changes into a thick glue-like liquid with viscous texture similar to that of sweet and sour sauce, a state referred to as *free* HA. Free HA hardly has any structure or elasticity and is thus incapable of providing support or projection in the tissue. If free HA is injected as the filler material, it will degrade within a week due to the activity of endogenous hyaluronidase or free radicals in the human tissues. Thus, to confer elasticity to the free HA and increase its duration in vivo, cross-linking is introduced between the HA polymers to stabilize the HA into a gel form. Cross-linking can be achieved either via physical or chemical methods. Each specific crosslinking procedure or gel technology results in gels whose properties depend on both physical and chemical factors. The physical factor enhances the effect of the chemical crosslinkers by entanglements between the HA polymers. This produces a tight-knit network of HA polymer chains (Fig. 2.7) that is held together by only a few chemical crosslinkers. For the chemical factors, the temperature at which the HA liquid (i.e., HA diluted in water) reacts with the crosslinking agent and the duration for which the HA reacts with the crosslinker are the most important parameters for binding the HA molecules to each other. A prime example of products whose properties are the result of physical factors is Restylane®. The NASHA™ technology used to generate the gels results in strong gels with a high G' but with less than 1% degree of modification (MoD), something that is of importance to assure a good biocompatibility.

While physical cross-linking plays an important part, the properties of a gel relies more on the introduction of cross-linking agents to interlink the HA molecules. Here, the cross-linking agent plays a role comparable to gluten in wheat flour. Unlike other grain, wheat flour mixed with water produces a dough that is bouncy, stretchy, and chewy, attributable primarily to the presence of gluten in the wheat protein. During the kneading of the dough, gluten in the wheat flour associates with starch to form a reticulated gluten membrane, which gives the dough its elasticity and allows it to hold its shape at rest and to stretch easily when pulled apart. In much the same fashion, cross-linking agents bind to individual HA polymer chains and join them together to build a tight network of cross-linked HA, converting the HA polymers from liquid to a gel form (Fig. 2.8). The HA gel mass thus produced effectively forms a united front against breakdown by free radicals. Finally, similar to how wheat flour is divided into hard, plain, and weak varieties depending on its gluten content, HA filler products can be classified as either firm (i.e., with high viscoelasticity) or soft (i.e., with low viscoelasticity) as determined by rheological measurments.

While various substances are available for use as cross-linking agents, including 1,4-butanediol diglycidyl ether (BDDE), divinyl sulfone (DVS), and biscarbodiimidie (BCDI), BDDE is the cross-linking agent by far the most widely used in the commercial production of HA fillers owing to its unrivaled low toxicity profile [5]. The

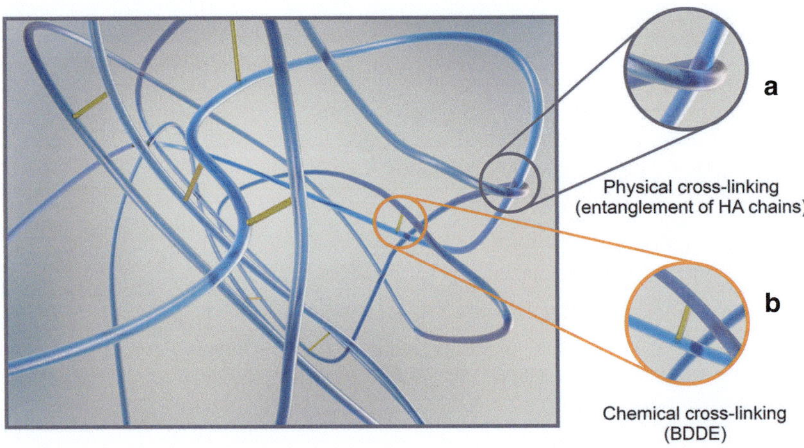

Fig. 2.7 A prime example of a physically cross-linked HA is NASHA technology incorporated in Restylane® (Photo: Courtesy of Galderma)

median lethal dose (LD50) of BDDE administered orally to rats is only 1134 mg/kg compared with 32 mg/kg for DVS. Strict standards apply against the amount of residual BDDE remaining in the product as remnants of unreacted BDDE can have a harmful effect on the human body. However, at the current limit of <2 μg, the residual BDDE in HA filler products amounts to only 1/25 million of the fatal dose in an adult of 50 kg [5]. Regardless, the industry remains committed to further minimizing the residual BDDE by increasing the reaction time or the reaction speed during the cross-linking reaction and by removing BDDE debris to the maximum during the cleaning and purification of the cross-linked HA gel. Meanwhile, during the cross-linking process, epoxide groups of BDDE react with the hydroxyl groups of HA under alkaline condition, forming derivatives of 1,4-butanediol di-(propane-2,3-diolyl) ether (BDPE) as shown in Fig. 2.9 [8]. In so doing, however, some BDDE molecules link with HA on both ends ("double-linked BDPE") while others join HA on one end only in the form of a pendant ("mono-linked BDPE") (Fig. 2.10).

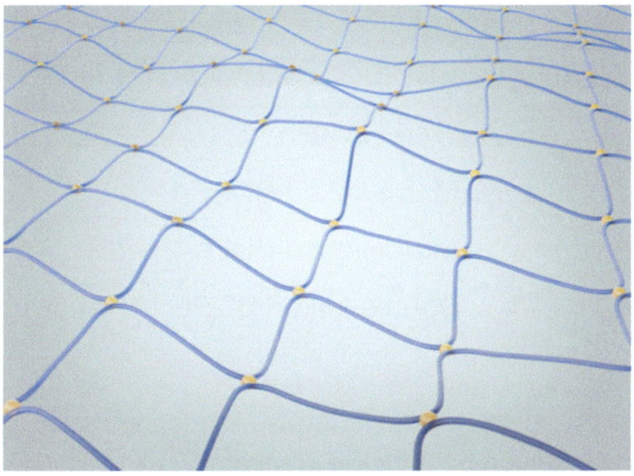

Fig. 2.8 Chemical cross-linking. Chemical cross-linking agents, 1,4-butanediol diglycidyl ether (BDDE) bind to individual HA polymer chains and join them together to build a tight network of cross-linked HA (OBT™ technology of Restylane®) (Photo: Courtesy of Galderma)

Fig. 2.9 During the cross-linking process, epoxide groups of BDDE react with the hydroxyl groups of HA under alkaline condition, forming derivatives of 1,4-butanediol di-(propane-2,3-diolyl) ether (BDPE)

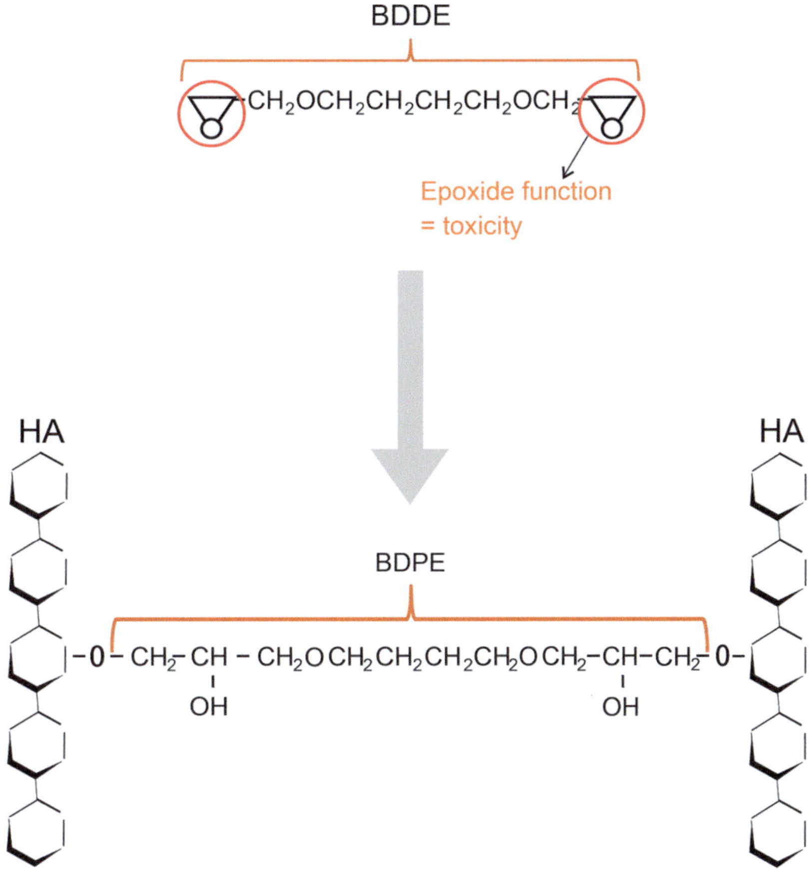

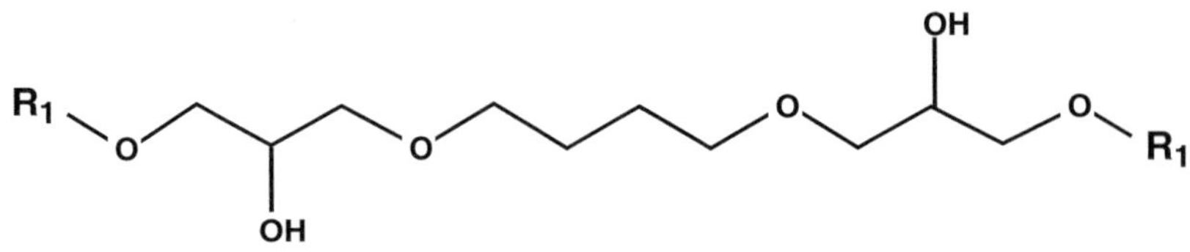

R_1	R_2	BDPE Classification
H	H	Free BDPE
HA	H	Mono-linked BDPE
H	HA	Mono-linked BDPE
HA	HA	Double-linked BDPE

Fig. 2.10 Some BDDE molecules link with HA on both ends (double-linked BDPE) while others join HA on one end only, in the form of a pendant (mono-linked BDPE)

A higher degree of cross-linking with BDDE is associated with prolonged duration of HA in the tissue, as well as greater elasticity and cohesiveness of the HA gel. Accordingly, the degree of cross-linking is a key factor in comparing the rheological properties of different HA products. The major parameters for describing the degree of cross-linking include degree of modification (MoD), degree of substitution (DS), degree of cross-linking (CrD), degree of cross-linking (DC), and effective cross-linker ratio (CrR), which are defined respectively as follows (Table 2.1) [8]:

(a) The degree of modification (MoD): the ratio between the sum of mono-linked (pendant-type) and double-linked BDPE and the total number of HA monomers (disaccharide units).
(b) The degree of substitution (DS): the ratio between the HA disaccharides bound with BDPE and the total number of HA monomers (disaccharide units).
(c) The degree of cross-linking represented by the acronym CrD: the ratio between BDPE residues that are double-linked and the total number of HA monomers (disaccharide units).
(d) The degree of cross-linking signified by the acronym DC: the number of HA disaccharides actually cross-linked relative to the total number of HA disaccharides.
(e) Effective cross-linker ratio (CrR): the ratio of double-linked BDDE in relation to the total BDPE.

In all of the above terms, the denominator is represented by the total number of HA monomer units (disaccharide units), while the numerator varies for each parameter. Simply put, MoD and CrD signify the ratio of BDPEs cross-linked with HA, while DS and DC represent the ratio of cross-linked HA disaccharide units vis-a-vis the total number of HA. Meanwhile, CrD represents the ratio of BDDE that is double-linked with HA (double-linked BDPE), whereas MoD covers the ratio of both the mono- (pendant- shaped) and double-linked BDPE.

By way of illustration, a CrD of 20% equates to a DC of 40%, as DC represents double the value of CrD. In each case, this implies that for each 10 HA monomers (or disaccharide units) in the gel, two BDDE molecules (CrD of 20%) or four HA disaccharide units (DC of 40%) have been cross-linked. Meanwhile, an MoD of 50% and CrR of 40% results in a DS of 70%, as this implies that for each 10 HA monomers (or disaccharide units), links have been formed with an average of five BDDE molecules (MoD of 50%), of which only two are double-linked BDDEs (CrR of 40%), and thus seven of the ten HA disaccharide units are connected to a BDDE (DS of 70%) (Fig. 2.11).

A high degree of cross-linking translates into greater gel hardness and prolonged longevity. Too much cross-linker content, however, hampers ease of injection due to product aggregation, undercuts HA hydrophilicity, and contributes only to causing immunogenic responses. Thus, an adequate balance of cross-linking is one of the

Table 2.1 Definitions of MoD, CrD, DS, and DC for modified HA fillers

	Definition based on number of…	
	…cross-linker units/HA units	…substituted HA units/HA units
Parameter	Degree of modification (MoD)	Degree of substitution (DS)
Definition	$\frac{n_{\text{linked cross-linkers}}}{n_{\text{HA disaccharides}}}$	$\frac{n_{\text{sustituted HA discaccharides}}}{n_{\text{HA disaccharides}}}$
Determination	From NMR	DS = MoD + CrD = MoD × (1 + CrR)
Parameter	Degree of cross-linking (CrD)	Degree of cross-linking (DC)
Definition	$\frac{n_{\text{doubled linked cross-linkers}}}{n_{\text{HA disaccharides}}}$	$\frac{n_{\text{cross-linked HA disaccharides}}}{n_{\text{HA disaccharides}}}$
Determination	CrD = CrR × MoD	DC = 2 × CrD = 2 × CrR × MoD

CrR: Effective cross-linker ratio. Modified from Ref. [8]

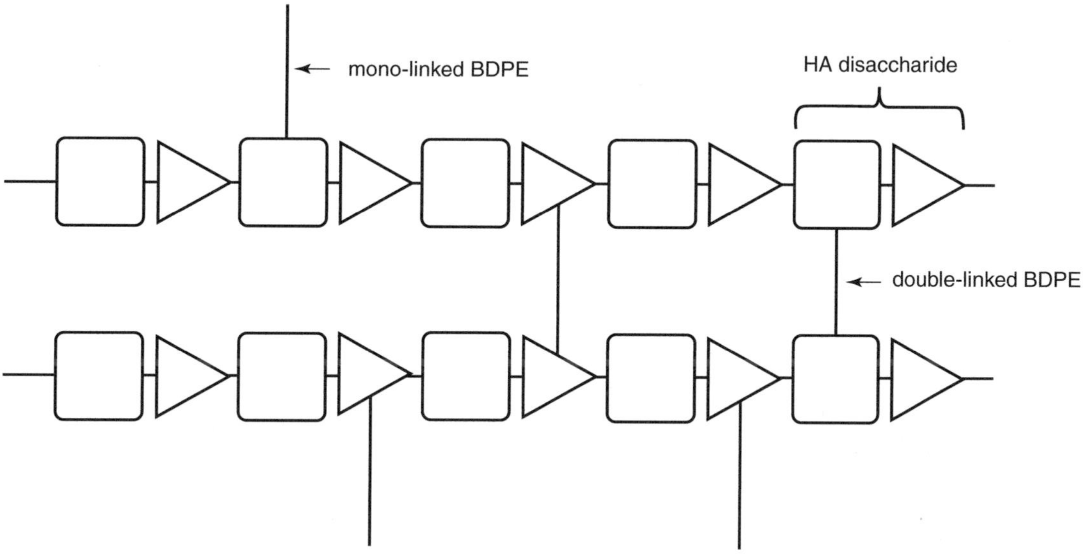

Fig. 2.11 A hypothetical structure of cross-linking between HA and BDDE including "double-linked BDPE" and "mono-linked BDPE" (Figure modified from Ref. [8])

essential elements of an ideal HA filler. In this regard, a product with a low CrR, comprised primarily of mono-linked BDPE rather than double-linked BDPE, tends to show a softer and more flexible rheological property.

2.2.2.3 Hyaluronic Acid Concentration

As a result of the thermal exposure during the sterilization process, all HA gels comprises both crosslinked gel and an extractable part, often denoted free HA. The free HA behaves as a lubricant for facilitating the introduction of HA particles into the tissue and does not provide structural support in and of itself. By way of example, while both Restylane®(Galderma) and Juvéderm® Voluma® (Allergan) have the same HA concentration of 20 mg/mL, and contains a sililar free HA concentration of between 20–30%.

Most commercial HA filler products currently on the market have HA concentrations within the range of 20–24 mg/mL. It is an accepted rule of thumb that a higher HA concentration correlates with higher elasticity and longer duration of effect. Among local Korean brands, Cleviel®

(Pharmaresearch Products, Korea), has a notably high HA concentration of 50 mg/mL for maximum elasticity and longevity. However, the downside of using a product with such high HA concentration is that it requires greater extrusion force during injection due to its hard, stiff texture; is not easily moldable after injection; and is harder to dissolve with exogenous hyaluronidase. Further, a higher HA concentration in HA fillers is known to be associated with an increase in the injected volume 2–4 weeks posttreatment due to the hydration of the cross-linked HA molecules [9]. In this respect, Juvéderm® Ultra™, with an HA concentration of 24 mg/mL and manufactured using the HYLACROSS™ technology, was particularly prone to causing undesired swelling or irregularity post-treatment due to the saturation of the HA molecules. Hence, subsequent releases of Juvéderm® fillers, which embody VYCROSS™ technology, have notably lowered their HA concentrations to avoid such problems. For example, Juvéderm® Voluma™ indicated for deep (subcutaneous) volume restoration contains 20 mg/mL of HA, Juvéderm® Volift™ for deep wrinkle correction contains 17.5 mg/m of HA, while Juvéderm® Volbella™ for fine lines and wrinkles including periorbital rhytids contains 15 mg/mL of HA in the product.

2.2.2.4 Monophasic vs. Biphasic HA

Often HA fillers are classified as monophasic and biphasic HA, based on their specific manufacturing processes. In the manufacturing of HA fillers, once the cross-linking reaction is complete, the HA gel is then transferred into a homogenizer or grinder where it is crushed into fine particles that can easily pass the needle. Biphasic HA is obtained at this stage by 'sieving' the HA gel through sizing screens of specified diameters, which produces HA particles of the desired size. By comparison, monophasic HA does not undergo particle sizing process and, as such, consists of a homogeneous gel containing particles of mixed shapes and sizes. Consequently, biphasic HA is firmer, more elastic and particulate in its feel with a granular consistency, while monophasic HA has a softer and smoother, more fluid texture with a soft cohesive consistency. In this respect, Restylane® SubQ™, which had the largest particle size among the Restylane® range of products, consisted of granules so large they were actually visible to the naked eye, measuring almost 1 mm in diameter [10].

However, scientifically speaking, categorizing HA fillers as monophasic or biphasic is not relevant, as all HA gels consist of gel particles when examined under the microscope (Fig. 2.12). As it happens, the term, 'monophasic HA filler' was initially advocated by Juvéderm® for the purpose of differentiating their soft HA filler from the originial NASHA™ filler, Restylane® with firm gel characteristics. However, the term monophasic HA gel actually represents an oxymoron since a gel, by definition, exists as a mixture of liquid phase within a solid phase, hence, at the very minimum, is biphasic in its physical property. By this logic,

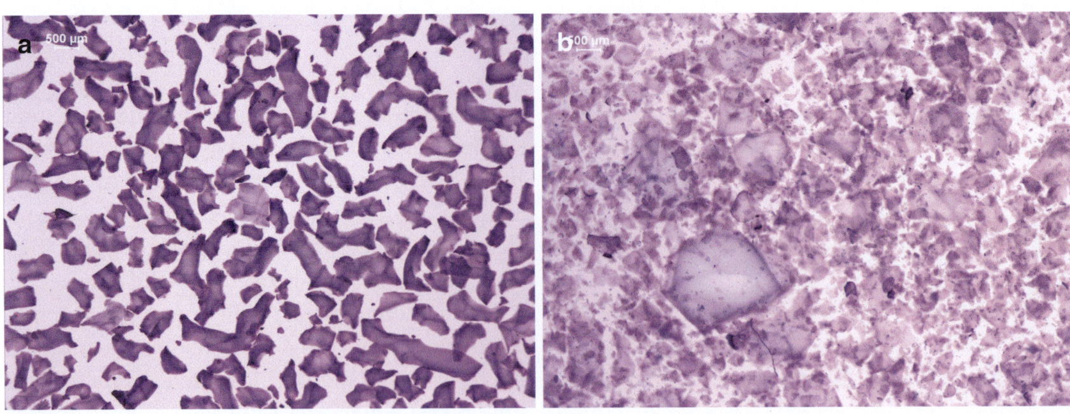

Fig. 2.12 Particles of HA fillers (Courtesy of Galderma). All HA gels consist of gel particles packed together. (**a**) Biphasic HA fillers. (**b**) Monophasic HA fillers

one may argue that a biphasic HA filler should more aptly be described as a triphasic gel [11]. Moreover, some HA fillers often classified as monophasic HA fillers such as Restylane® Volym e and Restylane® Refyne using OBT™ technology also demonstrate almost uniform particle size resulting from the 'sieving' process during the manufacture for optimal homogenicity. That notwithstanding, these terms are often adopted in clinical practice as a shorthand for characterizing different HA fillers to assist the understanding of treating physicians. Therefore, it bears noting that the terms, 'monophasic' and 'biphasic' as mentioned in this book is used for the purpose of convenience only. However, to best characterize HA fillers in a manner that facilitates the selection of a certain filler for a certain clinical indication, scientifically sound rheologic tests such as rheometry should be used.

In terms of their rheological properties, firm biphasic HA fillers tend to display higher elasticity and viscosity than soft monophasic HA (Table 2.2), which allows better retention of shape against external deformation and stronger lifting capacity [11]. Biphasic HA is, therefore, better suited for placement at the deeper planes where they can provide deep tissue lift or support for facial volume depletion but are less suitable for superficial injection in the dermis and are not easily moldable postinjection.

In contrast, monophasic HA tends to have lower elasticity and viscosity but demonstrates higher levels of cohesivity compared with biphasic HA which exist as individual grains of gel particles gathered together like sand. Cohesivity is yet another important rheological determinant that informs the ability of a product to resist external deformation. Significantly, in the study by Sundaram et al., Belotero® Balance™ and Juvéderm® Ultra Plus™ (both soft monophasic HA fillers) showed the highest cohesivity scores while Restylane® as a biphasic HA filler demonstrated the lowest cohesivity (Table 2.2). [13] Softer HA fillers with a lower G' and a higher cohesivty are more suitable than firm fillers for injection in areas of high facial movement such as the forehead, nasolabial folds, and cheek, as monophasic HA fillers can more effectively recover their original shape without dissociating upon deformation from facial muscular movements. In addition, owing to their lower viscosity, monophasic HA fillers can produce smooth results even when placed superficially in the dermis as they spread more easily through the tissue plane and can provide easy molding postinjection [14].

Due to its hydrophilic nature, HA filler can expand in volume within 2–4 weeks of placement and, in so doing, may cause unwanted lumpiness and irregularity, especially in areas with thin tissue coverage such as the periorbital region (Fig. 2.13). Such postinjection swelling from the hydration of HA molecules appears to occur more significantly in soft monophasic HA fillers than in firm biphasic HA fillers while other conditions such as HA concentration should be also considered (Fig. 2.14) [15]. The postinjection swelling of HA filler can be measured by 'the swelling factor' measurement which is indicative of a HA gel's hydration (saturation) status [17]. When near saturation (closes into equilibrium), a gel will not exhibit appreciable swelling after injection. Below equilibrium (unsaturated), a gel will readily take up water from the surrounding fluid until it reaches hydration equilibrium. Gel fluid uptake characteristics vary from product to product and are dependent on hyaluronic acid concentration and limited by the extent of crosslinking. In general, as the extent of crosslinking is increased in firm HA fillers with high G', swelling factor is decreased. Conversely, softer gels with a lower degree of crosslinking and lower G' products have higher swelling factor. It may be also postulated that this is partly due to the greater tendency of soft monophasic HA to spread in the tissue, which causes a larger gel surface area to come into contact with water in the tissue. This is in contrast with the less spreading biphasic HA fillers that integrate into the tissue in a more targeted manner and thus has more limited surface area per volume in the tissue. Notably, Juverderm® Ultra Plus™, based on the HYLACROSS™ technology with an HA concentration of 24 mg/m and Belotero® Volume™ incorporating the CPM™ technology with an HA concentration of 26 mg/m are monophasic HA products noted for their significant postinjection swelling (Table 2.2). Thus,

Table 2.2 Rheological properties, cohesivity levels, and clinical volumizing capacity of the nine HA fillers

Product reference	Lifting capacity	GS[a] cohesivity score	Shear-stress properties at 0.7 Hz			Static compression properties at 1.5 mm	Dynamic compression properties at 0.7 Hz		
			G' (Pa)	G'' (Pa)	tan δ	F_N (N')	E' (Pa)	E'' (Pa)	tan δ_c
BELOTERO® Balance	+	5	63 ± 3	34 ± 2	0.54 ± 0.04	0.51 ± 0.02	31,457 ± 1132	18,541 ± 472	0.59 ± 0.03
BELOTERO® Intense lidocaine	++	4	130 ± 3	52 ± 2	0.40 ± 0.02	1.16 ± 0.03	59,150 ± 1469	32,235 ± 622	0.54 ± 0.02
BELOTERO® Volume lidocaine	+++	3	300 ± 5	57 ± 1	0.19 ± 0.01	0.95 ± 0.03	111,044 ± 2250	58,047 ± 1880	0.52 ± 0.01
JUVEDERM® Volbella	+	2	174 ± 4	28 ± 1	0.16 ± 0.01	0.15 ± 0.01	12,003 ± 400	25,270 ± 1015	2.11 ± 0.08
JUVEDERM® Volift	++	2	279 ± 6	39 ± 2	0.14 ± 0.01	0.22 ± 0.01	21,994 ± 378	44,287 ± 1316	2.01 ± 0.05
JUVEDERM® Voluma	+++	2	314 ± 5	17 ± 1	0.06 ± 0.00	0.33 ± 0.02	41,747 ± 947	60,382 ± 1898	1.45 ± 0.02
RESTYL® ANE lidocaine	+	1	677 ± 13	136 ± 3	0.20 ± 0.01	0.23 ± 0.01	8,456 ± 256	32,469 ± 854	3.84 ± 0.17
Restylane® Lyft lidocaine	++	1	716 ± 9	110 ± 4	0.15 ± 0.01	0.30 ± 0.01	9,507 ± 216	35,184 ± 735	3.70 ± 0.04
JUVEDERM® Ultraplus XC	++	4	143 ± 5	36 ± 2	0.26 ± 0.02	0.98 ± 0.02	65,554 ± 1891	23,856 ± 330	0.36 ± 0.02

Mean ± SD

[a]Gavard-Sundaram Cohesivity Scale (Ref. [13]). Data modified from Ref. [12],

they are unsuitable for injection in thin-skinned areas of the face; even when used for contouring and sculpting, it is preferable to dilute the product with saline at a 6:4 ratio with six parts HA and four parts saline, respectively (see Sect. 3.1.3).

2.2.3 Choice of HA Filler

The three key factors to consider in choosing a filler product are safety, longevity, and price as the author has routinely highlighted in lectures since the early 2000s (Fig. 2.15). Among those, safety takes first priority, since injectable fillers essentially represent external substances introduced into the human body. On this score, HA outperforms all other types of soft tissue fillers currently on the market. Not only does it involve minimal risks of adverse reactions, but the injected HA filler is also readily reversible with injection of hyaluronidase should any problems occur, effectively restoring the patient back to the pretreatment condition. In light of recent concerns over the cases of inflammation from delayed-type hypersensitivity reactions to HA fillers, incidence of delayed type hypersensitivity has also become a significant safety criterion for selecting a HA filler product.

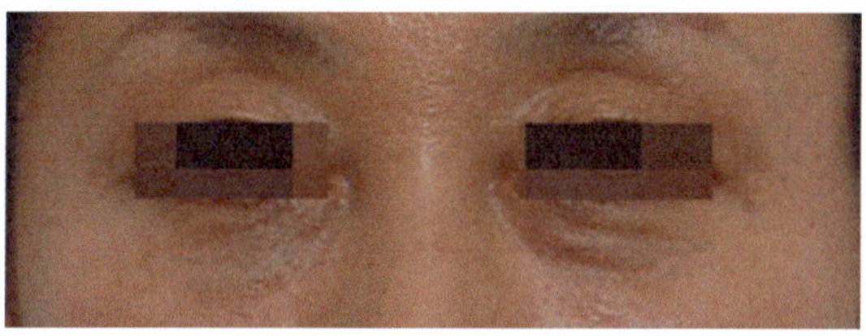

Fig. 2.13 Postinjection swelling at the tear trough occurred in the right side which was injected with monophasic HA filler (Juvederm® Ultra™), while the left side injected with biphasic HA filler (Restylane®) showed no postinjection swelling

While HA fillers were previously understood to last between 6 months and 1 year following their injection, it has been the author's observation that the duration of effect often extends beyond this suggested timeframe, lasting even longer up to 5–10 years with maintenance treatments repeated 2–3 times. While monophasic HA filler Juvéderm® Voluma and BELOTERO® Volume tend to outlast biphasic HA and variations seem to exist between different patients and different facial regions treated, there appears to be almost no significant difference in filler longevity among different HA filler brands as long as they have similar volumizing capacity. If anything, products containing too much cross-linker content for increased longevity tend to require more careful handling as

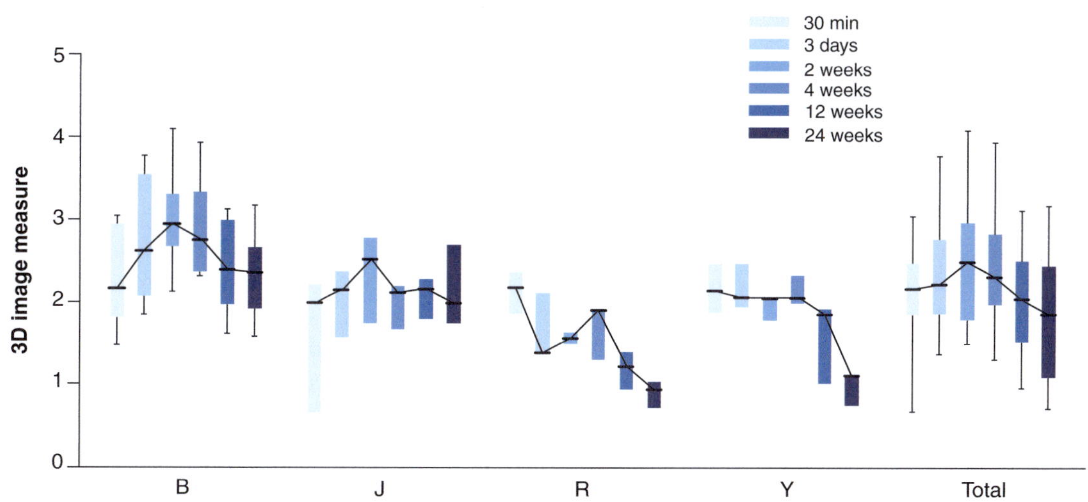

Fig. 2.14 Time trends in 3D image measurement according to filler type. No significant difference was observed between fillers B and J. The 3D measure were greater with filler B than with filler R at all times except for 30 min. Moreover, the 3D measures were greater with filler B than with filler Y at 2, 4, and 24 weeks. (B: Belotero® J: Juvéderm® R: Restylane® Y: YVOIRE®) (Cited from Ref. [15])

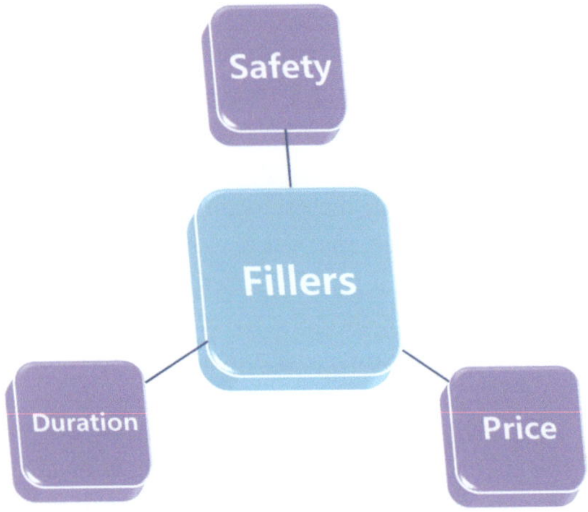

Fig. 2.15 The three key factors to consider in choosing a filler product

they are generally more resistant to dissolution with hyaluronidase.

Price is no doubt an important consideration for any practitioner concerned for his business's bottom line. However, with the drop in the price per mL of HA filler to below half that of the early 2000s, HA filler prices have come to represent significantly less of a concern for an average practitioner. That notwithstanding, the price of HA filler per syringe still matters in the case of full face volumization which requires at least 6–10 ml to be used in one session. In this respect, it is a welcome development that due to the fierce competition in the domestic market, Korean HA filler brands are now available at even 20–40 USD per 1 mL syringe while providing comparable quality, as their prices have fallen to 1/5–1/10 the price of imported HA fillers during the early 2000s. This has driven HA fillers to compare favorably with autologous fat graftautologotraua in Korea and to eventually replace fat for facial volumization.

Deciding among the vast array of HA filler products flooding the market can be overwhelming for the practitioner. However, selecting the right HA filler for a procedure is in many respects analogous to choosing the right golf club for a shot. Similar to how a driver that is great for driving is not necessarily best for putting a ball, there is an art to picking the perfect HA filler with the right rheologic property for the right indication. Also, just as a typical golfer's bag contains an assortment of golf clubs each of a different brand, such as an XXIO iron, a PING driver, and a Scotty Cameron putter, the practitioner may consider using a mix of different HA products from different manufacturers he feels most comfortable using. Personally, my favorite filler brand to use almost exclusively during the first 10+ years of practicing soft tissue filler treatments was Restylane®. Over the past 5–6 years, Belotero® HA fillers have been added as a favored choice. Essentially, the best choice of HA filler to use is a judgment call made by each practitioner based on his level of comfort with the product, the target area and plane of injection and the rheologic property of the product, that is, elasticity and cohesivity of HA, degree of HA concentration, and degree of cross-linking (Fig. 2.16), etc. Therefore, it is often the case that a combination of different HA filler brands can be used for treating different facial regions of a given patient, for example, by using Restylane® for the nose or tear trough in conjunction with Belotero® Volume for the anterior malar or sunken cheeks. Alternatively, different HA products within the same family of HA filler may be deployed in different subunits of a given facial area. A good example is the use of Belotero® Volume to volumize the body of the lips and Belotero® Balance to enhance the vermillion border.

Selecting HA filler Based on Facial region; As a general rule of thumb, the use of firm biphasic HA filler with higher G' such as Restylane® is advised in treating areas of thin overlying skin such as the periorbital region, including the lower pretarsal roll, tear trough, and upper eyelids, to avoid unfavorable postinjection swelling due to the water absorption by the HA molecules. For this reason, firm biphasic HA fillers with higher G' are also suitable for augmenting the nasal dorsum where the skin is thin as well. Generally speaking, products with higher G', large particle sizes or higher HA concentration are suitable for indications requiring volumetric augmentation as they provide better structural support regardless of softer monophasic or firmer biphasic HA filler. On the other hand, softer monophasic HA fillers with relatively higher G' and higher cohesivity such as

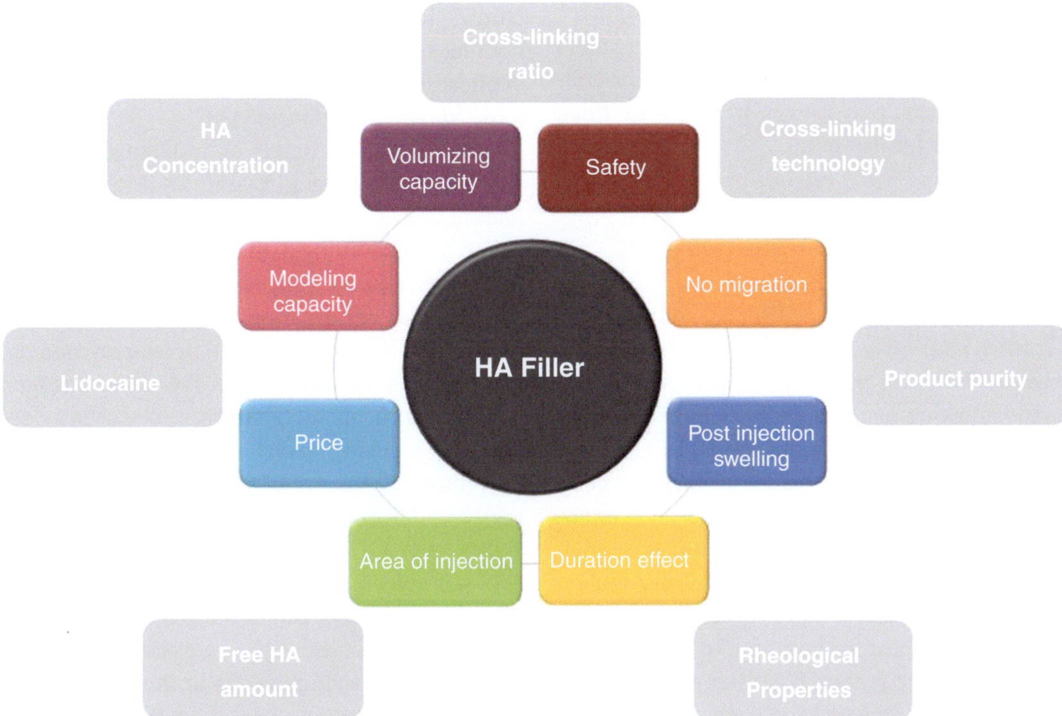

Fig. 2.16 Key factors in choosing HA filler products (Modifed from Merz Institute of Advanced Aesthetics)

Belotero® Volume, Juvéderm® Voluma and Restylane® Volyme are generally preferable for volumizing areas of high mobility such as the submalar depression, nasolabial fold, forehead and temples where substantial dynamic force is imposed by the underlying muscular movements. Treatment of the lips which require a soft, smooth texture consistent to the touch should be performed exclusively with softer monophasic HA products with lower G' such as Belotero® Intense, Restylane® Kysse, and Juverderm® Ultra XC. By contrast, a harder stiffer biphasic HA filler is preferred in areas such as the chin and nasal bridge where firm, crisp texture is desired.

Selecting HA filler Based on Skin Quality; For patients with thinner skin, where product palpability/visibility is an important consideration, products with lower G' values are generally most appropriate. Lower G' products such as BELOTERO® Intense, Restylane® Defyne, Juvéderm® Volift and Juvéderm® Ultra Plus XC are softer and more easily distributed in the tissue.

Selecting HA filler Based on Plane of Injection; In general, firmer products with higher G' values are indicated for deeper planes of injection and are applied to support a greater degree of correction, whereas lower G' (softer) products are indicated for more superficial planes of injection and less severe corrections. The higher G' products are suitable for indications requiring volumetric augmentation as they provide better structural support in the deep tissue. For areas such as the malar cheek, chin, and jawline, where the product can be placed against the bone for projection, a higher G' products such as BELOTERO® Volume, Restylane® Lyft and Juvéderm® Voluma will provide a greater advantage over a lower G' product because it will have greater resistance to the compression forces inherent in the deeper injection plane. Meanwhile, thinner, softer HA products with lower G' such as BELOTERO®

Soft, Restylane® Skinbooster Vital, Restylane® Fynesse, and Juvéderm® Volbella are better suited for making finer intradermal corrections or delicate refinements. See *Choice of Filler by Each Indication* for further detail.

2.2.4 Rheological Properties of HA Filler (Table 2.2)

It is often said *it's a poor craftsman that blames his tools*; however, part of being a master craftsman is knowing one's tools. In volumizing filler treatments, utilizing the right choice of HA for a given clinical indication marks the starting point for producing excellent aesthetic outcomes. Selecting the ideal HA is, in many respects, analogous to choosing the right golf club for a shot. Similar to how a driver that is great for driving is not necessarily best for putting a ball, there is an art to picking the perfect HA filler with the right rheologic characteristics for a given indication. Different regions of the face have varying levels of skin thickness and tension, muscle activity, and tissue density, for which each filler has its own place. In this respect, knowledge of each filler's rheological attributes is key to deciding which product to use and where. Rheology, which deals with the flow of matter, is especially pertinent to filler procedures as HA gels as biphasic materials demonstrate properties of both liquid and solid at the same time.

Rheology is defined as the study of flow-related properties, the understanding of which has been crucial for the manufacture and processing of materials across a wide array of industries ranging from paint, ink, ointment to adhesives, which exhibit both the viscose behavior of liquid and elastic behavior of a solid. HA fillers being gels also constitute a biphasic material consisting of both liquid and solid components. Thus, numerous studies have attempted to investigate the rheology of different HA fillers to establish their clinical behavior and compare their relative strengths and weaknesses in achieving the desired aesthetic outcome. Indeed, understanding these rheological properties can help predict the behavior of different HA fillers during and after implantation in the tissue, thus allowing the optimal selection of HA filler for a given clinical application, hence leading to the coining of the term "rheologic tailoring" [11].

Both during and after its implantation in the tissue, HA is subject to a complex array of deformation forces, to which different products behave differently according to their intrinsic rheological properties. During injection, the HA filler is subject to shear deformation as it is extruded from the syringe through the small needle or cannula. Once implanted in the tissue, the product is then exposed to mechanical stresses of varying vectors and intensity such as gravity, shearing by movement of the facial musculature, and compressive deformation exerted by the overlying skin tissue. Of these, lateral shearing arises in two possible scenarios. First is when the HA filler is placed between two different anatomical tissue layers, for example between the deep fat pad and the muscle plane as in the case of deep injection for hollow cheeks. In this case, each horizontal layer that interfaces the HA can apply a different level of shear stress on the implanted HA filler. Second is when the HA filler is injected within the same anatomical tissue layer, but the portion of the HA situated closer to the muscle surface is subject to a greater degree of shearing than the other parts. Meanwhile, compression represents a vertical deformation force applied on the HA filler not only when the face is in repose (i.e., static state) by the overlying skin tissues but also during facial movement (i.e., dynamic state) by the facial musculature. The amount of compression force acting on the injected HA is greater in the deep planes such as the supraperiosteal or subcutaneous layer than in the superficial dermal layer. The ability to resist the various deformation forces and retain the original shape without being displaced from the implanted location constitutes an essential element of a volumizing HA filler.

2.2.4.1 Elasticity

Elasticity represents the ability of the gel to recover its original shape after deformation, which is the most important rheologic property for the filler. For example, disposable earplugs made of polyurethane are characterised by high elasticity while honey is not. Also, while both are gels, molded gelatin demonstrates higher elasticity compared with chocolate pudding with a lower elasticity (Fig. 2.17). Elasticity of an HA filler can be expressed using different rheological parameters according to the type of deformation force applied. The elasticity of a gel under shear-stress (i.e., horizontal stress) is represented by the elastic modulus (*G'*), which measures the hardness or stiffness of a gel and thus its ability to resist deformation under applied shear pressure (Fig. 2.18a). On the other hand, the elasticity of a gel under compression (i.e., vertical stress) is measured by normal force (F_N) in static mode and by elastic modulus (E') during facial muscle movement, that is, in dynamic mode [12] (Fig. 2.18b). The severity of dynamic forces that contribute to the deformation of hyaluronic acid filler products implanted differs depending on the plane of injection. While the shear force is severer in the superficial (dermis) plane and the muscular layer, compression force becomes severer in the deeper planes (the deep subcutaneous fat layer and supraperiosteal layer) (Fig. 2.18c). Various factors may influence the *G'* and E' of an HA filler, including HA concentration, degree of cross-linking, the ratio of double-linked/pendant-type (mono-linked) BDPE in the gel, the proportion of free form HA in the gel, and the manufacturing process employed. Generally speaking, HA gels with higher HA concentration and degree of cross-linking have a high *G'*, while those with a higher composition of mono-linked BDPE or free-form HA in the gel are associated with a lower *G'*. Also, with the particle size being equal, biphasic HA gels generally have a higher *G'* in comparison to monophasic HA (Fig. 2.19). In terms of clinical implication, it follows that products with a high elastic modulus *G'* are not suitable for areas requiring a smooth, even feel such as the lips since the palpability of the hard, rubbery gel texture would be undesirable. Conversely, products with a higher *G'* can be expected to provide a more effective targeted lift given their tendency not to spread and retain the original shape in the implanted area (Fig. 2.20). Thus, they are regularly used in clinical practice for volume projection in the deep tissue planes. In short, a higher *G'* correlates to a material with a greater volumizing capacity as clinically proven in the controlled split-face study by Monheit et al. performed in 140 patients [17]. Similar observations have been obtained with respect to the compression parameters F_N and E', with higher F_N and E' values correlating with a higher volumizing capacity [12]. That said, it is relevant to note that harder stiffer products with higher elasticity require greater extrusion force during injection, as well as the use of larger, thicker needles or cannulas. Also, since these products do not provide easy molding and spread ability, they are better placed in the deep tissue planes rather than in the superficial layers.

2.2.4.2 Viscosity

Viscosity is defined as the ability of a fluid to resist deformation or its tendency to stick together without fragmenting when stressed. For example, refrigerated butter or peanut butter has high viscosity and thus does not spread easily on toast, whereas room temperature butter has low viscosity and thus glides easily along the surface when spread (Fig. 2.21). Viscosity is measured by viscous modulus (G'') or complex viscosity (η^*) in terms of shear deformability and by viscous modulus (E'') in terms of compressive deformation. Complex viscosity (η^*) describes the gel's ability to resist extrinsic shear deformation; in other words, the ability to resist being spread. When the shear force falls within a certain range (within the linear viscoelastic range), the η^* decreases in proportion to the increase in shear stress exerted [11]. Viscous modulus (G'')' is a measure of a gel's ability to dissipate energy when shear force is applied (Fig. 2.22). Within the linear viscoelastic range, G'' is known to be proportionate, if not entirely identical, to the complex viscosity (η^*). However, for biphasic HA fillers, η^* is considered to be a more accurate indicator than G'' for predicting their clinical behavior and is thus more widely used [11].

While HA fillers with higher viscosity require greater extrusion force as they do not inject smoothly, once implanted in the tissue, they can resist a greater amount of shearing stress without

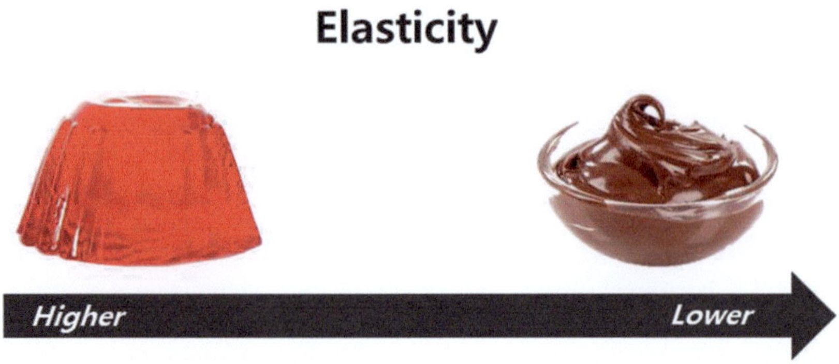

Fig. 2.17 Molded gelatin represents higher elasticity compared with chocolate pudding which has lower elasticity

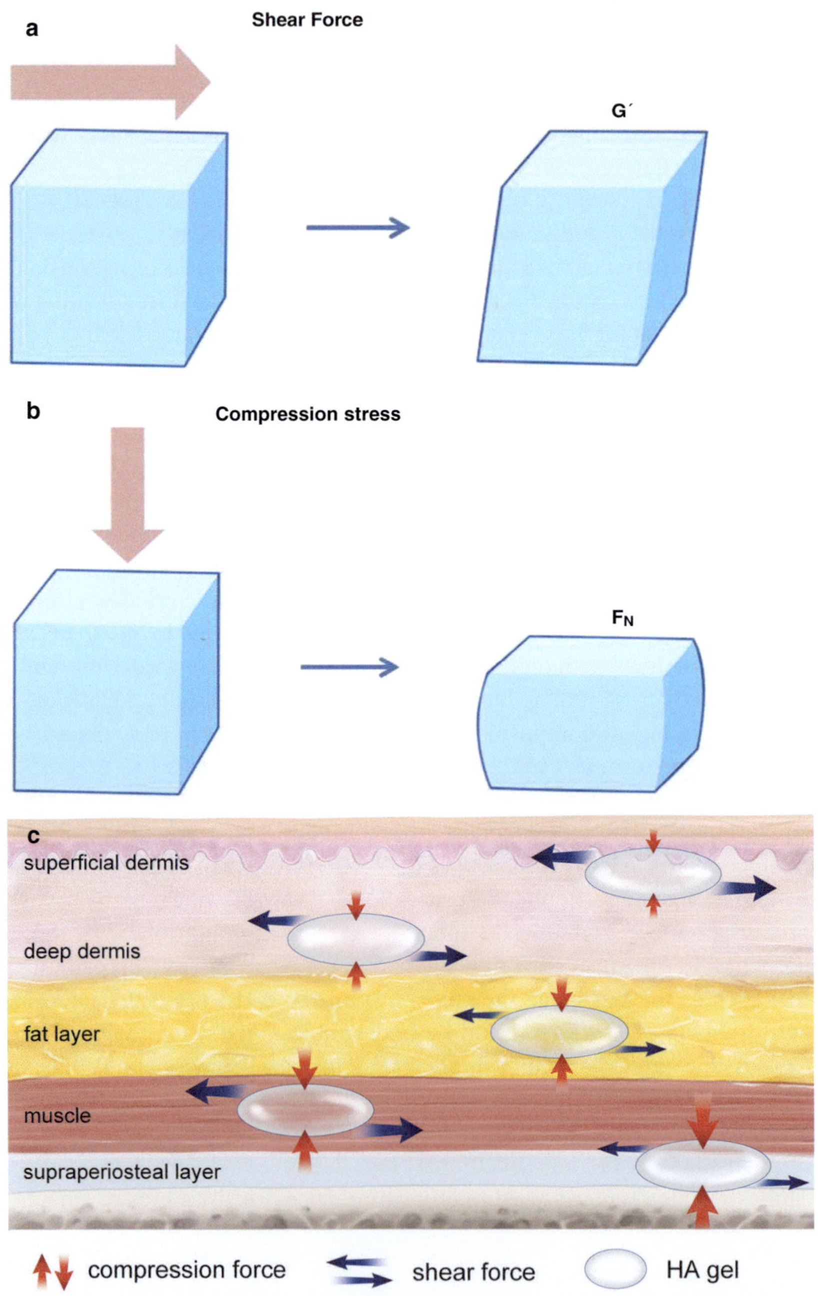

Fig. 2.18 (**a**) The elastic modulus (G'). The elasticity of a gel under shear-stress (i.e., horizontal stress) is represented by the elastic modulus (G'). (**b**) The elasticity of a gel under compression (i.e., vertical stress) is measured by normal force (F_N) in static mode. (**c**) Dynamic forces that contribute to deformation of hyaluronic acid filler products implanted in the superficial (dermis) and deep planes (deep fat pad and supraperiosteal) of soft tissues

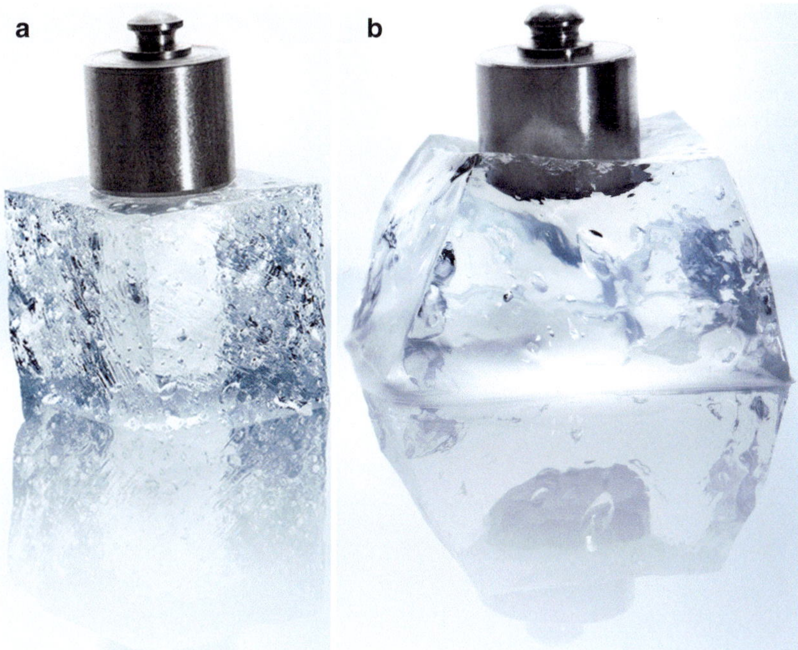

Fig. 2.19 Biphasic HA gels generally have a higher G' in comparison to monophasic HA (Courtesy of Galderma) (**a**) NASHA cube (Biphasic HA gel). (**b**) OBT cube (monophasic HA gel)

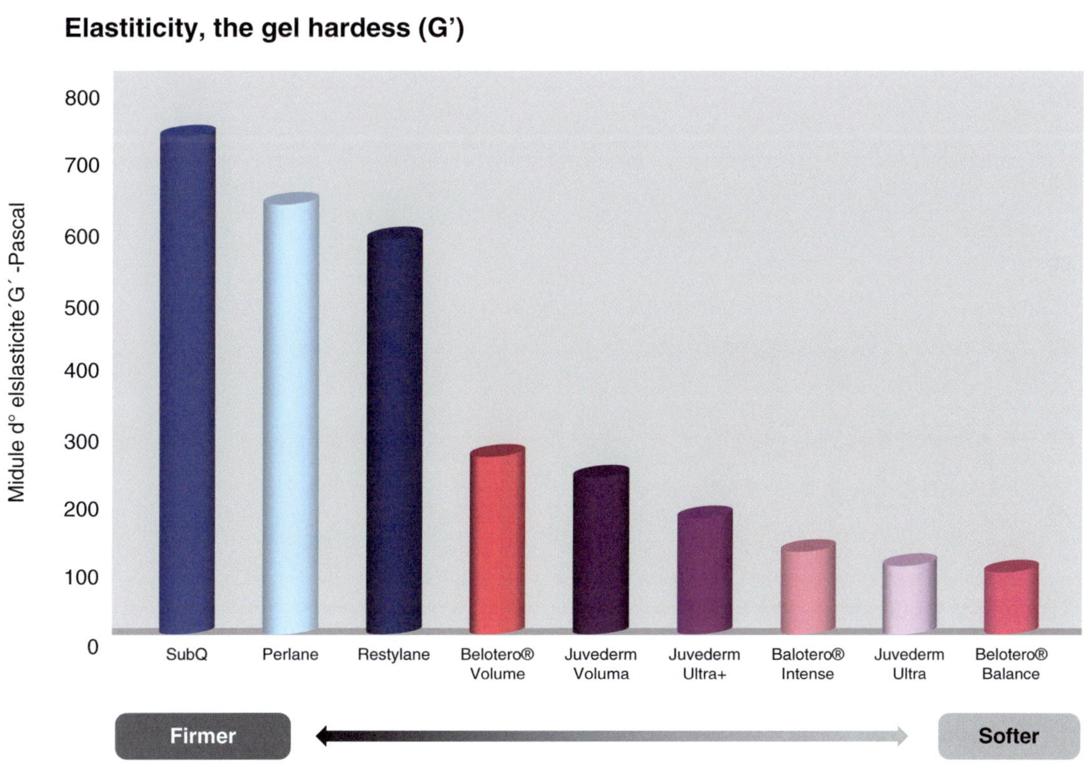

Fig. 2.20 *Elastic modulus (G′)*, Hardness of 9 HA fillers (Modified from Merz Institute of Advanced Aesthetics)

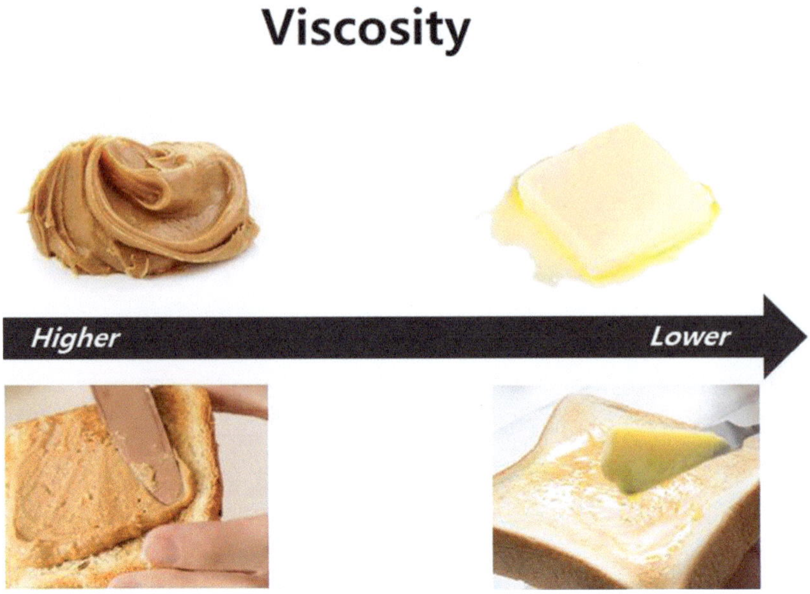

Fig. 2.21 Peanut butter has high viscosity and thus does not spread easily on toast, whereas room temperature butter has low viscosity and thus glides easily along the surface when spread. (Modified from Merz Institute of Advanced Aesthetics)

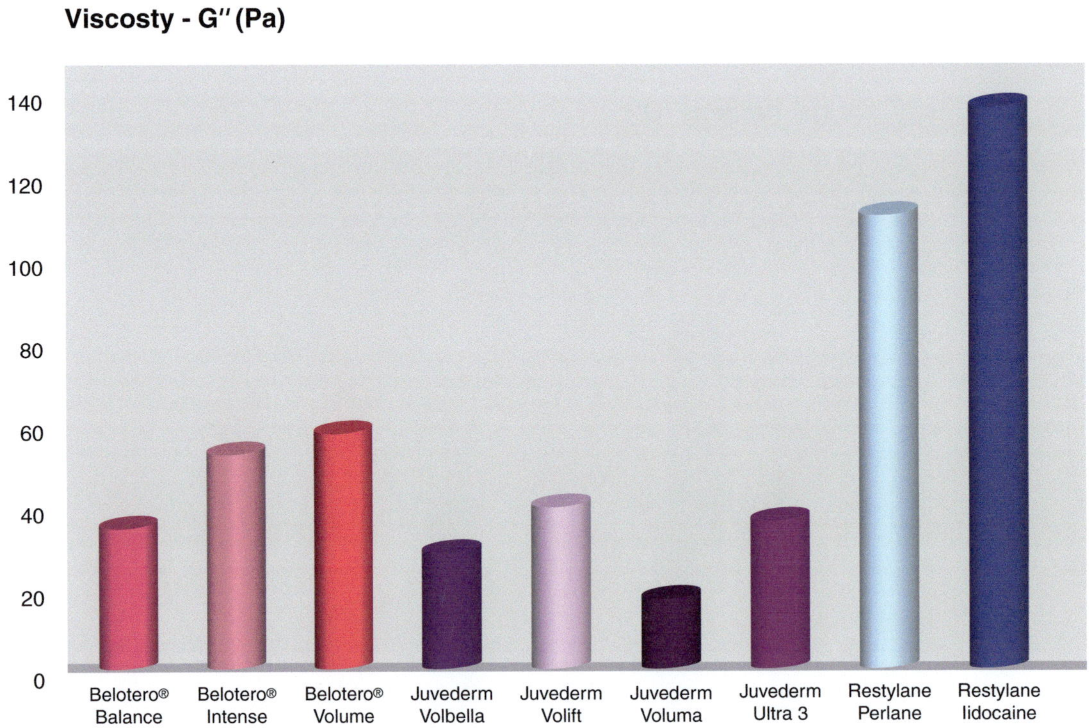

Fig. 2.22 Viscous modulus (G'')' of 9 HA fillers (Modified from Merz Institute of Advanced Aesthetics)

spreading, thus ensuring retention of shape and structural integrity. This makes them ideal for injection in areas of high facial muscle movement or in the deep tissue planes where they can provide deep volume projection. Conversely, more fluid HA fillers with less viscosity are easier to inject and flow more evenly through the tissue and are thus suitable for superficial placement in the dermis. In the study by Rosamilia et al. [18] based on the Belotero® range of HA fillers, Belotero® soft, a softer product with lower viscosity, was shown to spread more readily into the tissue compared to Belotero® Volume™, a less fluid product with higher viscosity. Meanwhile, biphasic HA fillers, being particulate in matter, are generally known to have a higher viscosity than monophasic HA [19]. Based on such rheological differences, when injected intradermally in the dermis, Belotero® Balance™ as monophasic HA has been shown to demonstrate more homogenous integration in the tissue compared with the micro bolus pattern of tissue integration of the biphasic Restylane® with higher viscosity [14].

2.2.4.3 Tan Delta (δ)

Since fillers are viscoelastic materials that exhibit the properties of both viscosity and elasticity, their behavior cannot be defined appropriately based on a parameter describing the characteristics of either a solid or fluid alone. This understanding has led to the proposal of various secondary rheologic calculations derived from the primary rheological parameters. Among these, tan delta (δ) is a relatively commonly used modulus, which measures the ratio of the viscous modulus G'' over the elastic modulus G' (G''/G') in a given material [11]. In other words, tan δ is a complex modulus that considers the overall balance of elasticity and viscosity of a given HA gel. A tan δ value of less than 1 denotes that the product is more elastic than viscous, while a tan δ greater than 1 signifies a predominance of viscosity over elasticity. Since most HA fillers tend to exhibit a more elastic than a fluid behavior, their tan δ values are typically less than 1, with some harder, more elastic fillers showing a tan δ value even lower than 0.2. Even within the same family of HA fillers, products indicated for deep volume correction tend to demonstrate lower tan δ values. Meanwhile, tan δ_C (E''/E') is the corresponding viscoelastic modulus for describing the gel behavior under applied compression force [12]. However, tan δ_C (E''/E') values appear to deviate from the tan δ (G''/G') values in that the tan δ_C was less than 1 for the Belotero® range of products and Hylacross™-based Juvéderm® Ultra™, that is, products with high tan δ values; 1–2 for VYCROSS™-based products; and greater than 3 for the Restylane® range of products whose tan δ value was the lowest among the tested products (i.e., less than 0.2). From this, it follows that HA behaves differently under shear-stress than under dynamic compression [11]. It is also relevant to note that HA placed in the deep tissue is exposed not only to shear stress but also to compression, with the amount of compression force being greater in the deep planes than in the superficial layer.

2.2.4.4 Cohesivity

Cohesivity describes a material's tendency not to dissociate due to the internal attraction of the molecules for each other. For example, honey is a highly cohesive material, while sand grains are far less cohesive (Fig. 2.23). The cohesivity of an HA filler represents the degree to which it remains intact in the tissue without dissociating following its implantation. For want of an objective evaluation protocol, the cohesivity of HA fillers is measured using a standardized 5-point visual scale referred to as the Gavard-Sundaram Cohesivity Scale (The "GS Cohesivity Scale"). [13] The GS Cohesivity Scale ranges between a value of 1 (fully dispersed) and 5 (fully cohesive) (Fig. 2.24). In general, with the particle size being identical, biphasic HA fillers tend to be less cohesive than monophasic HA fillers. As is turns out, Restylane® as a biphasic HA has a cohesivity score of 1 on the GS Cohesivity Scale, whereas the monophasic Belotero® Balance™ has the highest cohesivity of 5 [12, 13]. Even among monophasic HA fillers, significant variations exist in their cohesivity scores, reflecting differences in the underlying manufacturing process employed. For example, within the same Juvéderm family of HA fillers, Juvéderm® Ultra

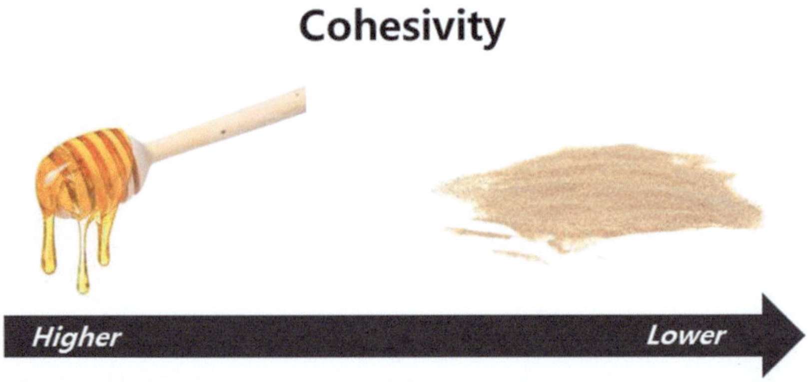

Fig. 2.23 Honey represents a highly cohesive material, while sand grains are far less cohesive (Courtesy of Merz Institute of Aesthetic Academy)

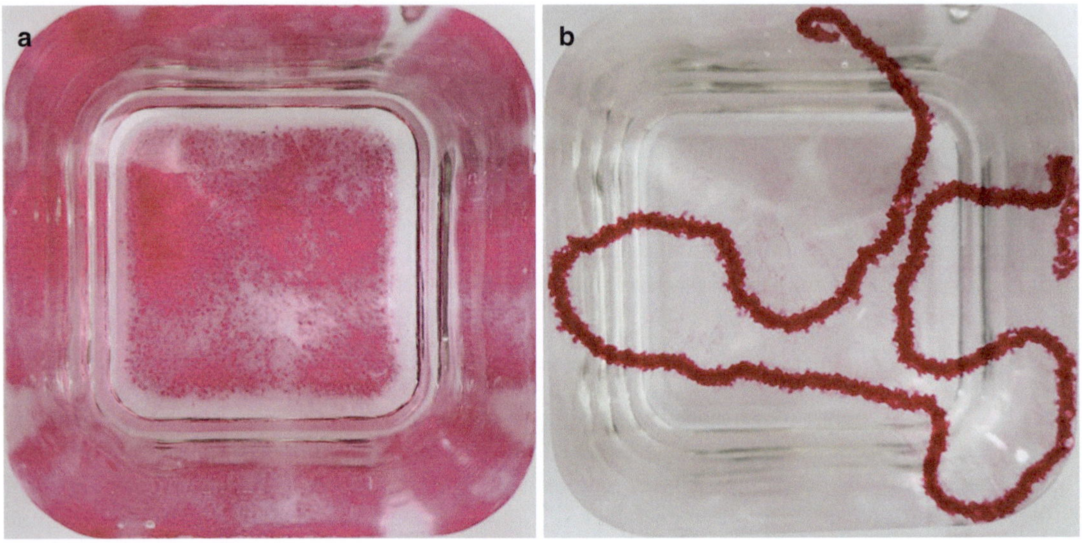

Fig. 2.24 The GS Cohesivity Scale*. (**a**) Restylane®; Score of 1 at 90 s (fully dispersed). (**b**) Belotero® Balance; Score of 5 at 90 s (fully cohesive). *Gavard-Sundaram Cohesivity Scale (Ref. [13])

Plus™ (Juvéderm® Ultra 3™) incorporating the HYLACROSS™ technology has a cohesivity score of 4, while Juvéderm® Voluma™ embodying the VYCROSS™ technology has a significantly lower cohesivity of 1 [12].

The most notable clinical significance of cohesivity lies in its ability to contribute to the lifting capacity of HA fillers, as with elasticity. This has been well elucidated in the split face nasolabial fold study comparing the treatment effect of Belotero® Intense vs. Restylane® Lyft in 20 subjects [20]. Needless to say, elasticity is the key factor in determining the lifting capacity of hyaluronic acid fillers. Given such, the above study is remarkable in that it demonstrated that Belotero® Intense with a *G'* of only 111 Pa (o.7 Hz) was able to yield volumizing effects comparable to that of Restylane® Lyft having a *G'* of 549 Pa. Thus, it can be postulated that, in spite of its lower *G'*, Belotero® Intense was able to effectively close the gap with Restylane® Lyft by virtue of its significantly higher cohesivity of 4 compared with Restylane® Lyft's score of 1. The influence of cohesivity on the volumizing capacity of the filler is particularly relevant when treating areas of high mobility such as the nasolabial folds, marionette lines, and the forehead. In the author's experience, low cohesivity products

Table 2.3 Clinical implications of rheological properties (see each indications)

Indications	Area	Appropriate rheological properties	Recommendation
Volumization under thin skin	Tear trough Palpebromalar groove	Biphasic, low to moderate viscoelasticity	Restylane®, Restylane® Skinbooster Vital
Intradermal injection Hydrolifting Fern pattern technique	Thick skin area	Monophasic or Biphasic with low viscosity	Belotero® Balance, Restylane® Skinbooster Vital, Juvéderm® Volbella
	Thin skin area (periorbital region and neck)	Monophasic with low viscosity	Belotero® Soft
Volumization and projection	Temporal region	Highest *G'* values within each product range	Restylane® Lyft, Restylane® Volym, Belotero® Volume, Juvéderm® Voluma Juvéderm® Volux
	Hyperdynamic areas Forehead, Nasolabial fold, Marionette line Chin	Monophasic with high elasticity and cohesivity	Belotero® Volume Juvéderm® Voluma Juvéderm® Volux
	Nasal dorsum	Biphasic with high elasticity	Restylane® Lyft
	Jawline, and lateral malar	Biphasic or monophasic with high elasticity	Restylane® Lyft, Restylane® Volume, Belotero® Volume, Juvéderm® Voluma
Double layering	Deep layer	Biphasic with high elasticity	Restylane® Lyft
	Superficial layer	Monophasic with high elasticity	Belotero® Volume

such as Restylane® SubQ are generally more susceptible to clumping or separation when sheared by the rigorous muscle activity in these areas, while Belotero® Volume tends to more effectively hold its ground and retain its original shape. Conceivably, such differences may also account for the equivalence in the lifting capacity between the Belotero® Intense and Restylane® Lyft, despite the much lower shear elastic modulus (*G'*) of the Belotero® range.

2.2.4.5 Clinical Implications (Table 2.3)

A direct head-to-head rheometric comparison can be elusive between products that have been formulated using different manufacturing processes. Indeed, the same product is often be found to show varying rheometric values in different studies depending on the underlying test parameters applied. Therefore, when evaluating the rheology of different HA gels, it is more relevant to compare products within the same brand family rather than across different families. Rheometric values of products belonging to different brands may be useful only to the extent they may help elucidate a general tendency or pattern.

Thicker, firmer fillers with high viscoelasticity are generally harder to inject and thus require the use of thicker needles or cannulas. For example, even though Belotero® Volume as a monophasic gel may even pass a 30-G needle as extrusion of monophasic HA is not constrained by the size of the injection tool, the product apparently feels much stiffer when extruded through a 25-G cannula than when passed through a thicker 23-G cannula.

Soft, fluid products with low viscoelasticity such as Restylane® Vital, Belotero® Soft, and Juvéderm® Volbella are suitable for superficial injection in the dermis as they will spread more readily through the tissue plane. Generally speaking, soft monophasic HA fillers with lower G' such as Belotero® Soft, and Juvéderm® Volbella flows more evenly and integrates homogeneously into the tissue, thus creating less irregularity or Tyndalling than biphasic HA that are thicker and stiffer in texture. On the other hand, their higher spreadability means that soft monophasic HA fillers present significantly more surface area to free radicals and endogenous hyaluronidase enzymes than firm biphasic HA, resulting in more rapid degradation. Indeed, in the author's experience, when Restylane® and Belotero® were used for intradermal injection in the nasolabial folds (via fern pattern technique) or in the facial skin (via hydro lifting technique), Restylane® appeared to provide longer duration, lasting for more than 1 year while Belotero® Balance seemed to last for a shorter period. This observation is in agreement with the findings from the study by Tran et al., which compared the biointegration of different HA fillers in the dermis based on their viscoelastic properties. According to the study, while Belotero® Balance was shown to provide more homogeneous integration within the tissue, it appeared to have less of the product remaining 118 days later than Restylane® [14].

Hence, the author's preferred approach when performing hydrolifting treatments is to use Belotero® Balance in patients with photoaged or thin skin, or in areas of the face with thin tissue coverage such as the periorbital region, and Restylane® or Restylane® Vital in patients with normal skin thickness.

Meanwhile, where the aim is to provide volume and projection, it is more preferable to choose a thicker, firmer HA filler such as Restylane® Lyft, Belotero® Volume, and Juvéderm® Voluma that have the highest *G'* values within each product range. Restylane® Lyft, as a biphasic HA filler with high elasticity, and thus a rather hard gel texture, is better suited for placement in areas where the bone lies just under the skin, such that palpability of the hard product does not become an issue. A further consideration in using Restylane® Lyft is that owing to the relatively low cohesivity of the Restylane® range of HA fillers, it is usually better placed in areas of low mobility such as the nasal dorsum, jawline, and lateral malar where the product is not submitted to intense contraction of the surrounding musculature. Notably, the temporal region can be treated using either a biphasic or a monophasic HA, despite the repetitive contraction of the temporalis m, since the thick temporalis fascia overlying the implanted filler prevents the creation of visible irregularities. Meanwhile, a strong monophasic HA with high cohesivity such as Belotero® Volume is usually most suitable in the hyperdynamic areas of the forehead, the cheeks, chin, nasolabial folds, marionette lines, and anterior malar.

Monophasic HA fillers, being soft fillers with less viscoelasticity, are ideal for placement in areas such as the lips and cheeks that must be soft and smooth in their feel. On the other hand, firmer and more elastic biphasic HA fillers are better suited for implantation in areas where the underlying bone is directly palpable, such as the nasal dorsum, jawline, and the malar, While, by extension, the forehead may also be considered an area suitable for treatment with biphasic HA, in practice, that is not the case. Instead, given the dynamic muscle activity and limited space available for filler placement in the area, softer monophasic HA with a higher cohesivity and more homogeneous tissue integration represents a better option for forehead augmentation. On the other hand, biphasic HA fillers are better suited for placement in areas of thin overlying skin such as the periorbital region, including the lower pretarsal roll and the tear trough, owing to the tendency of monophasic HA fillers with lower G' to retain water when implanted in these regions.

Meanwhile, when HA filler is injected in boluses into the dermis or subdermis, it can produce the so-called Tyndall effect (Fig. 2.25), a bluish discoloration that is visible to the eye caused by preferential scattering of light by the superficially implanted HA filler. This phenomenon, which should more accurately be termed "Rayleigh scattering", occurs when light passing through air or liquid is scattered by the dispersed air or water particles whose sizes are smaller than the wavelength of light [21]. As it happens, light of shorter wavelength is scattered much

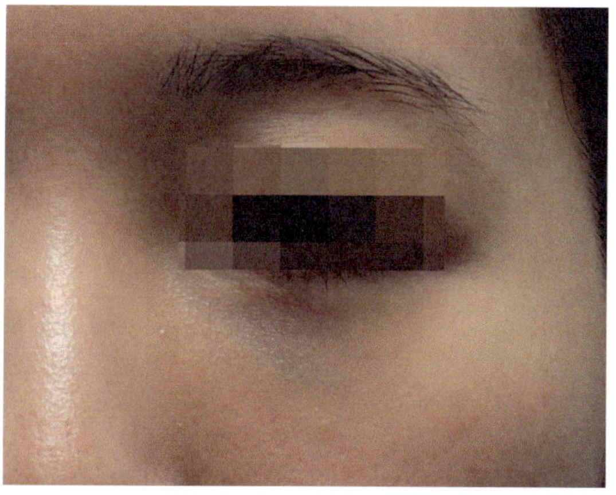

Fig. 2.25 Tyndall effect after injection of HA fillers for tear trough correction

more strongly; thus, blue light, which has a short wavelength, is preferentially reflected back to the eye. This explains why the sky appears blue, as does the water in a clear pond. By comparison, a Tyndall effect, in its true sense, is what is seen when light produces a visible beam while traveling through a colloidal substance that has particle sizes ranging between 1 and 1000 nm in diameter [22]. It is for this reason that the car headlight flashed into fog will produce a luminous beam. Hence, while Rayleigh scattering should be the proper term, considering that the term Tyndall effect is more routinely used for describing the unsightly bluish hue appearing in implanted HA fillers, we will refer to the phenomenon as the Tyndall effect for the sake of our present discussion. A Tyndall effect occurs most often if the HA filler is placed too superficially in the dermis or in large volumes at the subcutaneous level in delicate thin-skinned areas of the face such as the pretarsal roll or the tear trough. While it has been proposed in this regard that Belotero® tends to produce less Tyndalling when implanted in the thin-skinned periorbital region such as in the pretarsal roll and the tear trough, care is warranted in interpreting these findings. The underlying hypothesis supporting the finding is that unlike biphasic HA, which has a microbolus distribution pattern when injected in the dermal tissue, Belotero® has low viscosity and soft consistency which allows it to spread through the dermis in a more fluid, homogeneous pattern, with no discrete filler particles causing potential scattering of blue light [11]. However, it bears pointing out that, in clinical practice, tear trough correction is performed by placing a fine layer of volume *subdermally* using the retrograde linear thread technique, as opposed to an intradermal injection in the superficial dermis. On this basis, it is hard to conclude Belotero® confers a particular benefit over other products for tear trough correction. The same applies to when it is used for pretarsal roll augmentation, in which volume is actually placed at the subcutaneous level during the retraction of the needle.

Instead, in my own practice, I have anecdotally observed cases of Tyndalling after injecting Belotero® Volume™ in large volumes (>1 mL) in the single earlobe. Based on such clinical experience, it is the author's view that no product can be absolutely free from the risk of Tyndalling when deposited in areas of thin tissue coverage or in large volumes in the subcutaneous tissue. Granted, Belotero® has been shown to produce less Tyndalling in the superficial dermis. However, when it comes to tear-trough or pretarsal roll augmentation, the target depth of injection is *not* in the superficial dermis. If anything, the hydrophilicity of monophasic HA may serve only to contribute to the risk of Tyndalling in these areas; and as such, biphasic HA fillers may instead represent a better option, though this point remains a subject of a future split-face clinical study.

Restylane®, as a biphasic HA, has a rather hard, rubbery gel texture reflecting its high *G'* and viscosity and possesses great tissue lifting capacity as a firm, less spreading filler. While its high viscoelasticity inhibits smooth injection flow and its low gel spread makes it less moldable on injection, its high tissue lifting capacity makes the product ideal for placement in the deep tissue plane where it can provide good structure and projection.

When used for double-layering technique, biphasic HA such as Restylane® can be combined with the placement of monophasic HA in the superficial layer for optimum results. Monophasic HA fillers provide better malleability and thus are ideally suited for superficial layering. For instance, when augmenting the infraorbital ante-

Table 2.4 Volumizing HA fillers with higher volumizing capacity

Trade name	Restylane® Lyft™	Restylane® Volyme™	Juvéderm® VOLUMA™	Juvéderm® VOLUX™	Belotero® Volume™
Manufacturer	Galderma (Sweden)	Galderma (Sweden)	Allergan (France)	Allergan (France)	Merz (Switzerland)
Manufacturing technology	NASHA™	OBT™	Vycross™	Vycross™	CPM™
Monophasic or Biphasic	Biphasic	Monophasic	Monophasic	Monophasic	Monophasic
HA concentration	20 mg/mL	20 mg/mL	20 mg/mL	25 mg/mL	26 mg/mL
MoD(%)	less than 1%[a]	6–8%	4%	6–7%	5.1%[a]
Needle	29G ½″	27G ½″	27G ½″	27G ½″	27G ½″ 30G ½″
Injection level	Subcutaneous/ Supraperiosteal/ Deep dermis	Subcutaneous/ Supraperiosteal	Subcutaneous/ Supraperiosteal/ Deep dermis	Subcutaneous/ Supraperiosteal	Deep dermis/ Subcutaneous/ Supraperiosteal

Trade name	YVOIRE® Y-Solution™720	YVOIRE® Contour™	Neuramis® Volume™	e.p.t.q.® S500™
Manufacturer	LG Chem (Korea)	LG Chem (Korea)	Medytox (Korea)	JETEMA (Korea)
Manufacturing technology	S-HICE™	HICE™	SHAPE™	2CM™
Monophasic or biphasic	Biphasic	Biphasic	Monophasic	Monophasic
HA concentration	20 mg/mL	22 mg/mL	20 mg/mL	24 mg/mL
MoD(%)	3.3%	2.0%	not disclosed	1.89(%)
Needle	27G½″	23G½″	27G½″	27G½″
Injection level	Subcutaneous/ Supraperiosteal	Subcutaneous/ Supraperiosteal	Deep dermis Subcutaneous	Subcutaneous/ Supraperiosteal areas

[a]Yang B, Guo X, Zang H, Liu J. Determination of modification degree in BDDE-modified hyaluronic acid hydrogel by SEC/MS. Carbohydr Polym. 2015 Oct 20;131:233–9.

rior malar, it is more practicable to first place a biphasic HA in the deep tissue plane for overall volume and lift and to refine any remaining surface depressions with a monophasic HA in the superficial plane (Table 2.4).

2.3 Major HA Filler Products

2.3.1 Restylane®: The Golden Standard of HA Fillers (Fig. 2.26)

Restylane® (Galderma, Sweden) is the first HA filler approved by the FDA in the US in 2003, following its CE certification in Europe in 1996. Today, Restylane® is considered the gold standard of HA fillers based on its globally established safety and efficacy profile. As of 2020, more than 40 million treatments have been performed worldwide using Restylane®. Significantly, Restylane® represents the first HA filler to embody the nonanimal stabilized hyaluronic acid (NASHA™) technology. While the use of non-animal HA is no longer a distinguishing feature among the commercial HA fillers available today, as most are based on nonanimal HA derived from bacterial fermentation, back when Restylane® was first launched, NASHA™ was a truly innovative feature, such that it was incorporated into the product name, as existing HA gels had all been based on rooster comb

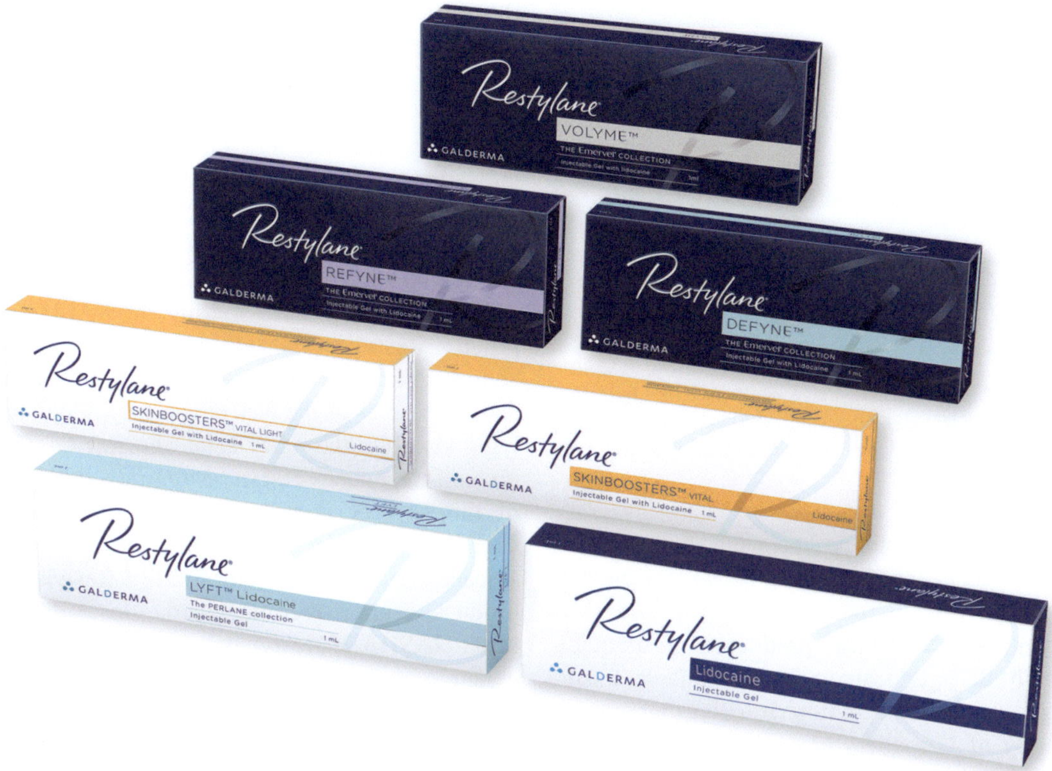

Fig. 2.26 Restylane® products

extracts. Meanwhile, the term "stabilized" in NASHA signifies the characteristics of Restylane® as a strong HA gel with a low degree of modifcation consisting only of gel particles of the same size.

Utilizing the patented NASHA™ technology for stabilizing the HA gel instead of chemical cross-linking with BDDE allows Restylane® to achieve less than 1% of MoD (degree of modification) in the final product (Fig. 2.7). Consequently, it is able to minimize potential complications arising from the modification of HA by the cross-linking agent and thus assures optimum biocompatibility. Meanwhile, each product within the Restylane® family represents an elastic biphasic HA filler containing gel particles of its own specified size (Fig. 2.27). In ascending order of the gel particulate size, the product range includes Restylane® Skinbooster Vital Light, Restylane® Skinbooster Vital, Restylane®, and Restylane® Lyft (previously Restylane® Perlane) (Table 2.5). While Restylane® SubQ had also been included in the portfolio mix, featuring the largest particulate size, it was subsequently discontinued in 2018. Meanwhile, it is also significant to note that Restylane® had embraced the so-called 'tissue-tailored concept', by which products are tailored to different clinical indications and depths of injection as early as the beginning of the 2000s during its inception, which has since become a standard feature of most HA filler brands today. Accordingly, Restylane® Skinbooster Vital, for example, which consists of smaller gel particles, is indicated for superficial injection in the dermis for the treatment of fine lines and loss of elasticity; Restylane® Lyft with a larger gel particulate size is commonly used for deep injections directly above the periosteum or in the subcutaneous tissue for restoration of volume deficit; Restylane® Skinbooster Vital Light featuring the finest particle size is targeted for use in delicate, fine-skinned areas, including the periorbital and neck regions. Meanwhile, the classic Restylane® has

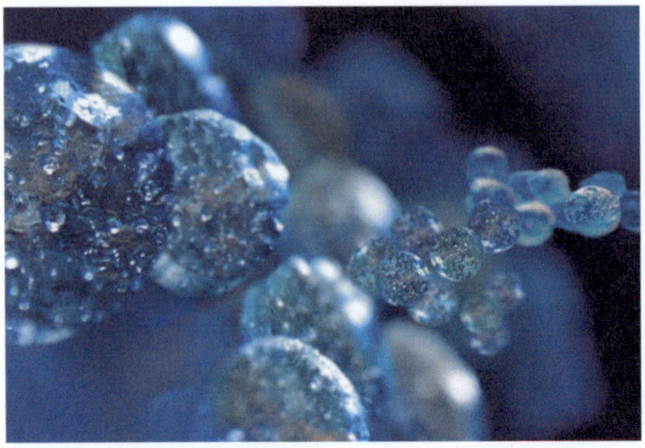

Fig. 2.27 Microscopic image of Restylane® Lyft (left bigger particles) and Restylane® (R) superscript) demonstrating NASHA™ gel particles with different sizes (Courtesy of Galderma)

an intermediate particle size, which makes it suitable for injection in the deep dermis for the correction of average folds.

In 2009, Restylane® products with the addition of 0.3% lidocaine became available, ensuring greater patient comfort. In 2010, the Emervel family of HA fillers incorporating the OBT™ (optimal balance technology) technology was approved in the EU, which in 2016 was renamed and integrated into the Restylane® brand, thus expanding the scope and versatility of the Restylane® product range (Fig. 2.8). OBT™ products are soft (monophasic) HA fillers with the same HA concentration of 20 mg/mL, but with differences in the degree and type of cross-linking, as well as particle size. The MoD of OBT™ fillers is within a range of 6–8% and varies depending on the product. While products using the OBT™ technology are often classified as soft monophasic HA, they also demonstrate near constant particle size as the result of 'sieving' undertaken during their manufacture for optimal homogenicity. The products with small particle size and with a low cross-linking are designed for superficial injection (e.g., Restylane® Fyness), whereas the products with lager particle size and with high cross-linking are designed for deeper and volumizing injection (e.g., Restylane® Volyme™). They are characterized as having a softer and more flexible gel texture than NASHA™ products. Products incorporating the OBT™ technology include Restylane® Fyness, Restylane® Kysse, Restylane® Refyne, Restylane® Defyne, and Restylane® Volyme™.

Ranging from very soft to very firm HA fillers, the Restylane® range of products is extremely versatile, and finds it use in most indications. The firm NASHA™ product Restylane® Lyft™ possesses a higher tissue-supporting capacity, which makes it suitable for use for volume restoration. Owing to its relatively low postinjection swelling, the NASHA™ product Restylane® also becomes the filler of choice for treating the nasal dorsum, tear trough, and other areas of the face covered by thin overlying skin. On the other hand, the soft OBT™ product Restylane® Refyne is optimized for use in the superficial dermis to avoid potential irregularities due to its malleability and spreadability. Also, the soft OBT™ Restylane® products are recommended instead of firm NASHA™ Restylane® Lyft™ for use in dynamic treatment areas such as the marionette lines and the forehead .

2.3.2 Juvéderm®: The First Original Soft HA Filler (Fig. 2.28)

Juvéderm® (Allergan, France) was CE approved in Europe in 2004 and approved by the FDA in the US in 2006. Juverderm® is the first original soft (monophasic) HA filler developed using the HYLACROSS™ technology in response to the firm HA filler, NASHA™ range of products (Table 2.6). Whereas Restylane® as firm (biphasic) HA filler, is a gel displaying granular consistency, Juvéderm® has a smooth and homogeneous gel texture characteristic of monophasic HA. As a smooth, spreading filler with low viscoelasticity, Juverderm® provides greater ease of injection and easy molding, which makes it particularly suitable for placement in the superficial plane. Despite its low viscoelasticity Juverderm® is also ideal for volumizing and contouring by virtue of its high cohesivity. Within the Juvéderm® range of products, Juvéderm® Ultra™ and Juvéderm® Ultra Plus™ are formulated using the HYLACROSS™ technology with the same HA concentration of 24 mg/mL, though featuring different percentages of cross-linking, with 6% for

Table 2.5 Restylane® products

Trade name	Restylane® Lyft	Restylane® Lidocaine	Restylane® Skinbooster Vital	Restylane® Skinbooster Vital Light
Manufacturing Technology	NASHA™	NASHA™	NASHA™	NASHA™
Monophasic or biphasic	Biphasic	Biphasic	Biphasic	Biphasic
HA concentration	20 mg/mL	20 mg/mL	20 mg/mL	12 mg/mL
Lifting capacity	+++	++	+	+
Size of Needle	29G ½	29G ½	29G ½	29G ½
Injection level	Subcutaneous/ Supraperiosteal/ Deep dermis	Mid to deep dermis	Superficial to mid dermis	Superficial to mid dermis
Particular Size	650 μm	300 μm		

Trade name	Restylane® Fynesse™	Restylane® Refyne™	Restylane® Defyne™	Restylane® Volyme™	Restylane® Kysse™
Manufacturing technology	OBT™	OBT™	OBT™	OBT™	OBT™
Monophasic or biphasic	Monophasic	Monophasic	Monophasic	Monophasic	Monophasic
HA concentration	20 mg/mL	20 mg/mL	20 mg/mL	20 mg/mL	20 mg/mL
Lifting capacity	+	++	+++	++++	+++
Size of Needle	30G ½	30G ½	27G ½	27G ½	30G ½
Injection level	Upper dermis	Mid to deep dermis	Deep dermis/ Subcutaneous	Subcutaneous/ Supraperiosteal	Upper dermis

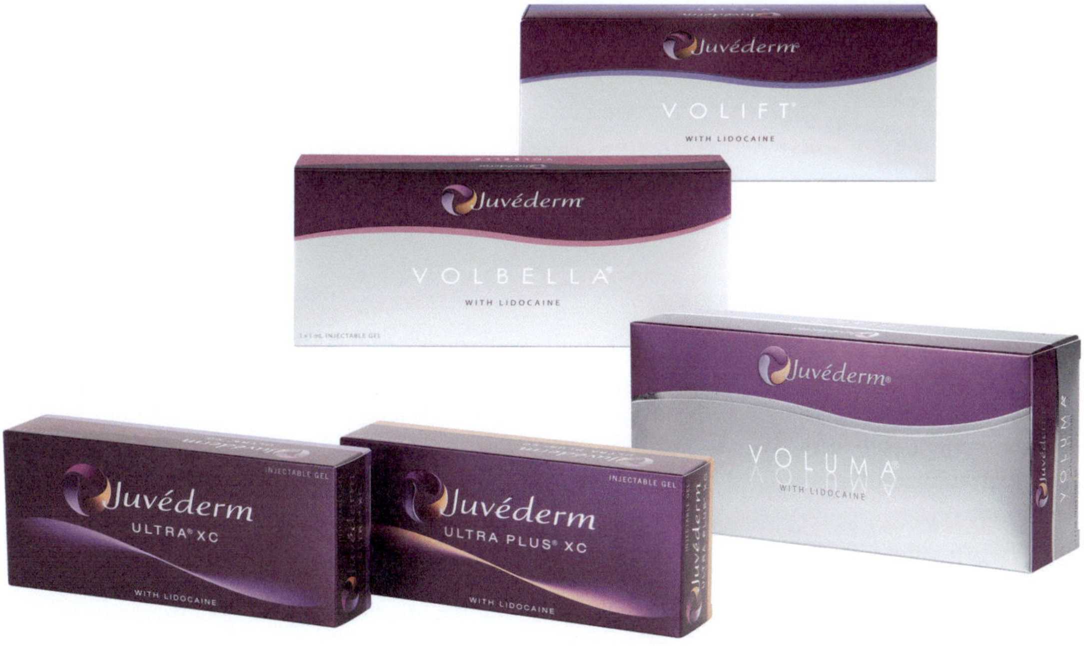

Fig. 2.28 Juvéderm® products

Table 2.6 Juvéderm products

Trade name	Juvéderm® VOLITE™	Juvéderm® VOLBELLA™	Juvéderm® VOLIFT™	Juvéderm® VOLUMA™	Juvéderm® VOLUX™
Manufacturing technology	Vycross™	Vycross™	Vycross™	Vycross™	Vycross™
Monophasic or biphasic	Monophasic	Monophasic	Monophasic	Monophasic	Monophasic
HA concentration	12 mg/mL	15 mg/mL	17.5 mg/mL	20 mg/mL	25 mg/mL
Lifting capacity	+	++	+++	++++	++++
Size of needle	32G ½′	30G ½′	30G ½′	27G ½′	27G ½′
Injection level	Intradermal	Superficial/ intradermal/ lips mucosa	Deep dermis/ lips mucosa	Subcutaneous/ Supraperiosteal/ deep dermis	Subcutaneous/ Supraperiosteal

Trade name	Juvéderm® Ultra XC	Juvéderm® Ultra Plus XC
Manufacturing technology	Hylacross™	Hylacross™
Monophasic or biphasic	Monophasic	Monophasic
HA concentration	24 mg/mL	24 mg/mL
Cross-linking level	6%	8%
Needle	30G ½’	27G ½’
Injection level	Middermis	Middermis and/or deep dermis

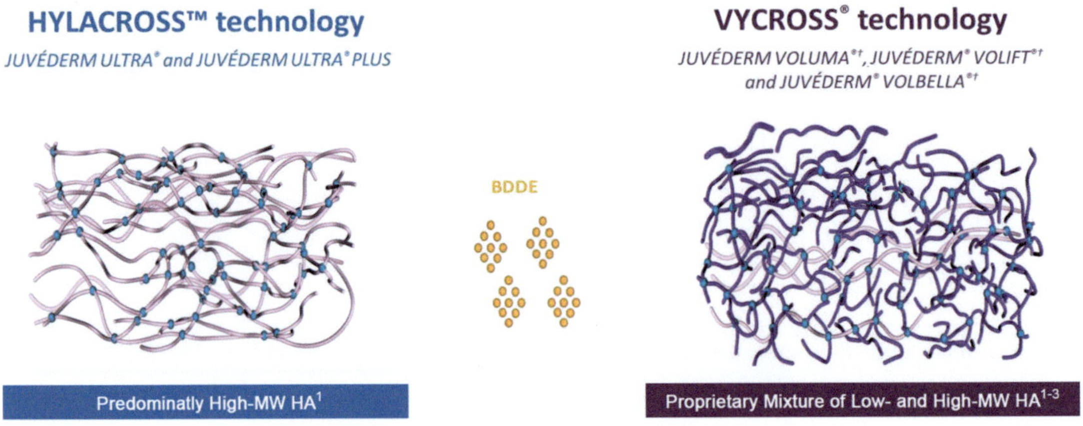

Fig. 2.29 HYLACROSS™ vs. VYCROSS™ technology (Courtesy of Allergan)

Juvéderm® Ultra™ and 8% for Juvéderm® Ultra Plus™. Due to its higher percentage of cross-linking, Juvéderm® Ultra Plus™ provides greater cohesivity and tissue lifting capacity and thus is commonly utilized for adding of volume in the deep plane [9].

However, due to their high HA concentration (24 mg/mL) and use of high-molecular-weight HA, HYLACROSS™ products are much more susceptible to hydration (i.e., swelling of the gel) and can draw in twice as much water as products built on VYCROSS™ technology [9]. Lumpiness and irregularity have thus been noted as common side effects of HYLACROSS™ products on account of such post-injection swelling.

To address such a drawback, VYCROSS™ was introduced as an evolution for delivering both reduced swelling and enhanced stability. To achieve this, VYCROSS™ combines both high- and low-molecular-weight HA to produce an HA gel matrix that integrates more efficiently into the tissue at lower HA concentrations (Fig. 2.29). Having a mixture of low-molecular-weight HA (short chains) and high-molecular-weight HA (long chains) during cross-linking can create a tighter and more efficient binding among HA molecules than would be possible based on the use of high-molecular-weight HA alone. The efficiency of the VYCROSS™ cross-linking technology can be best illustrated by an analogy to mixing up a bowl of spicy mixed noodles (*bibim-myeon* similar to *bibimbap* (Korean mixed rice) but with cold noodles) after pouring the sauce over it. Here, one would find that cutting up portions of the noodle with scissors allows the sauce to blend in more thoroughly and evenly and into the noodle strands. Likewise, VYCROSS™ is an efficient method for producing more thoroughly cross-linked and densely-packed HA molecules that provide greater stability with minimum hydration.

As with other major HA filler families, the VYCROSS™ range also includes a complementary mix of products designed to match different clinical indications based on varying gel properties.

Juvéderm® Voluma™, 20 mg/mL, which represents the very first product formulated using the VYCROSS™ technology, has the highest HA concentration (20 mg/mL) and elasticity within the VYCROSS™ range, which allows it to provide maximal tissue lift when placed in the deep tissue planes as a volumizing HA filler. In 2013, Juvéderm® Voluma™ was FDA-approved for correction of midface volume deficit. Noted for its ability to produce long-lasting results, Juvéderm® Voluma™ also became the first HA filler to receive FDA approval for 24 months duration of correction. Juvéderm® Volift™, which contains a lower HA concentration of 17.5 mg/mL, has intermediate rheological properties that fall somewhere between those of Juvéderm® Voluma™ and Juvéderm® Volbella™ and shows 30% less hydration than Juvéderm® Voluma™ [9].

Juvéderm® Volift™ is suited for injection in the deep dermis or the subcutaneous plane, not only for filling in etched-in lines and wrinkles such as the nasolabial folds and perioral lines but also for volume augmentation in areas such as the forehead. Meanwhile, Juvéderm® Volbella™ is a soft spreading filler with an HA concentration of 15 mg/mL, thus possesses the lowest viscoelasticity and cohesivity within the product range. Juvéderm® Volbella™ is appropriate for injection in the dermis for softening superficial wrinkles and tear trough deformities as well as for adding subtle volume to the lips.

All of the products within the Juvéderm® family, including not only Juvéderm® Ultra™ and Juvéderm® Ultra Plus™ but also the entire VYCROSS™ range, are currently available with 0.3% lidocaine to provide comfort during treatment, with each formulation having been duly approved by the USFDA. Juvéderm® Ultra is Juvéderm® Ultra XC without lidocaine and Juvéderm® Ultra Plus is Juvéderm® Ultra Plus XC without lidocaine.

2.3.3 Belotero®: HA Filler with a Reputation for Safety (Fig. 2.30)

The Belotero® range of products is manufactured and marketed by Merz Pharmaceuticals GmbH (Germany) and was originally developed by Anteis S.A., Switzerland, under the trade name Esthélis® (Table 2.7). Belotero® obtained CE certification in 2005 and was approved by the US FDA in 2011. Though a relative latecomer to the market, Belotero® has been widely recognized over the years for its favorable safety and efficacy profile as a monophasic HA filler. The Belotero® product line is built on the Cohesive Polydensified Matrix (CPM™) technology involving a second application of HA molecules to cross-link with the residual BDDE remaining after initial cross-linking. This results in a highly cohesive yet fluid gel matrix unique to Belotero®, where varying degrees of cross-linking coexist within the same gel substance (Fig. 2.31). The presence of high-density zones in the gel confers volumizing capacity and longevity to the product, while the less viscose low-density zones provide greater ease of injection and more homogenous product distribution/integration into the tissue. Containing several density grades within the same product also allows it to maintain better resilience and structural integrity against outside deformation forces applied by the facial musculature subsequent to its injection. Studies show that products incorporating the CPM™ technology are signifi-

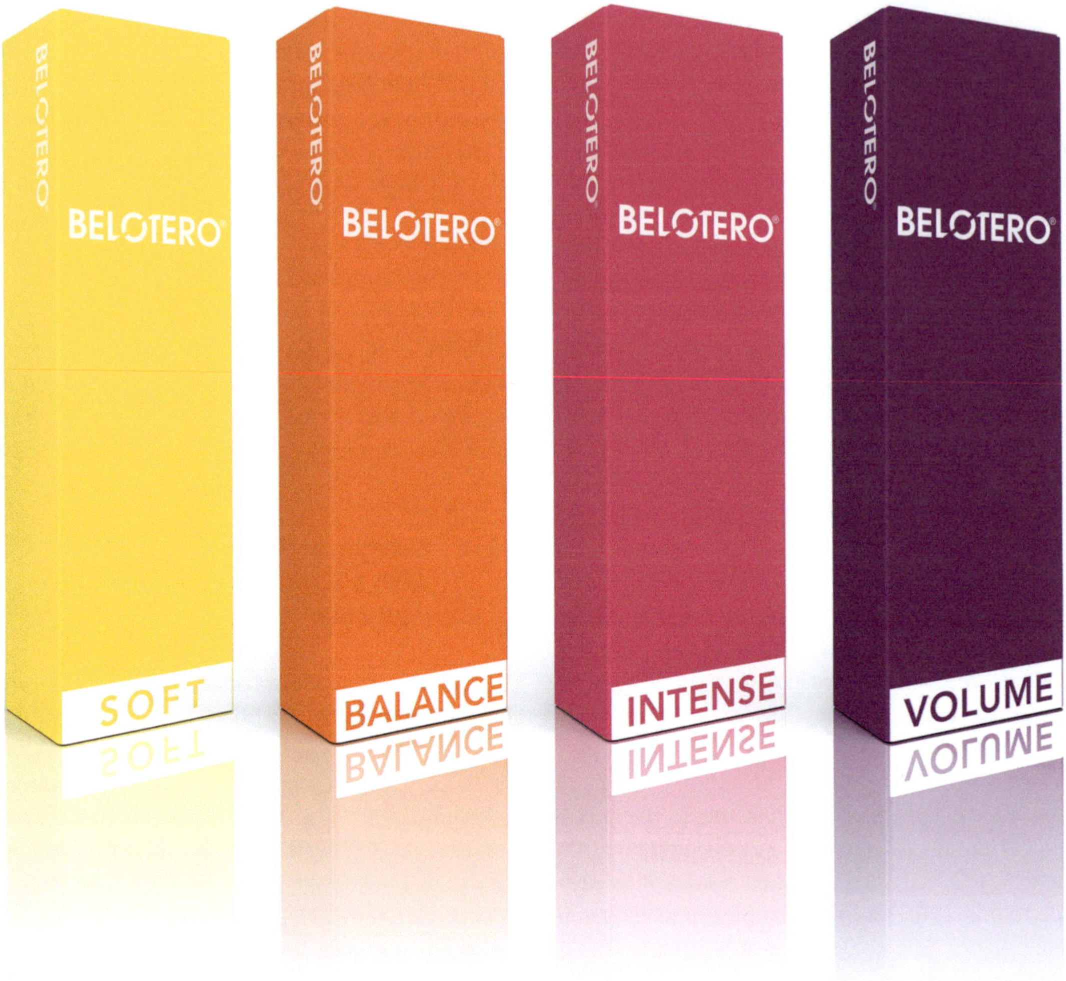

Fig. 2.30 Belotero® products

Table 2.7 Belotero® products (particle size and MoD is not disclosed by the company)

Trade name	Belotero® Soft™	Belotero® Balance™	Belotero® Intense™	Belotero® Volume™
Monophasic or biphasic	Monophasic	Monophasic	Monophasic	Monophasic
HA concentration	20 mg/mL	22.5 mg/mL	25.5 mg/mL	26 mg/mL
Lifting capacity	+	++	+++	++++
Size of Needle	30G ½	30G ½ 27G ½	27G ½	27G ½ 30G ½
Injection level	Superficial to mid-dermis	Mid to deep dermis	Deep dermis Subcutaneous	Deep dermis Subcutaneous Supraperiosteal

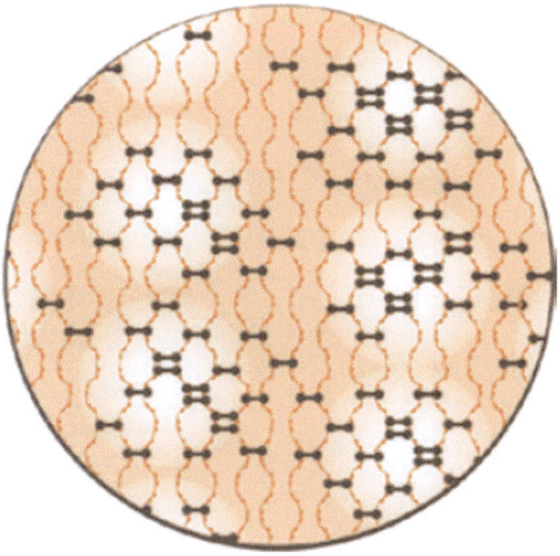

Fig. 2.31 Belotero® CPM™ technology (Courtesy of Mertz)

cantly more cohesive than those based on VYCROSS™ or NASHA technologies [13]. CPM™ products are also shown to demonstrate higher elastic modulus E' and normal force F_N than VYCROSS™ or NASHA products under applied compressive pressure [15]. It is for these reasons that Belotero® is able to demonstrate volumizing capacity comparable to that of NASHA products, despite having a significantly lower G'. Notably, cohesivity plays a significant role in the HA filler's volumizing effect as it allows the product to maintain its volume and shape even in dynamic treatment areas such as nasolabial folds, marionette lines, and the forehead.

Apart from its proven efficacy, another advantage of Belotero® lies in its favorable safety and tolerability profile. By virtue of its lower viscosity, Belotero® penetrates the dermis in a more diffuse and distributed manner, which allows it to create a smooth, even result with less Tyndalling. Most significantly, there have been no reported cases of granulomas from Belotero® injection since its release in 2005. It also involves the lowest incidence of delayed immune-related complications among available HA fillers to date.

The Belotero® range also includes a spectrum of products suited to varying indications and depth of injection. Belotero® Volume™ has the highest HA concentration (26 mg/mL) and the highest degree of cross-linking among the CPM™ products, and thus the highest shear elastic modulus G' and elastic modulus E'. It is thus suitable for placement in the deep tissue plane for restoration of facial volumes. Belotero® Intense™ has an HA concentration of 25.5 mg/mL and intermediate viscoelasticity that falls between that of Belotero® Volume™ and Belotero® Balance™. Nonetheless, it is still ideal for facial volume restoration as its F_N (normal force) and cohesivity are higher than those of Belotero® Volume™. It is thus indicated for injection in the deep dermis or the subcutaneous tissue for correction of deeper lines (e.g., nasolabial folds) or, alternately, for adding of volume in the lips or the forehead. Belotero® Balance has an HA concentration of 22.5 mg/mL and low viscosity and elasticity but has the highest cohesivity among the CPM™ products. As a soft, spreading filler, Belotero® Balance™ has an even and diffuse integration into the tissue, which makes it suitable for superficial injection in the dermal plane. It is appropriate not only for correction of moderate lines but also for hydro lifting injections in the dermis for improved skin elasticity, as well as for accentuating the vermillion border. Finally, Belotero® Soft™ has the lowest HA concentration (20 mg/mL) and degree of cross-linking among the CPM™ products and thus demonstrates the lowest viscoelasticity. Conversely though, it is these very characteristics that confer a soft, spreadable texture, which makes it ideal for use in the superficial dermis or in areas of thin tissue coverage such as the periorbital region and the neck.

2.3.4 YVOIRE®: Korea's First HA Filler (Fig. 2.32)

YVOIRE® is Korea's first HA filler developed in 2011 with the HICE™ (High Concentration Equalized) cross-linking technology) (Table 2.8). LG Chem (Korea)'s YVOIRE® products are biphasic HA filler, classified according to the particle size of the hyaluronic acid to suit their purpose and use. HICE™ cross-linking technology is LG Chem's own unique manufacturing tech-

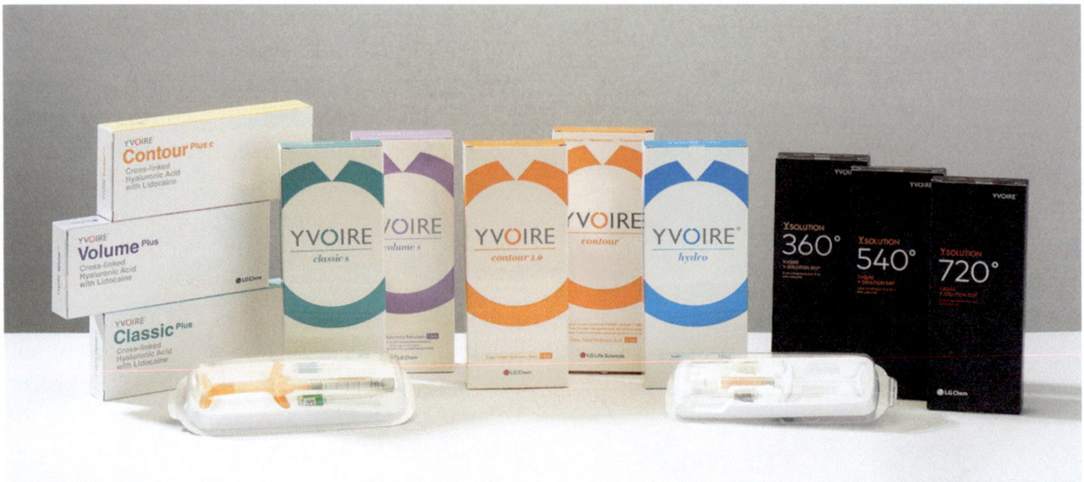

Fig. 2.32 YVOIRE® products

Table 2.8 YVOIRE® products

Trade name	Y-Solution™ 360	Y-Solution™ 540	Y-Solution™ 720	YVOIRE® Classic S™	YVOIRE® Classic Plus™
Manufacturing technology	S-HICE™	S-HICE™	S-HICE™	HICE™	HICE™
Monophasic or biphasic	Y-phasic	Y-phasic	Y-phasic	Biphasic	Biphasic
HA concentration	12 mg/mL	20 mg/mL	20 mg/mL	22 mg/mL	20 mg/mL
Lifting capacity	+	+++	++++	++	++
Size of Needle	29G ½″	27G ½″	27G ½″	27G ½″ 30G ½″	27G ½″ 30G ½″
Injection level	Upper dermis	Deep dermis	Subcutaneous/ Supraperiosteal	Deep dermis	Deep dermis
Particle size	230μm	360μm	360μm	400μm	400μm

Trade name	YVOIRE® Volume S™	YVOIRE® Volume Plus™	YVOIRE® Contour™	YVOIRE® Contour Plus C™
Manufacturing technology	HICE™	HICE™	HICE™	HICE™
Monophasic or biphasic	Biphasic	Biphasic	Biphasic	Biphasic
HA concentration	22 mg/mL	20 mg/mL	22 mg/mL	20 mg/mL
Lifting capacity	+++	+++	++++	++++
Size of Needle	27G ½″	27G ½″	23G 1″	23G 1″
Injection level	Deep dermis Subcutaneous	Subcutaneous/ Supraperiosteal	Subcutaneous/ Supraperiosteal	Subcutaneous/ Supraperiosteal
Particle size	900μm	900μm	1300μm/ 350μm	1300μm/ 350μm

nology, which can obtain high cross-linking efficiency even if small amounts of cross-linking agent is added by evenly dispersing cross-linking agents and high concentrations of high-molecular-weight HA. As a result of the cross-linking technology, YVOIRE® is a filler product that has been steadily used for more than 10 years and is recognized for its high elasticity and safety by using the least amount of cross-linking agent. From the hyaluronic acid raw material to the final product, LG Chem directly conducts the research and handles the manufacturing process. Hyaluronic acid raw material used in YVOIRE® has been listed on Drug master file (DMF) of US FDA and certified by European EDQM (European Directorate for the Quality of Medicines & Healthcare) ensuring overseas recognition of the relevant safety and technologies in overseas countries.

YVOIRE® Classic™/Classic plus™ has the smallest particles (350–400μm) and low elasticity and is suitable for wrinkle improvement. YVOIRE® Volume™/Volume plus™ which has larger particles (800–900μm) than Classic has higher elasticity suitable universally for most volumizing needs. When YVOIRE® Classic™ or YVOIRE® Volume™ were applied in the randomized, split-face designed, evaluator-blind studies with 58 and 57 subjects with moderate-to-severe NLFs compared to Restylane® or Lyft™, respectively, the nasolabial fold-correcting effects and safety profiles were comparable ($p < 0.05$) [23]. YVOIRE® Contour™/Contour plus™ which is suitable for areas requiring lifting capacity has the highest elasticity. As YVOIRE® Contour/Contour plus has a dual particle composition which allows the voids between the large particles (1400μm) to be filled with smaller particles (350μm, it provides constant injection force, resulting in a smooth and natural facial appearance. In the randomized, split-face, evaluator-blind clinical study with 83 subjects for anteromedial malar augmentation, there were no statistical difference ($p < 0.05$) in the effectiveness and safety profiles of YVOIRE® Contour when compared to Restylane® Sub-Q at 26 and 52 weeks after treatment [23]. Plus products contain lidocaine to reduce pain caused by injection. HA concentration of products without lidocaine is 22 mg and HA concentration of plus products with lidocaine is 20 mg. Immediately after treatment, more than 90% of subjects who were treated with YVOIRE® Classic plus or YVOIRE® Volume™ plus reported reduced pain when compared with those who were treated with YVOIRE® Classic or YVOIRE® Volume™, respectively in the randomized, split-face, evaluator-blind studies. That said, the clinical effectiveness and safety profiles of YVOIRE® Classic plus™ or Volume plus™ were comparable to those of YVOIRE® Classics or Volume™ s, respectively [27].

YVOIRE® Y-solution™ was developed to increase cohesivity, usually lower in biphasic fillers. To satisfy both high elasticity and cohesivity, YVOIRE® Y-solution™ embodies the S-HICE™ (Superior, Stable High Concentration Equalized) cross-linking technology that is more advanced than HICE™ to achieve higher cohesivity. S-HICE™ is an upgraded technology that increases the sustainability and cohesiveness between particles in the form of small particles through various particlization processes. Based on the S-HICE™ cross-linking technology, YVOIRE® Y-solution™ is Y-phasic™ filler with high lifting capacity achieved by combining the advantages of a monophasic filler with a high cohesivity and a biphasic filler with high elasticity. YVOIRE® Y-solution™ was first launched in Korea in 2018 with three products in its lineup including Y-solution 360™, Y-solution 540™, and Y-solution 720™. All YVOIRE® Y-solution™ products contain lidocaine and its HA concentration is, respectively, 12 mg, 20 mg, and 20 mg with MoD being 2.4%, 3.5%, and 3.3% respectively.

2.3.5 Neuramis®: Representative Korean Soft HA Filler (Fig. 2.33)

Neuramis® is a range of monophasic hyaluronic acid fillers developed by Medytox Inc. (Korea) (Table 2.9). Since the first product Neuramis® Deep obtained CE marking in 2011, a spectrum of products containing lidocaine were

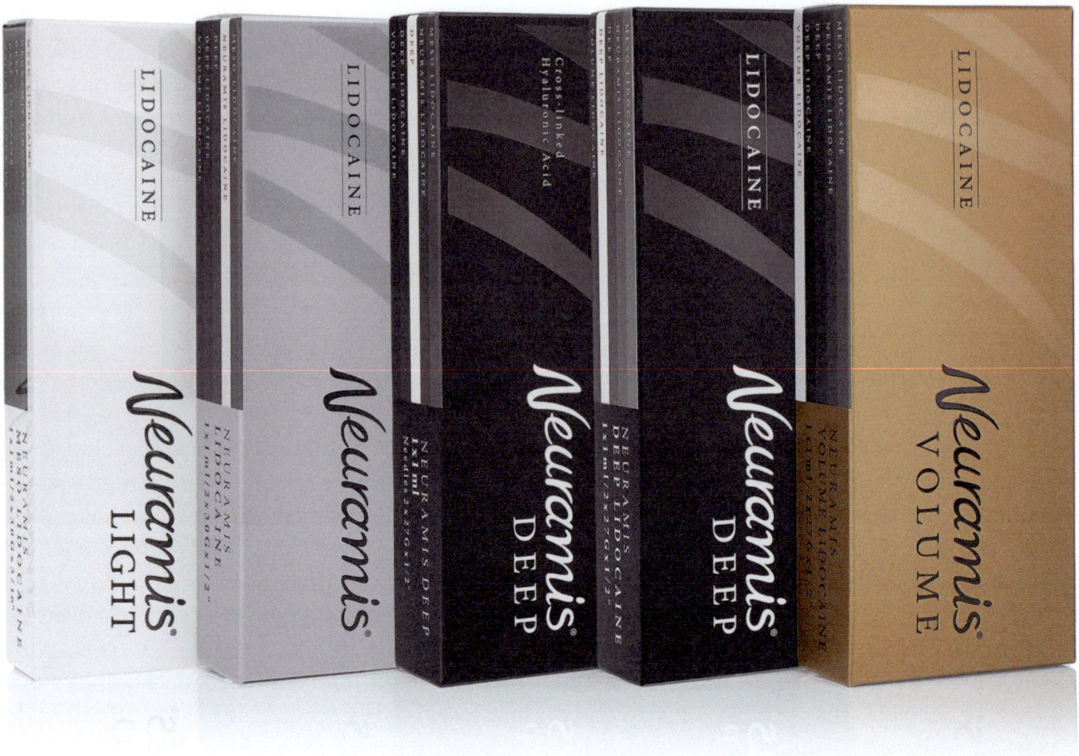

Fig. 2.33 Neuramis® products

Table 2.9 Product specification of Neuramis® lidocaine series

Trade name	Neuramis® Light Lidocaine™	Neuramis® Lidocaine™	Neuramis® Deep Lidocaine™	Neuramis® Volume Lidocaine™
Manufacturing technology	SHAPE™	SHAPE™	SHAPE™	SHAPE™
Monophasic or biphasic	Monophasic	Monophasic	Monophasic	Monophasic
HA concentration	20 mg/mL	20 mg/mL	20 mg/mL	20 mg/mL
Lifting capacity	+	++	+++	++++
Size of Needle	30G × 3/16″	30G × 1/2″	27G × 1/2″	27G × 1/2″
Injection level	Superficial to mid dermis	Mid to deep dermis	Mid to deep dermis	Subcutaneous Supraperiosteal

developed, namely, Neuramis® Light Lidocain, Neuramis® Lidocaine, Neuramis® Deep Lidocaine™, and Neuramis® Volume Lidocain™. Currently, Neuramis® Deep™ and Neuramis® Deep Lidocain™, and Neuramis® Volume Lidocaine™ have obtained CE certificate. Through a unique manufacturing process referred to as "SHAPE™ (Stabilized Hyaluronic Acid & Purification Enhancement)" technology, tailored cross-linking of hyaluronic acid is formed resulting in a highly cohesive hyaluronic acid gel. No uncross-linked hyaluronic acid is added, and the final products contains hyaluronic acid at the concentration of 20 mg/mL. For the safety and quality of the products, it uses only highly qualified hyaluronic acid registered in FDA Drug Master Files and European Directorate for the Quality of Medicines and Healthcare. Hyaluronic acid concentration of all products is 20 mg/mL.

Neuramis® lidocaine series offers four products with different degrees of cross-linking to suit various needs (Table 2.9). Neuramis® Light Lidocaine™ is a lightly cross-linked hyaluronic acid intended to be injected in the dermis for the improvement of fine wrinkles. Neuramis® Lidocaine™ and Neuramis® Deep Lidocaine™ are intended to be used for the restoration of tissue in mid to deep dermis. In a randomized spilt-face clinical trial, Neurmis® Deep Lidocaine™ demonstrated significantly better correction of the nasolabial folds, compared with Restylane® Lyft™ for up to 24 weeks ($p < 0.05$) [29]. Neuramis® Volume Lidocaine™ is the most heavily cross-linked hyaluronic acid product intended to be injected into subcutaneous and/or supraperiosteal layer. In a randomized, double-blinded, comparative study, Neuramis® Volume Lidocaine™ showed similar results compared with Juvederm® voluma™ for the efficacy and safety in restoration of mid-facial volume deficit in 88 subjects [30].

2.3.6 e.p.t.q.®: HA Filler with a Top Priority on Safety (Fig. 2.34)

e.p.t.q.® (epitique) (JETEMA, Korea), a monophasic hyaluronic acid filler was developed in 2017 by applying *2CM*™ (2 Crosslinking Method) technology and acquired a CE marking for e.p.t.q.® lidocaine in 2020. 2CM™ Technology employs not only a chemical cross-linking but

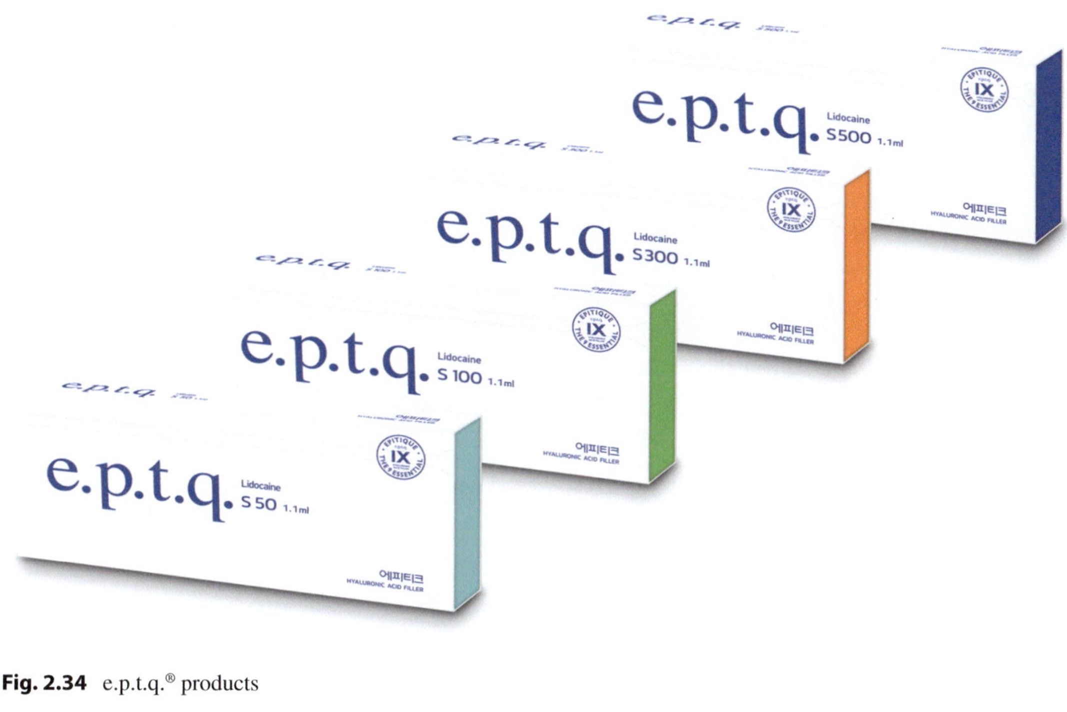

Fig. 2.34 e.p.t.q.® products

Table 2.10 e.p.t.q. products

Trade name	e.p.t.q.® Lidocaine S100™	e.p.t.q.® Lidocaine S300™	e.p.t.q.® Lidocaine S500™
Manufacturing technology	2CM™	2CM™	2CM™
Monophasic or biphasic	Monophasic	Monophasic	Monophasic
HA concentration	24 mg/mL	24 mg/mL	24 mg/mL
Lifting capacity	+	+++	++++
Size of Needle	27G 1/2″	27G 1/2″	27G 1/2″
Injection level	Dermis	Deep dermis	Subcutaneous
Particle size	310μm	310μm	310μm
MoD (%)	1.18	1.53	1.89

also a physical cross-linking so that maximum cross-linking efficiency can be achieved with a minimum amount of BDDE to create a rigid and stable hive structure. e.p.t.q.® has a modification degree (MoD) in the 1% range with minimal input of cross-linkers for excellent safety, but still retains high cohesiveness. Leveraging a grinding technology called the *Downing Process*, e.p.t.q.® has fine and uniform particles. Thanks to these fine particles, e.p.t.q.® can be injected with thin needles (30G). Typically, products containing large-sized gel particles should not be used with thin needles due to the potential effects on particle size and rheological equilibrium [31].

e.p.t.q.® is categorized by its viscoelasticity: S100, S300, S500 (Table 2.10) [29]. All three have a hyaluronic acid concentration of 24 mg/mL and contain lidocaine to ease the pain. While e.p.t.q.® is a monophasic filler with softer gel formulation, it has uniform particle size with excellent molding. In addition, owing to the manufacturing process focusing on the safety issue such as minimum cross-linker content (MoD of 1% range), the incidence of inflammatory reaction from delayed type hypersensitivity seems to be as low as less than 0.1% based on the author's experience using 2,000 syringes for last 2 years.

2.4 Other Types of Injectable Fillers

2.4.1 Collagen Fillers

As a key component of the dermal matrix responsible for the skin's strength and resilience, collagen was the first material ever to be used as soft tissue fillers. The first collagen-based fillers approved for use by the USFDA in the early 1980s were the bovine-based ZYDERM®1 (bovine collagen 35 mg/mL), ZYDERM® 2 (bovine collagen 65 mg/mL), and ZYPLAST® (bovine collagen 35 mg/mL, cross-linked with glutaraldehyde) (Allergan. CA, US) fillers [3]. The Japanese version, that is, Koken Atelocollagen® (Koken Co. Japan), was also derived from a bovine source. Due to their animal origin, however, these bovine collagen fillers required a skin allergy test to be performed 4 weeks prior to treatment, though a negative testing did not rule out the risk of an allergic response. With the subsequent advent and dominance of HA fillers, however, bovine collagen fillers soon went out of use globally, which led Allergan to eventually end the production of ZYDERM® and ZYPLAST® in 2010. Meanwhile, EVOLENCE® (Johnson & Johnson.

New Jersey, US) is a porcine collagen filler (porcine collagen 30 mg/mL), which obtained USFDA approval in 2008 [3]. The benefits of EVOLENCE® were that they were cross-linked, therefore provided longer-lasting results over the previous collagen fillers and did not require allergy testing. Despite these advantages, however, Johnson & Johnson was also compelled to discontinue EVOLENCE® in 2009 due to the declining market interest in collagen-based fillers. Meanwhile, COSMODERM® and COSMOPLAST® (Allergan, CA) are human tissue-derived collagen fillers approved by the USFDA in 2003 but were subsequently discontinued in 2010.

Comment: While collagen fillers broke new ground by pioneering the market for injectable dermal fillers, their value today is mostly historical, as they have been rendered practically obsolete by the risk of immunogenic reactions and the short duration of effect lasting for only 3–6 months. That said, it should be accepted that collagen fillers provided good moldability and spread easily into the tissues while being free of problems of Tyndalling, which made them ideal for treating fine wrinkles in delicate thin-skinned areas such as the periorbital region.

2.4.2 Permanent Injectables

2.4.2.1 PMMA (Polymethyl Methacrylate)

Polymethyl Methacrylate (PMMA) is a substance routinely used in orthopedic surgical practice as bone cement for the human body (Fig. 2.35). BellaFill® is (Suneva Medical Inc., US) a PMMA-based permanent filler containing smooth-surfaced PMMA microspheres ranging 30–50μm in size designed to avoid macrophage phagocytosis [31, 31] (Fig. 2.36). In 2006, injectable PMMA was approved by the USFDA under the trade name ArteFill® (Artes Medical, US) upon which ArteFill® became the first permanent soft tissue filler to obtain USFDA approval. ArteFill® was rebranded as BellaFill® in 2014. BellaFill® is composed of PMMA microspheres suspended in 3.5% bovine collagen at a 1:4 ratio [30]. Over time, collagen is reabsorbed and PMMA microspheres acts as a scaffold to biostimulate collagen

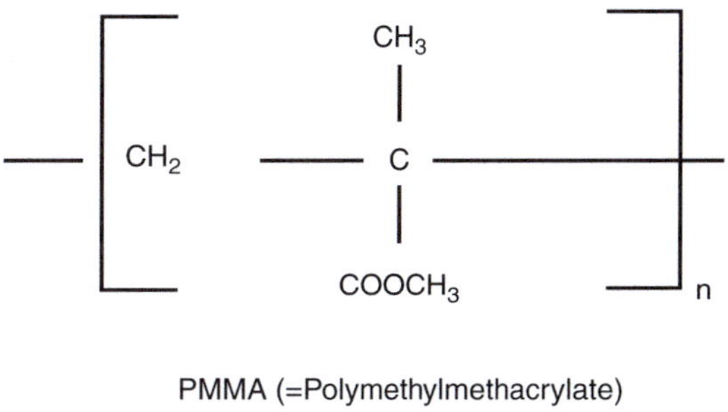

Fig. 2.35 PMMA molecular formula

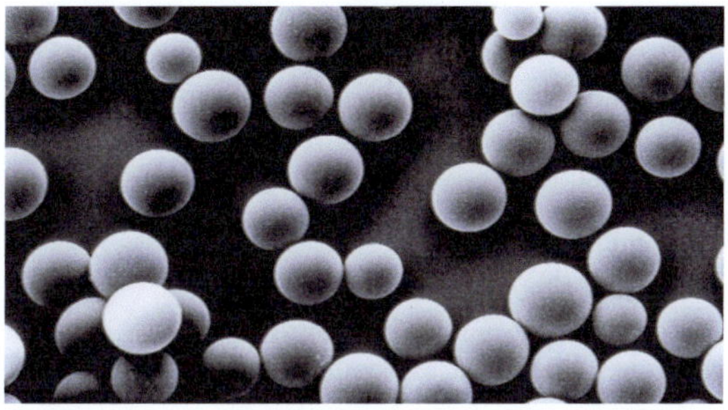

Fig. 2.36 BellaFill® is a PMMA-based permanent filler containing smooth-surfaced PMMA microspheres ranging 30–50μm in size. (Courtesy of Artes Medical)

synthesis. To the extent the product contains bovine collagen as the carrier substance, it is necessary to perform a skin allergy test before treatment with BellaFill®. Side effects, though rare, include foreign body reaction, granuloma, contour deformity, and inflammation [30]. Caution must be taken in its use since PMMA is a synthetic compound not reversible with a reversal agent should problems occur.

Comment: Permanency of fillers implies that any potential complications arising from such fillers are also permanent. To avoid life's unpleasant surprises, practitioners, except perhaps for the most daring, are well-advised to stay away from these permanent solutions.

2.4.2.2 PAAG (Polyacrylamide Gel)

Polyacrylamide gel (PAAG) is a high polymer used as an ingredient in the manufacture of soft contact lenses (Fig. 2.37). Permanent soft tissue filler containing PAAG was developed for the first time in 1980 in Ukraine under the tradename Interfall® and was awarded CE certification in 2001 in Denmark under the tradename Aquamid®

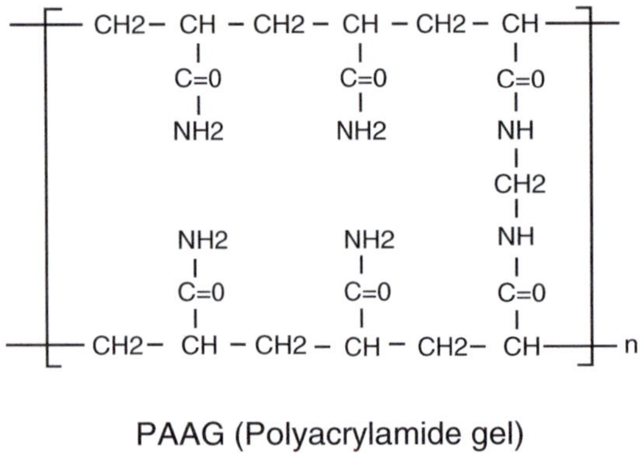

Fig. 2.37 PAAG molecular formula

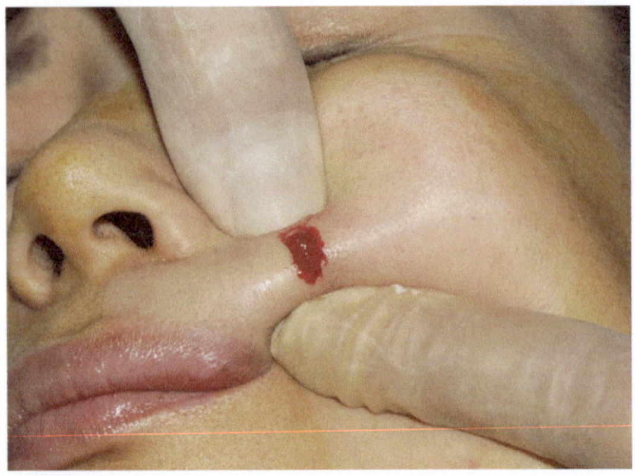

Fig. 2.38 Removal of Aquamid® by squeezing out

(Contura International A/S, Denmark). Aquamid® is a hydrogel product combining 2.5% cross-linked polyacrylamide and 97.5% water and is reputed to have natural texture and favorable biocompatibility [31]. Granuloma, contour deformation, and product migration have been often observed, however, following its application [33]. Fortunately, the product can be removed even several years post-treatment by administering saline 2–3 times the volume of the injected PAAG, followed by 3–5 min of intense massage and puncture with an 18-G needle or incision, after which the product can be substantially squeezed out (Fig. 2.38) [32, 33]. In the wake of the negative publicity surrounding the complications from Amazing gel® (FuHua High Molecular weight company, China) injections for breast augmentation, PAAG has largely fallen out of favor and is practically no longer in use. While Aquafilling® (Czech), consisting of PAAG (2%) and water (98%) was introduced to the market a few years ago claiming to be reversible with normal saline, Aquafilling® injections, as with Aquamid®, *cannot* be dissolved away simply using a reversal agent (Fig. 2.39).

2.4.3 Collagen-Stimulating Fillers

Prior to 2000, soft tissue fillers were developed primarily for use as volumizers or filling agents,

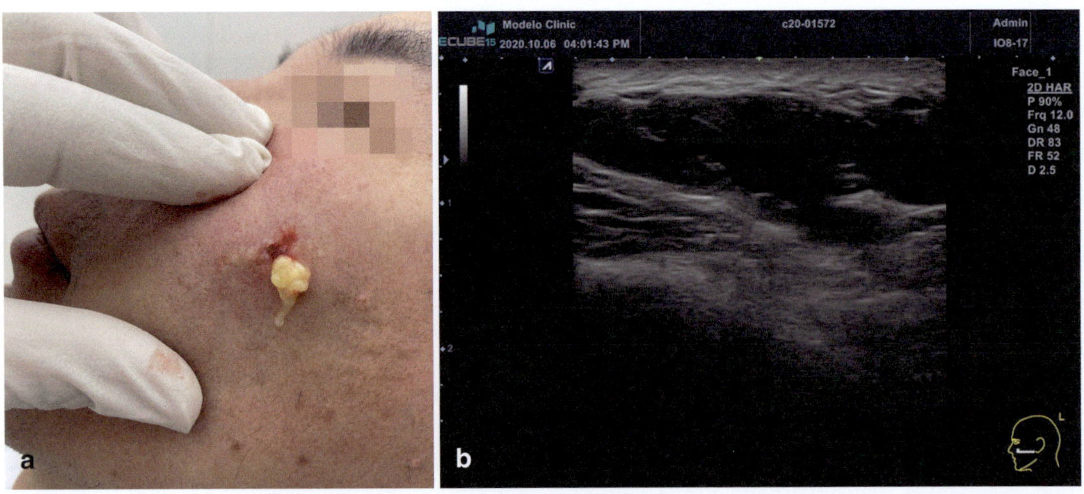

Fig. 2.39 (**a**) Removal of Aquafilling® by squeezing out. (**b**) Sonography of Aquafilling®

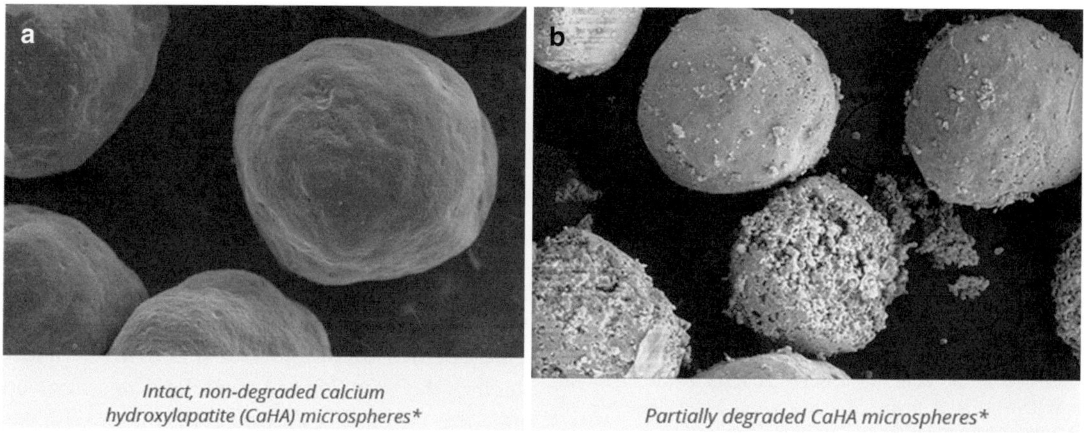

Fig. 2.40 The scanning electron microscope of the CaHA (Courtesy of Merz Institute of Advanced Aesthetics). (**a**) The CaHA is composed of smooth microspheres ranging 25–45μm in diameter. (**b**) Partially degraded CaHA microspheres

with collagen-based or HA fillers injected to provide replacement volume for facial deflation. From 2000 onwards, however, the prevailing trend in soft tissue filler development shifted away from replacement fillers toward biodegradable high polymers capable of inducting collagen biostimulation in the injected area while they themselves were slowly degraded in the body. These collagen-stimulating fillers, also referred to as biostimulating fillers, are known to provide better longevity compared with HA fillers. Key examples include calcium hydroxylapatite (CaHA), PLLA, PDLLA, PCA, and PDO-based fillers. On the flip side, however, the use of biostimulating fillers presents associated risks and challenges, including individual variability in collagen synthesis, nodule formation from overproduction of collagen, and surface irregularity from elevated nodules. Most significantly, results of collagen-stimulating fillers remain irreversible in case of misplacement or complications. Accordingly, their use should be avoided in unforgiving facial areas with thin overlying skin, such as the periorbital region or the labial mucosa.

2.4.3.1 Calcium Hydroxylapatite (CaHA) Filler

Calcium Hydroxylapatite ($Ca_{10}(PO_4)_6(OH)_2$) or CaHA is the main mineral of which the teeth and bones are composed. Similar in composition to gallstones or urinary stones, it has been long used in orthopedic surgical procedures or dental applications as dental filling material or dental regeneration material. Calcium hydroxylapatite fillers consist of 30% CaHA and 70% sodium carboxymethylcellulose (CMC), glycerine, and sterile water. The CaHA is composed of smooth microspheres ranging 25–45μm in diameter designed to avoid macrophage phagocytosis (Fig. 2.40). Once placed in the soft tissue, CaHA microspheres elicit neocollagenesis at the injection site while they themselves slowly disintegrate into calcium and *phosphate* ions, and are completely removed from the system [34] (Fig. 2.41). Meanwhile, the gel carrier, sodium carboxymethylcellulose (CMC), provides initial volume during the first few weeks or months of injection, after which it gradually dissipates away, leaving in its place new collagen to fill the space [35].

Radiesse® (Merz, Germany) was the first CaHA filler to be approved by the USFDA in *2001* for use in vocal fold insufficiency treatment and bone void filling (Fig. 2.42). In 2006, it received US FDA approval for the correction of severe facial wrinkles and/or facial lipoatrophy in individuals with human immunodeficiency virus (HIV). Though composed principally of calcium, Radiesse® does not ossify or calcify in the soft tissue or the periosteum into which it has been placed [36]. There have been no reported cases of bone generation occurring as a result of Radiesse® injection in the soft tissue [34]. This is because,

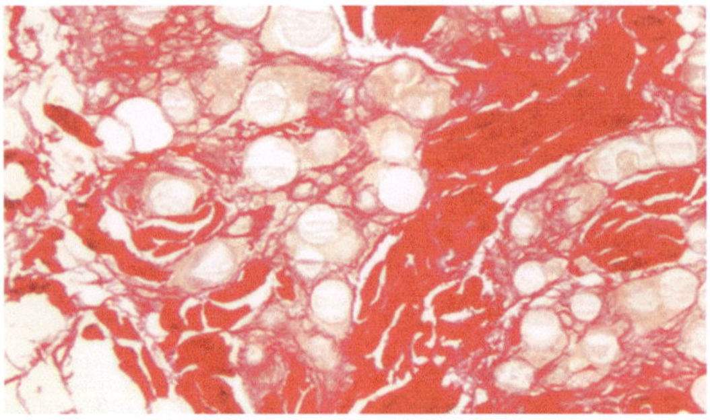

Fig. 2.41 Calcium hydroxyl apatite microspheres act as scaffolds while eliciting neocollagenesis at the injection site (Sirus Red stain) (Courtesy of Merz Institute of Advanced Aesthetics)

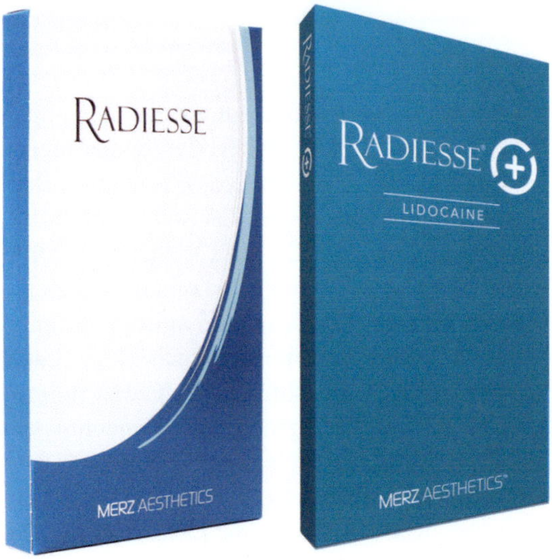

Fig. 2.42 Radiesse® products

theoretically, new cell growth into the implanted CaHA is consistent with the surrounding tissue, and new cells do not differentiate into other cell types [34].

While Radiesse® is known to provide longevity lasting for several years, the patient may initially perceive the effect as being temporary and short-lived as the gel carrier deflates after the first few weeks or months of injection. In such case, it is helpful to provide a touch-up injection 1–2 months posttreatment [36]. It also bears noting that Radiesse® injections can be highly painful as the product's pH levels (6.8–8.0) fall outside the pH range of the human body. Reconstituting 1.3 mL Radiesse® with 0.2 mL lidocaine before the injection can significantly help to reduce the pain [36]. Radiesse® also tends to cause greater initial swelling than HA fillers, perhaps due to its gel carrier substance. Hence, it is best to avoid large volume injections of Radiesse® into the same site during a single session. Instead, it is preferable to use a stepwise approach with treatments spaced 2–4 weeks apart until the desired outcome is reached. A notable complication of Radiesse® is the formation of hard nodules when injected as boluses in places such as the thin-skinned periorbital region or lip mucosa. Surgical removal or treatment with triamcinolone local injection is required in case nodules are formed [37]. Conversely, granuloma formation due to foreign body reaction is not that frequent in Radiesse® compared with other permanent fillers, PLLA or even HA fillers [37–39]. Complaints of contour irregularity or overcorrection within the first 2 weeks of treatment can be addressed by puncturing the injection site using an 18-G needle and manually extracting the product out through the puncture site. However, in case substantial time has passed since the initial treatment, this is no longer an option, and surgical removal or triamcinolone injections becomes the only available option.

Comment: Radiesse® was acclaimed as a new milestone in facial volumization when it first came to market. However, its initial popularity and versatility were soon limited by drawbacks such as significant initial swelling, potential nodule formation upon bolus injection, and the risk of overgrowth of collagen fibers which may deter cannula advancement during subsequent second or third treatments. Moreover, as the product could not be dissolved away with a reversal agent, facial volumization with Radiesse® left no room for errors. These factors combined to restrict the widespread use of Radiesse® in facial volumization applications. However, the collagen biostimulating effect of Radiesse® has been popularly used for *skin-tightening* purposes by diluting the product two- to three-fold with saline and lidocaine and injecting it superficially into the subdermis [40]. Examples include rejuvenation of crepey skin in the neck and the dorsum of the hand.

2.4.3.2 PCL Filler (Fig. 2.43)

Polycaprolactone (PCL) is a type of bioresorbable polymer that has long been used in the medical field as resorbable surgical sutures (Fig. 2.44). Polycaprolactone (PCL)-based soft tissue filler is marketed as Ellansé™ (AQTIS Medical, Netherlands). Ellansé™ represents a biodegradable high polymer filler consisting of 30% PCL suspended in 70% carboxymethylcellulose (CMC) as the gel carrier. Similar to Radiesse®, PCL-based Ellansé™ consists of smooth microspheres with particulate size ranging 25–50μm to avoid macrophage phagocytosis. When injected, PCL microspheres promote new collagen formation in the surrounding tissue and gradually break down into water and CO_2, after which they are eliminated from the system. The gel carrier, sodium carboxymethylcellulose (CMC), provides immediate volume correction during the initial weeks or months and dissipates in 3 months, to be replaced by new collagen. In sum, apart from the differences in the active ingredient, Ellansé™ shares many similarities with Radiesse® in terms of the composition, mechanism of action, indication, and complications.

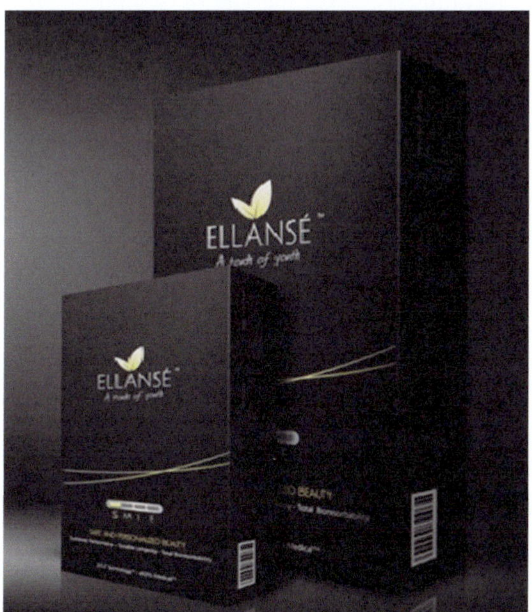

Fig. 2.43 Ellansé™ products

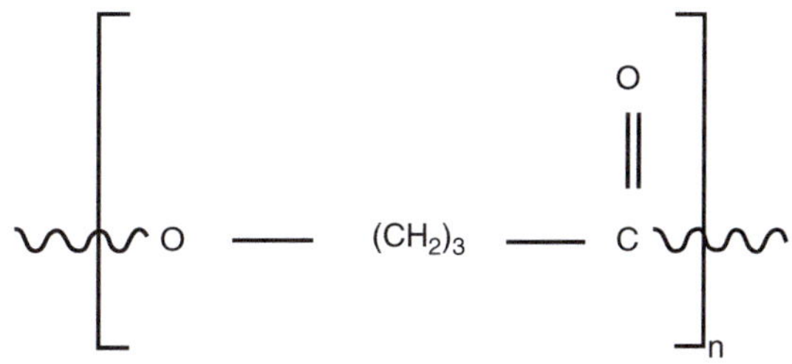

Fig. 2.44 PCL molecular formula

2.4.3.3 PLLA (Poly-L-Lactic Acid) (Fig. 2.45)

Poly-L-lactic acid (PLLA) is a bioresorbable biocompatible polymer that has been widely used in the medical practice since the 1970s as absorbable surgical sutures or as intra-bone implants, pins, and plates in orthopedic surgery or dental procedures (Fig. 2.46). Sculptra® (Galderma, Switzerland) is a formulation consisting of freeze-dried powder of poly-L-lactic acid (PLLA). It received CE certification in 1999 and obtained USFDA approval for the treatment of facial lipoatrophy in patients with human immunodeficiency virus (HIV) in 2003 [41]. Subsequently in 2009, it was FDA approved for the correction of facial wrinkles and folds in the US market. Once placed in the tissue, PLLA gradually breaks down to lactic acid monomers over the course of 24 months via nonenzymatic hydrolysis [42]. In the process, it creates controlled inflammation at the injected area to elicit collagen production [43]. The lactic acid is subsequently metabolized to carbon dioxide and water and naturally excreted from the body [44]. The PLLA microparticles present in the product are in the form of irregular crystals instead of smooth microspheres. Sculptra® only contains PLLA particles 40–60μm in diameter to avoid macrophage phagocytosis [44]. Other components present in the powder apart from PLLA include Mannitol and Sodium. Sculptra® is available in a 367.5 mg dose vial, with each vial containing PLLA 150 mg, sodium carboxymethylcellulose (CMC) 90 mg and mannitol 127.5 mg. CMC is included to ensure even distribution of PLLA particles [45] while mannitol is added to produce a firm, homogenous cake in the final process of freeze-drying [46].

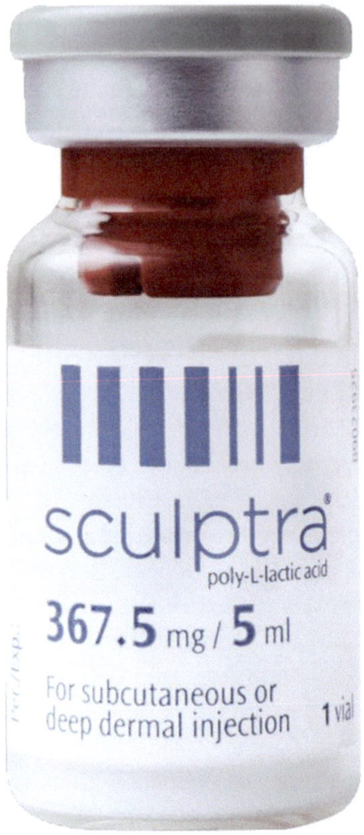

Fig. 2.45 Sculptra® products

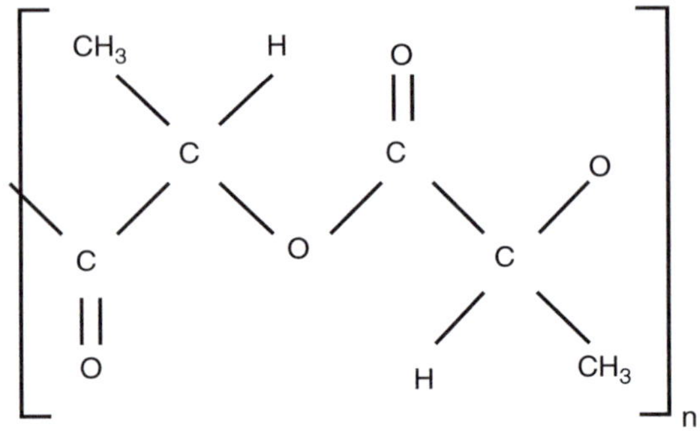

Fig. 2.46 PLLA molecular formula

Unlike Radiesse® or EllanséTM, which incorporate gel carriers, Sculptra® comes in the form of freeze-dried powder and thus requires reconstitution with sterile distilled water (hereinafter "distilled water") 2–72 h prior to use [47, 48]. Given the presence of Mannitol in the powder, distilled water rather than saline should be used to ensure adequate osmolarity. Although the recommended reconstitution volume is 5 mL per vial [48, 49], the prevailing trend among injectors is to use a higher reconstitution volume of 10 mL to minimize the risk of nodule formation [50]. Rather than reconstituting with distilled water alone, it is preferable to add 1–2 mL of 1% lidocaine to 8–9 mL of distilled water for diluting the product to minimize discomfort during the injection [50]. Regarding the reconstitution time, it is advisable to reconstitute the product at least 1 day prior to use. The wisdom of reconstituting the product in advance with distilled water and leaving the reconstituted material to sit for sufficient hydration is to ensure uniform dispersion of the aggregated PLLA microparticles in the mixture and prevent clumps of product from causing nodules. While storage of up to 3 days after hydration is described in the pharmacopeia, the reconstituted Sculptra® can be stored for up to 3–4 weeks at refrigeration, provided necessary safeguards are in place to prevent contamination [50]. PLLA in itself is insoluble in water and thus becomes suspended when reconstituted with distilled water. CMC and mannitol, on the other hand, are soluble and, following reconstitution with distilled water, undergo hydration. Thus, it is recommended that the vial of Sculptra®, once hydrated with distilled water, is gently agitated just before injection to ensure even and homogenous dispersion of PLLA. The suspension is then transferred from the vial into a 1 mL syringe for injection into the tissue. To avoid bruising and inadvertent intravascular injection of Sculptra®, it is recommended to use a 23-G cannula for delivering the product evenly into the deep subcutaneous or supraperiosteal plane. The one area reserved for using a 21-G needle is the temporal region covered by thick fascia, which cannot be easily penetrated with a cannula.

The injection volume required to cover the entire face, including the anteromedial malar, anterior cheek (buccal hollows), and temporal fossa, ranges from 1 vial up to 2 vials per session depending on the extent of facial volume loss [48]. By facial regions, the volume of product injected is 1–2 mL for the anteromedial malar,

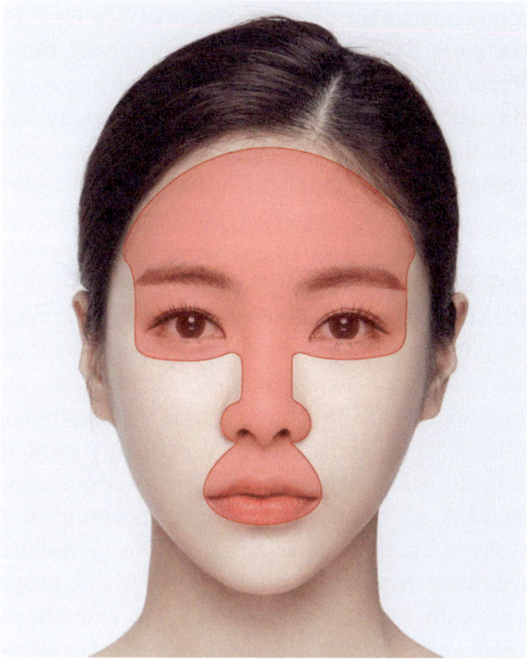

Fig. 2.47 PLLA should be avoided in thin-skinned areas such as the periorbital region, the forehead and the nose, and in dynamic areas such as the perioral region and the lip vermillion

2–4 mL for the anterior cheek, and 1–3 mL for the temple per side. As a general rule of thumb, one vial per session should suffice in case the temples do not require treatment. Where treatment is necessary also in the temples or severe facial volume deflation is present, up to two vials may be needed in a single session. To avoid the appearance of nodules, it is critical to refrain from superficial injections or injection in thin-skinned areas such as the periorbital region. Accordingly, the forehead and the nose with thin overlying skin are not suited for treatment with Sculptra®. PLLA should also be avoided in dynamic areas such as the perioral region and the lip vermillion (Fig. 2.47). Immediately upon completing the injection, it is helpful to thoroughly massage the treated areas to distribute the PLLA evenly throughout the tissue to avoid nodule formation. In addition, it is recommended that patients be instructed to massage the treatment areas for 5 min, 5 times a day, for 5 days after treatment (5-5-5-regimen) [51].

The immediate postinjection volume effect from Sculptra® is attributable to the direct volume replacement provided by the reconstituted material including distilled water, which disappears within 2–3 days starting from the very next day. New collagen production from PLLA injection kicks in 4 weeks from treatment and reaches the peak after the third month, with the collagen biostimulation from the injection lasting for more than 25 months. Treatment with Sculptra® typically requires around three injection sessions spaced 3–4 weeks apart for the best effect [51].

However, unlike other volumizing fillers such as HA, which allow customization of the desired volume by the physician or patient, the result of Sculptra® is subject to individual variability in new collagen formation in the treated area. Therefore, the risk exists that results may not be visible even after completing the full three rounds of treatment. Treatment with Sculptra® thus requires corresponding effort on the part of the patient to maximize collagen formation, for example, by avoiding weight loss, eating a healthy diet rich in protein, and maintaining regular, quality sleep. Concerning adverse reactions, a common complication of Sculptra® is nodule formation due to uneven placement of product in the tissue or the aggregation of PLLA microparticles in the injected product. The best prevention strategy is to use a thin and uniform suspension diluted to 10 mL and to make sure it is injected evenly in the tissue. It also helps for the patient to periodically massage the treated areas during the first week. It bears noting that nodules are more prone to occur in thin-skinned regions including the periorbital and forehead regions. They typically appear in the size of a lentil or pea 1–2 months after injection and persist until resolved in less than a year. In the interim, a vigorous deep massage may be attempted to mechanically crush the nodules apart [52, 53]. If there is no improvement, it may be worthwhile to consider subcising the clumped-up PLLA particles with a needle following intralesional injection of saline in the treated area. Meanwhile, granulomas represent

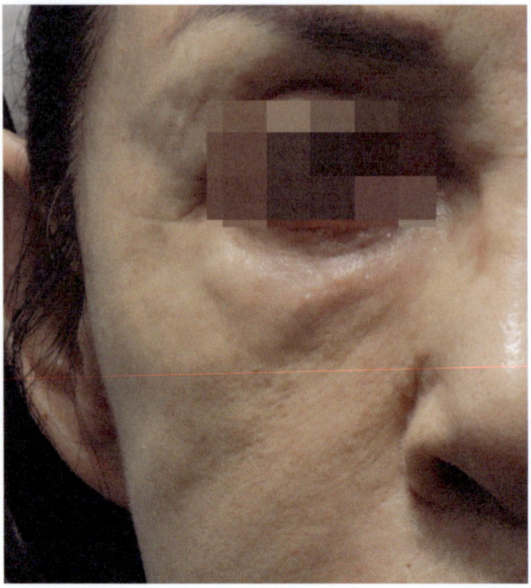

Fig. 2.48 Granuloma in the infraorbital area due to the inappropriate injection of Sculptra®

another complication of Sculptra®, which should be distinguished from nodules (Fig. 2.48). Granulomas typically occur 3–6 months postinjection as a result of excessive foreign body reaction [51, 53]. Though they appear in the form of nodules or papules, histologically, they represent foreign body granulomas. The granuloma may be accompanied by skin discoloration, edema, and erythema. Possible treatments for granulomas include injections of intralesional triamcinolone or 5-FU [54]. If the granuloma does not respond to intralesional injections, following up with surgical removal is advised. Vigilance is required as granulomas left untreated can persist for more than 10 years.

Comment: As a biostimulator that offers to stimulate the body's own collagen production, Sculptra® can be a compelling alternative for patients who seek rejuvenation but are reluctant to use injectable fillers due to their aversion to implanting a foreign substance in their face. The drawback, however, is that results of Sculptra® depend heavily on the body's reaction to build natural collagen, which may vary significantly among individuals; thus, outcomes may be limited if not almost negligible in some patients. Granted, this seeming weakness may translate, in marketing-speak, as an advantage of Sculptra® in building subtle yet natural volume over time. Recently, the PLLA has also been used as a biostimulator, enhancing not only skin elasticity but also the appearance of pores, scars, skin tone, and complexion via superficial injection into the subdermis [42].

2.4.3.4 P-D,L-LA (Poly-D,L-Lactic Acid)

PDLLA (poly-D,L-lactic acid) is a stereoisomer of polylactic acid comprised of D-and L-lactic acids arranged in alternating order to form an irregular chain structure. Unlike PLLA (poly-L-lactic acid) consisting only of tightly packed L-lactic acids, the D- and L-isomers comprising PDLLA are spaced farther apart, resulting in a weaker intermolecular linkage. This gives the resulting material, PDLLA, a soft, friable property with reduced hardness and an amorphous shape, unlike the PLLA particles that are crystalline in shape [55].

Lenisna® (VAIM, Korea) and Juvelook® (VAIM, Korea) are products containing reticulated foamy microspheres of PDLLA obtained by dissolving the amorphous PDLLA particles in a mixture of DMSO (dimethylsulfoxide) and EC (ethylene carbonate) and microspraying the content (Fig. 2.49). Lenisna® and Juvelook® received CE certification in 2020 and was approved for use in Europe. A notable advantage of Lenisna® and Juvelook® is that they contain HA in place of CMC, albeit in a non-cross-linked form, which allows these products to provide immediate volume correction during the initial period of treatment.

A vial of Lenisna® contains 200 mg of freeze-dried power of PDLLA (PDLLA 170 mg, HA 30 mg), while Juvelook® comes in a 50-mg dose vial (PDLLA 42.5 mg, HA 7.5 mg.) That said, Juvelook® does not simply represent a smaller repackage dosage unit of Lenisna®, as it is formulated specifically to contain only PDLLA microspheres sized 50μm or smaller. Consequently, the average particle size of Juvelook® is 24μm (20–50μm) in diameter compared with 51μm (50–80μm) of Lenisna®. This allows Juvelook® to be placed directly into the dermis to produce skin regeneration without concerns of nodule forma-

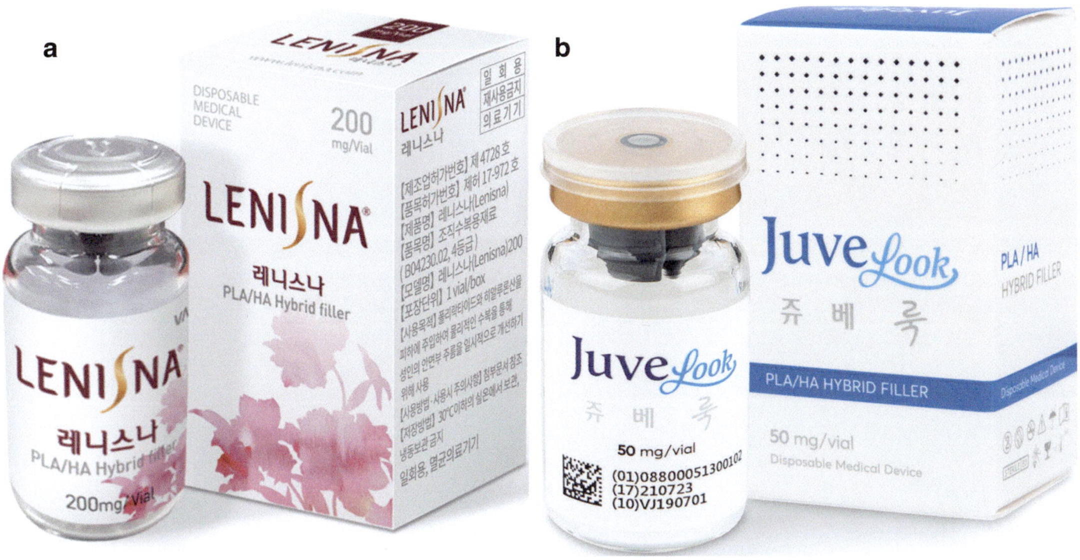

Fig. 2.49 PDLLA products. (**a**) Lenisna®. (**b**) Juvelook®

tion, which distinguishes it from Sculptra®, though it provides reduced longevity and volume projection compared with Lenisna® [55].

The microspheres present in Lenisna® and Juvelook® are comprised of a multi-pore spongiform structure, causing them to undergo a more rapid process of hydrolysis from within (Fig. 2.50). As a consequence, when hydrolyzed, these products progressively break down into lactic acid monomers within a span of 1–1.5 years. As with PLLA, PDLLA also creates inflammation in the injected area during its degradation, eliciting collagen production, albeit at reduced duration and amount compared with PLLA. However, this point can simultaneously serve as a strength, as it implies a lower risk of nodularity and granuloma formation. Lenisna® is suitable for volume replenishment, similar to Sculptra®, via injection in the deep subcutaneous plane; by comparison, Juvelook®, consisting of finer particles, is designed primarily for skin regeneration via intradermal injection in the skin.

As with Sculptra®, Lenisna®, and Juvelook® come as freeze-dried powder which is not suspended in a gel carrier but instead requires reconstitution with sterile distilled water before injection. Considering that the power contains mannitol, distilled water rather than saline should be used for the reconstitution to ensure adequate osmolarity. Regarding the dilution volume, Lenisna® is reconstituted with 6 mL of distilled water, to which 1 mL lidocaine is added; while Juvelook® is reconstituted with 4 mL of distilled water, to which 1 mL lidocaine is added [56]. Given Lenisna® and Juvelook® consist of multipore microspheres and saturate more easily than Sculptra®, they can be used right away following 30–60 min of hydration. Nonetheless, it can be helpful to use a vortex generator to agitate the vial for approx. 20 min before injection or to reconstitute the product 1 day or preferably 1 week prior to use. The reconstituted products can be stored for up to 3–4 weeks in a refrigerator, provided care is taken to avoid contamination.

Immediately before use, it is recommended to gently shake the hydrated vial of Lenisna® or Juvelook® to obtain an even and homogenous suspension. The suspension is then transferred from the vial into a 1-mL syringe for injection into the tissue. To avoid bruising and inadvertent intravascular injection, it is recommended to use a 23-G cannula for delivering the product evenly into the deep subcutaneous or supraperiosteal plane. The one area reserved for using a 21-G needle is the temporal region, covered by

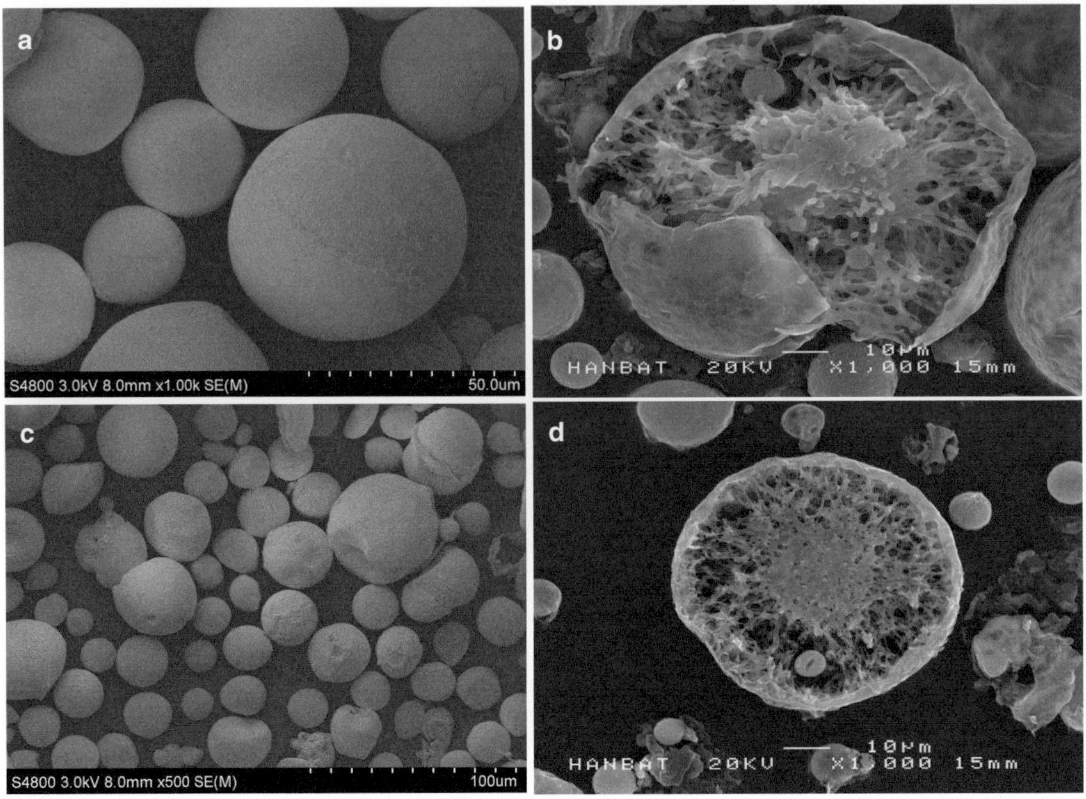

Fig. 2.50 The scanning electron microscope of the PDLLA (Courtesy of Vaim)

thick fascia that is hard to penetrate with a cannula. When using the product for volume replacement, it is recommended to use 0.7 mL of reconstituted Lenisna® further diluted with 0.3 mL of saline [56]. This produces an effect comparable to using Sculptra® reconstituted to 10 mL. The volume of product injected per treatment area (per side) is 1–2 mL for the anteromedial malar, 2–4 mL for the anterior cheek, and 1–3 mL for the temple. One vial per session should suffice if the temples do not require treatment. Where no treatment is necessary for the temples or where severe facial volume deflation is present, up to two vials may be needed for a single session. Combination with cross-linked HA may be considered in patients who desire instant volume addition or wish to avoid repeat treatments. In such case, the use of 0.7 mL of reconstituted Lenisna® further diluted with 0.3 mL of cross-linked HA is advised [56].

The relevant injection volume should be equivalent to 1.5–2 times the amount that would have been injected using only cross-linked HA. While results may appear insufficient initially, the volume becomes progressively evident after the fourth week, as collagen production from PDLLA injection starts to kicks in. One advantage of Lenisna® is the minimal risk of nodule formation even when placed superficially into the skin. This gives the product greater versatility, to be applied not only for facial volume replenishment but also for skin tightening. When used for skin rejuvenation, it is recommended to add 0.5 mL of saline to 0.5 mL of the reconstituted Lenisna® for placement into the subdermis. Immediately upon completing the injection, it is helpful to massage the treated areas to distribute the PDLLA evenly throughout the tissue, although more softly than when massaging in Sculptra®. Patients should be instructed to rub the treatment areas for 3 min, 3 times a day, for 3 days after treatment (3-3-3-regimen) [56].

The biggest advantage of Juvelook® its ability to be placed directly in the dermis to provide skin tightening, as it involves minimal risk of nodularity even when placed very superficially in the skin. The PDLLA injected in the dermis can act as a biostimulator, enhancing not only skin elasticity but also the appearance of pores, scars, skin tone, and complexion as is the case with PLLA [57]. Juvelook® may be used either alone or in combination with cross-linked HA or other skin-boosting ingredients such as PDRN, placenta extracts, and exosome. Caution is required in areas of reduced dermal thickness, such as the periorbital region. That being said, nodules formed by Juvelook® are known to resolve within a month upon repeated massage using a radiofrequency device, as the application of heat combined with strong pressure can be effective in removing PDLLA microspheres that have a multi-porous structure and a melting point of 55–60 °C, more than 10 °C lower than that of PLLA.

References

1. Glogau RG. Fillers: paradigm shifts produce new challenges. In: Carruthers J, Carruthers A, editors. Soft tissue augmentation. Philadelphia: Elsevier; 2018. p. 3–6.
2. Fraser JR, Laurent TC, Laurent UB. Hyaluronan: its nature, distribution, functions and turnover. J Intern Med. 1997;242(1):27–33.
3. Soo-Keun L. Textbook of botulinum toxin and filler. 2nd ed. Seoul: Hanbibook Co; 2018. p. 233–42.
4. Stern R. Hyaluronan catabolism: a new metabolic pathway. Eur J Cell Biol. 2004;83(7):317–25.
5. Lim CY. Are the hyaluronic acid fillers safe? Filler Toxin. 2014;1(2):6–9.
6. Choi S, Choi W, Kim S, Lee SY, Noh I, Kim CW, Choi S. Purification and biocompatibility of fermented hyaluronic acid for its applications to biomaterials. Biomater Res. 2014;18:6–16.
7. Roh NK. The truth nobody tells about fillers. Filler Toxin. 2017;4(2):45–9.
8. Kenne L, Gohil S, Nilsson EM, Karlsson A, Ericsson D, Helander Kenne A, Nord LI. Modification and cross-linking parameters in hyaluronic acid hydrogels—definitions and analytical methods. Carbohydr Polym. 2013;91(1):410–8.
9. Humphrey S, Fotzgeral R. Juvederm family. In: Carruthers J, Carruthers A, editors. Soft tissue augmentation. Philadelphia: Elsevier; 2018. p. 67–70.
10. Narins RS, Mariwalla K. NASHA Family. In: Carruthers J, Carruthers A, editors. Soft tissue augmentation. Philadelphia: Elsevier; 2018. p. 17–24.
11. Sundaram H, Cassuto D. Biophysical characteristics of hyaluronic acid soft-tissue fillers and their relevance to aesthetic applications. Plast Reconstr Surg. 2013;132(4 Suppl 2):5S–21S.
12. Molliard GS, Albert S, Mondon K. Key importance of compression properties in the biophysical characteristics of hyaluronic acid soft-tissue fillers. J Mech Behav Biomed Mater. 2016;61:290–8.
13. Sundaram H, Rohrich RJ, Liew S, Sattler G, Talarico S, Trévidic P, Molliard SG. Cohesivity of hyaluronic acid fillers: development and clinical implications of a novel assay, pilot validation with a five-point grading scale, and evaluation of six U.S. Food and Drug Administration-approved fillers. Plast Reconstr Surg. 2015;136(4):678–86.
14. Tran C, Carraux P, Micheels P, Kaya G, Salomon D. In vivo bio-integration of three hyaluronic acid fillers in human skin: a histological study. Dermatology. 2014;228(1):47–54.
15. Park KY, Kim JM, Seok J, Seo SJ, Kim MN, Youn CS. Comparative split-face study of durational changes in hyaluronic acid fillers for mid-face volume augmentation. Dermatol Ther. 2019;32(4):e12950.
16. Fagien S, Bertucci V, von Grote E, Mashburn JH.Rheologic and Physicochemical Properties Used to Differentiate Injectable Hyaluronic Acid Filler Products. Plast Reconstr Surg. 2019;143(4):707e–720e.
17. Monheit GD, Baumann LS, Gold MH, Goldberg DJ, Goldman MP, Narins RS, Bachtell N, Garcia E, Kablik J, Gershkovich J, Burkholder D. Novel hyaluronic acid dermal filler: dermal gel extra physical properties and clinical outcomes. Dermatol Surg. 2010;36(Suppl 3):1833–41.
18. Rosamilia G, Hamade H, Freytag DL, Frank K, Green JB, Devineni A, Gavril DL, Hernandez CA, Pavicic T, Cotofana S. Soft tissue distribution pattern of facial soft tissue fillers with different viscoelastic properties. J Cosmet Dermatol. 2020;19(2):312–20.
19. Monheit G, Kestemont P, Sundaram H. Hyaluronic acid fillers on the horizon: roundtable discussion. J Drugs Dermatol. 2012;11(8):s26–8; discussion s28.
20. Buntrock H, Reuther T, Prager W, Kerscher M. Efficacy, safety, and patient satisfaction of a monophasic cohesive polydensified matrix versus a biphasic nonanimal stabilized hyaluronic acid filler after single injection in nasolabial folds. Dermatol Surg. 2013;39(7):1097–105.
21. Mandelson B. Rayleigh scattering. https://en.m.wikipedia.org/wiki/Rayleigh_scattering.
22. Rootman DB, Lin JL, Goldberg R, Rootman DB. Does the Tyndall effect describe the blue hue periodically observed in subdermal hyaluronic acid gel placement? Ophthal Plast Reconstr Surg. 2014;30(6):524–7.

23. Yang SD, Shin S, Lee J, Yang SD. Two randomized controlled trials of hyaluronic acid fillers for the correction of nasolabial folds. Plast Reconstr Surg Glob Open. 2020;8(7):e2975.
24. Huh CH, Eom Y, Yang SD, Shin JW, Seo KK. A randomized, active-controlled, 52-week study of hyaluronic acid fillers for anteromedial malar region augmentation. Plast Reconstr Surg Glob Open. 2020;8(2):e2648.
25. Choi SY, Han HS, Yoo KH, Lee JS, Kim BJ, Lee YW. Reduced pain with injection of hyaluronic acid with pre-incorporated lidocaine for nasolabial fold correction: a multicenter, double-blind, randomized, active-controlled, split-face designed, clinical study. J Cosmet Dermatol. 2020;19:3229–33. https://doi.org/10.1111/jocd.13421.
26. Joo HJ, Woo YJ, Kim JE, Kim BJ, Kang H. A randomized clinical trial to evaluate the efficacy and safety of lidocaine-containing monophasic hyaluronic acid filler for nasolabial folds. Plast Reconstr Surg. 2016;137(3):799–808.
27. Jung JM, Lee WS, Kim HT, Moon YS, Paik SH, Lee WJ, Chang SE, Lee MW, Won CH, Kim BJ. A multi-center, randomized, double blinded, comparative study of two hyaluronic acid fillers for temporary restoration of mid-face volume in Asians. J Cosmet Dermatol. 2020;19(7):1619–26.
28. Won L, et al. Soft tissue filler properties can be altered by a small-diameter needle. Dermatol Surg. 2020;46(9):1155–62.
29. LEE W, et al. Clinical application of a new hyaluronic acid filler based on its rheological properties and the anatomical site of injection. Biomed Dermatol. 2018;2:22.
30. Khetarpal S, Dover JS. Introduction to permanent fillers: pors and cons. In: Carruthers J, Carruthers A, editors. Soft tissue augmentation. Philadelphia: Elsevier; 2018. p. 67–70.
31. Sadick NS. Bellafill. In: Carruthers J, Carruthers A, editors. Soft tissue augmentation. Philadelphia: Elsevier; 2018. p. 79–84.
32. Ono S, Ogawa R, Hyakusoku H. Complications after polyacrylamide hydrogel injection for soft-tissue augmentation. Plast Reconstr Surg. 2010;126(4):1349–57.
33. Kavoussi H, Ebrahimi A. Delayed gel indurations as an adverse effect of polyacrylamide filler and its easy treatment. Dermatol Res Pract. 2012;2012:539153.
34. Radmanesh M, Radmanesh R, Bahadoram M. Successful removal of polyacrylamide hydrogel by pulsed fiberoptic 1444-nm Nd-YAG laser. J Cosmet Laser Ther. 2013;15(6):342–4.
35. Drobeck HP, et al. Histologic observation of soft tissue responses to implanted, multifaceted particles and discs of hydroxylapatite. J Oral Maxillofac Surg. 1984;42:143–9.
36. Sheinin RC, Mahmould BH, Ozog DM. Radiesse and radiesse with lidocaine. In: Carruthers J, Carruthers A, editors. Soft tissue augmentation. Philadelphia: Elsevier; 2018. p. 41–8.
37. Voigts R, Devore DP, Grazer JM. Dispersion of calcium hydroxylapatite accumulations in the skin: animal studies and clinical practices. Dermatol Surg. 2010;36(Supplement s1):798–803.
38. Pavicic T. Calcium hydroxylapatite filler: an overview of safety and tolerability. J Drugs Dermatol. 2013;12(9):996–1002.
39. Tzikas TL. A 52-month summary of results using calcium hydroxylapatite for facial soft tissue augmentation. Dermatol Surg. 2008;34(Suppl 1):9–15.
40. Sadick NS, Katz BE, Roy D. A multicenter, 47-month study of safety and efficacy of calcium hydroxylapatite for soft tissue augmentation of nasolabial folds and other areas of the face. Dermatol Surg. 2007;33(Suppl 2):S122–6; discussion S126–7.
41. Goldie K, Peeters W, Alghoul M, Butterwick K, Casabona G, Chao YYY, Costa J, Eviatar J, Fabi SG, Lupo M, Sattler G, Waldorf H, Yutskovskaya Y, Lorenc P, Goldie K. Global consensus guidelines for the injection of diluted and hyperdiluted calcium hydroxylapatite for skin tightening. Dermatol Surg. 2018;44(Suppl 1):S32–41.
42. Beleznay K, Fitzgerald R, Humphrey S. Poly-L-lactic acid. In: Carruthers J, Carruthers A, editors. Soft tissue augmentation. Philadelphia: Elsevier; 2018. p. 49–56.
43. Brown SA, Rohrich RJ, Baumann L, Brandt FS, Fagien S, Glazer S, Kenkel JM, Lowe NJ, Monheit GD, Narins RS, Rendon MI, Werschler WP. l. Subject global evaluation and subject satisfaction using injectable poly-L-lactic acid versus human collagen for the correction of nasolabial fold wrinkles. Plast Reconstr Surg. 2011;127(4):1684–92.
44. Fitzgerald R, Bass LM, Goldberg DJ, Graivier MH, Lorenc ZP, Lin MJ, Dubin DP, Goldberg DJ, Khorasani H. Practices in the usage and reconstitution of poly-L-lactic acid. J Drugs Dermatol. 2019;18(9):880–6.
45. Stein P, Vitavska O, Kind P, Hoppe W, Wieczorek H, Schürer NY. The biological basis for poly-L-lactic acid-induced augmentation. J Dermatol Sci. 2015;78(1):26–33.
46. Drugs.com. Sodium Carboxymethylcellulose. https://www.drugs.com/inactive/carboxymethylcellulose-sodium-452.html. Accessed 16 Apr 2019.
47. Schierle CF, Casas L. Nonsurgical rejuvenation of the aging face with injectable poly-L-lactic acid for restoration of soft tissue volume. Aesthet Surg J. 2011;31(1):95–109.
48. Sculptra®Aesthetic. Product Labeling. Instructions for Use. L.P. Fort Worth, TX: Galderma Laboratories; September 2014.
49. Palm M, Chayavichitsilp P. The "skinny" on Sculptra: a practical primer to volumization with poly-L-lactic acid. J Drugs Dermatol. 2012;11(9):1046–52.
50. Lowe NJ, Maxwell CA, Lowe P, Shah A, Patnaik R. Injectable poly-l-lactic acid: 3 years of aesthetic experience. Dermatol Surg. 2009;35(Suppl 1):344–9.
51. Lin MJ, Dubin DP, Goldberg DJ, Khorasani H. Practices in the usage and reconstitution of poly-L-lactic acid. J Drugs Dermatol. 2019;18(9):880–6.

52. Redaelli A, Forte R. Cosmetic use of polylactic acid: report of 568 patients. J Cosmet Dermatol. 2009;8(4):239–48.
53. Lee JM, Kim YJ. Foreign body granulomas after the use of dermal fillers: pathophysiology, clinical appearance, histologic features, and treatment. Arch Plast Surg. 2015;42(2):232–9.
54. Graivier MH, Bass LM, Lorenc ZP, Fitzgerald R, Goldberg DJ, Lemperle G. Differentiating non-permanent injectable fillers: prevention and treatment of filler complications. Aesthet Surg J. 2018;38(suppl_1):S29–40.
55. Blanco MD, Sastre RL, Teijón C, Olmo R, Teijón JM. Degradation behaviour of microspheres prepared by spray-drying poly(D,L-lactide) and poly(D,L-lactide-co-glycolide) polymers. Int J Pharm. 2006;326(1–2):139–47.
56. Jung WK. Sculptra vs. Esthephil vs. Etreville vs. Lenisa vs. Juvelook. Filler Toxin. 2020;6(1):35–9.
57. Bohnert K, Dorizas A, Lorenc P, Sadick NS. Randomized, controlled, multicentered, double-blind investigation of injectable poly-L-lactic acid for improving skin quality. Dermatol Surg. 2019;45(5):718–24.

3 Hyaluronic Acid (HA) Filler Injection Procedure

3.1 Preparation Prior to the Injection

3.1.1 Preparation of Tray

Tray Setup: Filler, needle, cannula, gauze, betadine balls, chlorohexidine gauze, boric acid gauze, Tegaderm® transparent film.

Prepare two sterile (or disposable) trays, one containing HA filler(s) only and the other containing the remaining instruments, including the needle, cannula, gauze, betadine balls, chlorohexidine gauze, boric acid gauze, and Tegaderm® film (Fig. 3.1). The purpose of such segregation is to prevent the potential contamination of remnants of HA fillers that have been prepared for injection, given that the precise amount of HA filler to be used in a procedure cannot be calculated in advance. Use only sterile forceps to transfer the HA filler from one tray to the other.

3.1.2 Dispensing

It can be helpful to divide the 1-mL syringe of HA filler into volumes of 0.2, 0.3, and 0.5 mL in preparation for cases where a full 1-mL syringe is unlikely to be used (Fig. 3.1). The HA filler is dispensed by transferring each subdivision into an empty 1-mL syringe (Beckton Dickinson®) using a three-way. As a general rule, filler dispensed into smaller volumes should be consumed within the same day to prevent contamination.

3.1.3 Dilution of HA Filler

HA fillers have a propensity to draw water from surrounding tissues over time and expand. Due to this nature, the HA filler may demonstrate an incremental increase in volume 2–4 weeks postinjection vis-a-vis the initial injection volume. Monophasic HA fillers tend to show a higher degree of water absorption compared with biphasic HA fillers. As such, dilution is advised when using monophasic HA fillers to limit unfavorable swelling due to their water retention capacity. The ideal dilution ratio between the monophasic HA filler and the diluent is approximately 1:0.6. The diluent is prepared by admixing a 0.5 mL saline solution with 0.1 mL lidocaine 2%. Syringes respectively containing the HA filler and the diluent are connected onto a three-way or a "transfer," and the liquid is pumped back and forth between the two syringes in a piston movement at least 20 times to ensure thorough mixture (Fig. 3.2).

3.1.4 Disinfection

Whilst rare, acute bacterial infection following HA filler injection can occur. However, to an even

K. K. Seo, *Facial Volumization with Fillers*, https://doi.org/10.1007/978-981-33-6212-3_3

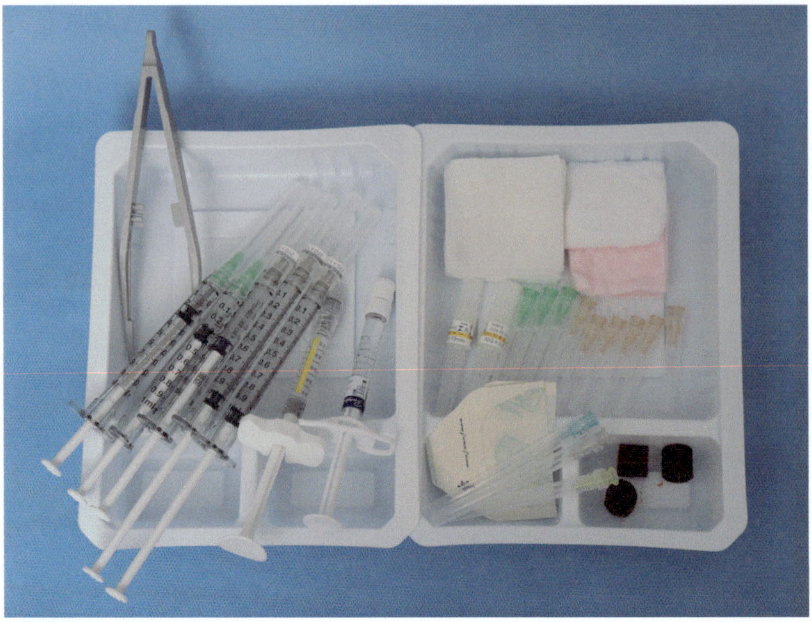

Fig. 3.1 Preparation of tray

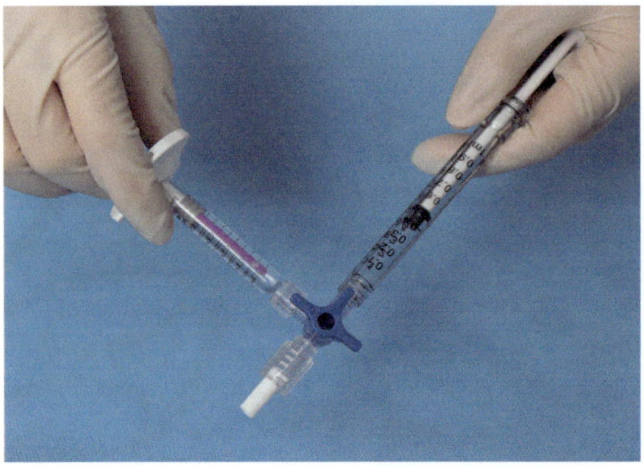

Fig. 3.2 Dilution of HA filler (Bellotero® Volume) with normal saline

lesser extent, there can also be incidences of delayed inflammatory nodules due to the introduction of nonpathogenic resident skin flora into the tissue, or formation of biofilms from nonspecific mycobacteria occuring months after the treatment. To avoid such adverse events, meticulous preparation and disinfection of the skin are required prior to the injection of HA filler. As the first step, make-up should be thoroughly removed from the patient's face, after which the skin is to be disinfected with betadine balls. Further cleansing is performed with chlorohexidine and boric acid balls. Note, however, that disinfecting the skin does not necessarily guarantee full sterility. Hence, vigilance is still required to ensure that the needle or cannula does not come into contact with the skin surface during the procedure. This risk is notably higher when injecting with a long cannula, as the instrument may inadvertently brush against the skin during its entry and advancement, becoming contaminated with any remaining resident bacteria on the skin. Placing a Tegaderm® transparent film dressing, over the cannula entry point helps to avoid such risk (Fig. 3.3). Where the procedure involves making multiple punctures on the skin or multiple back-and-forth strokes of the needle or cannula, the instrument should be replaced as frequently as possible during the procedure to minimize the risk of contamination.

3.1.5 Anesthesia

3.1.5.1 Topical Anesthetic Cream

Local anesthetic cream containing lidocaine applied for more than 20–30 min can help mitigate pain caused by the needle pucture during the procedure. In patients who are sensitive to pain, it may be beneficial to keep the numbing cream on the skin for around 1 hour. A local anesthetic cream applied around the cannula entry point 20–30 mins in advance can be instrumental in reducing pain during the puncture of the entry point with a needle.

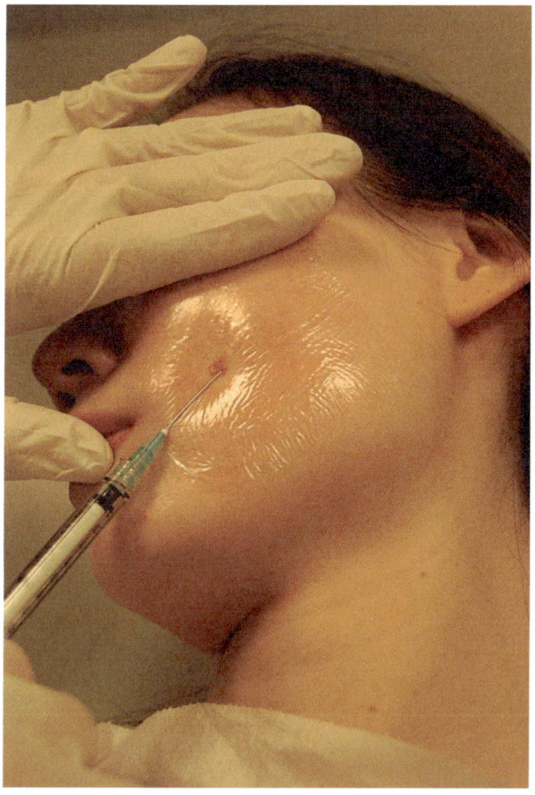

Fig. 3.3 3 M Tegaderm® transparent film dressing over the cannula entry point

3.1.5.2 Nerve Block

Nerve blocks allow the HA filler to be injected almost painlessly by blocking the specific sensory nerve(s) supplying the target area. The use of nerve blocks may be helpful in minimizing pain during the augmentation of the forehead, lower pretarsal roll, lips, or the chin. However, given that most fillers in use today come premixed with lidocaine if not reconstituted in the office with local anesthesia, a nerve block is not always a prerequisite to an HA filler procedure. One possible exception is forehead augmentation, which can be extremely painful in the absence of nerve blocks as the procedure involves the scraping of the periosteum with a cannula as the HA filler is delivered. The target nerves and the injection points are summarized in Fig. 3.4 [1]. As shown in Table 3.1, the supraorbital nerve and the supratrochlear nerve are targeted for forehead augmentation, infraorbital nerve blocked for pretarsal roll augmentation, mental nerve block used for chin augmentation, and infraorbital and mental nerves targeted for lip augmentation and hydrolifting around mouth and chin.

Anesthesia of the forehead is provided by supraorbital and supratrochlear nerve blocks, which are performed as follows. For the supraorbital nerve block, palpate the supraorbital foramen (or notch) located at the medial aspect of the supraorbital rim from which the supraorbital nerve emerges, and inject 1 mL of 2% lidocaine into the frontal bone lying immediately above the said notch or foramen. Where the supraorbital foramen or notch cannot be palpated by hand, inject the local anesthetic instead into a point 20–25 mm lateral to the median sagittal plane (Fig. 3.4a, b) [1]. The supratrochlear nerve may on occasion arise out of the supraorbital foramen or notch in tandem with the supraorbital nerve. However, to provide for cases where the supratrochlear nerve makes a separate emergence, it is best to inject 1 mL lidocaine additionally 1 cm medial to the supraorbital notch, as the supratrochlear nerve usually runs approximately 5–10 mm medial to the said notch (Fig. 3.4c) [1].

Meanwhile, an infraorbital nerve block for lip augmentation can be administered either from inside or outside the oral cavity. In the extraoral approach, 2% lidocaine 1 mL is injected 1 cm inferior to the lower orbital rim along the mid pupillary line to block the infraorbital nerve arising from the infraorbital foramen. In the intraoral approach, the needle is inserted superiorly into the mucosa above the maxillary second premolar teeth (Fig. 3.4d) [2]. A mental nerve block for lip fillers can also be performed either extraorally or intraorally. In the extraoral approach, 1 mL of lidocaine is injected 1 cm superior to the lower margin of the mandible along the mid pupillary line to block the mental nerve exiting from the mental foramen. Alternatively, in the intraoral approach, the injection is made inferoposterior to the lower second premolar teeth Fig. 3.4e) [2].

3.1.5.3 Anesthetic Injection of the Cannula Entry Point

When volumizing the nose, lips, forehead, and ears, etc. with HA filler, it is advisable to inject a local anesthetic containing approximately 0.05 mL of 2% dental lidocaine with epinephrine 1:100,000 at the cannula entry point 2–3 min prior to the procedure, as it helps to reduce bleeding while puncturing the entry point with a needle. The relevant cannula entry points for each facial region are discussed in the respective sections.

3.1.5.4 Intravenous Anesthesia/ Sedation

Intravenous anesthesia or sedation may be undertaken in patients with exceptionally low pain threshold or fear of needles. Propofol (10 mg/mL) is most commonly used for inducing sedation, with an initial loading dose of 7–10 mL (70–100 mg) followed by a maintenance infusion of 4–12 mg/kg/h or approximately 50–70 mL/h [3]. When propofol is administered in intermittent bolus doses, 3–4 mL is injected every 3–5 min.

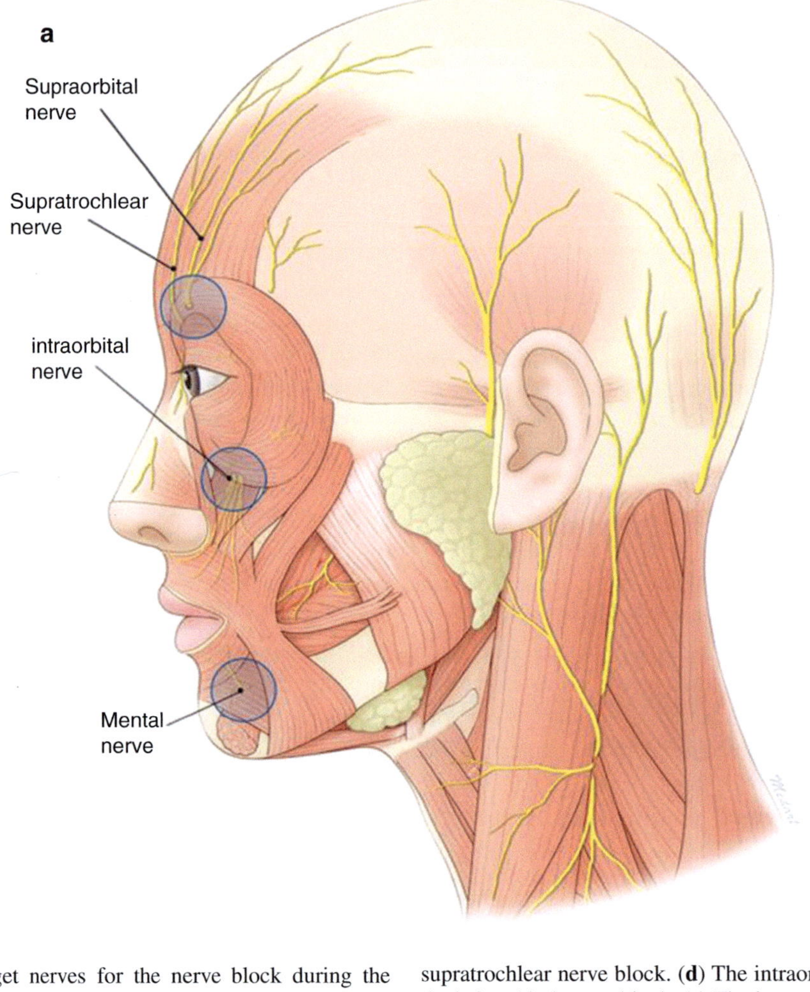

Fig. 3.4 Target nerves for the nerve block during the filler injection. (**a**) Target nerves and injection points of the nerve block. (**b**) The supraorbital nerve block. (**c**) The supratrochlear nerve block. (**d**) The intraoral approach of the infraorbital nerve block. (**e**) The intraoral approach of the mental nerve block

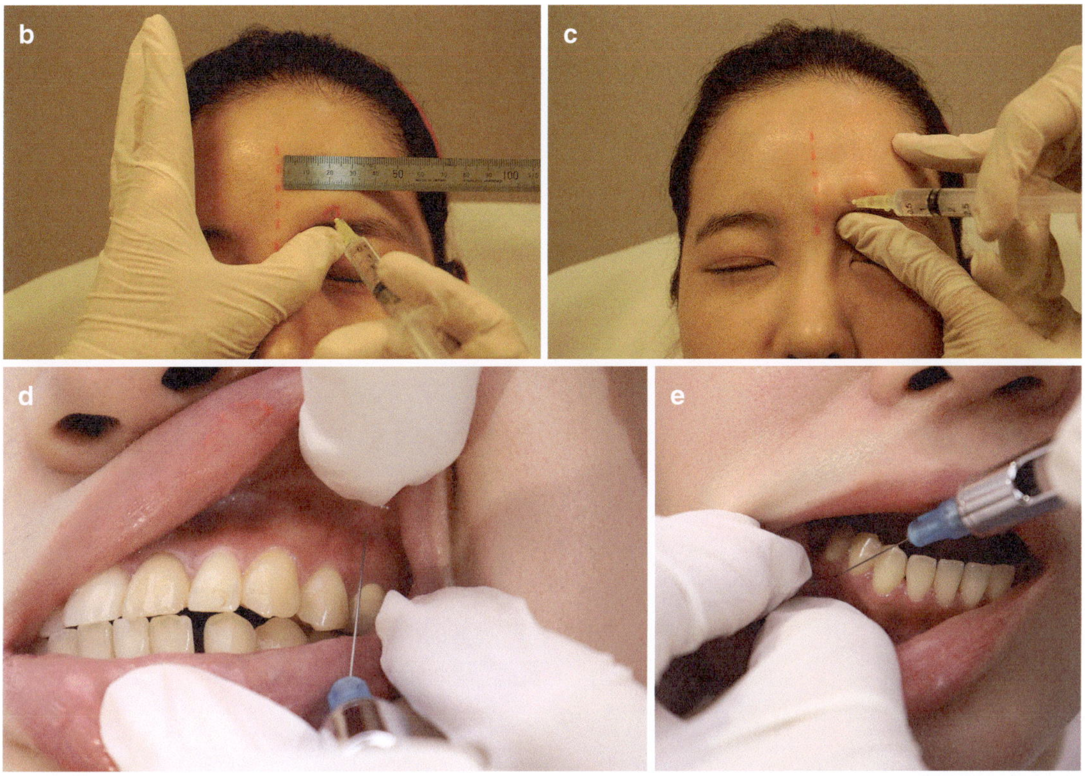

Fig. 3.4 (continued)

Table 3.1 Target nerves of the nerve block depending on the indications of filler injection

Indication	Target nerves
Forehead augmentation	Supraorbital nerve and supratrochlear nerve
Pretarsal roll augmentation	Infraorbital nerve
Lip augmentation	Infraorbital nerve and mental nerve
Chin augmentation	Mental nerve
Hydrolifting around mouth and chin	Infraorbital nerve and mental nerve

The use of intravenous anesthesia can be beneficial in procedures such as forehead augmentation, as it obviates the need to perform nerve blocks and helps to avoid the superfluous creation of volume by the local anesthetic agent. The corresponding drawback, however, is that the patient is typically semi-awake upon recovery and is therefore not in the best condition to adequately assess the post-treatment results.

3.1.5.5 Distraction Method

According to the gate theory of pain, divergence prevents effective transmission of the pain signals by jamming up the nerve pathway with other stimuli. This explains why nurses tend to tap the patient's buttocks just before administering an intramuscular injection. Likewise, tapping the patient's face with a finger or having the patient or an assistant hold a vibration tool against the patient's face to distract the patient's attention during HA filler injection can be a useful way to alleviate pain. Similarly, engaging the patient in constant conversation during the procedure can help to draw the patient's mind away from the immediate pain.

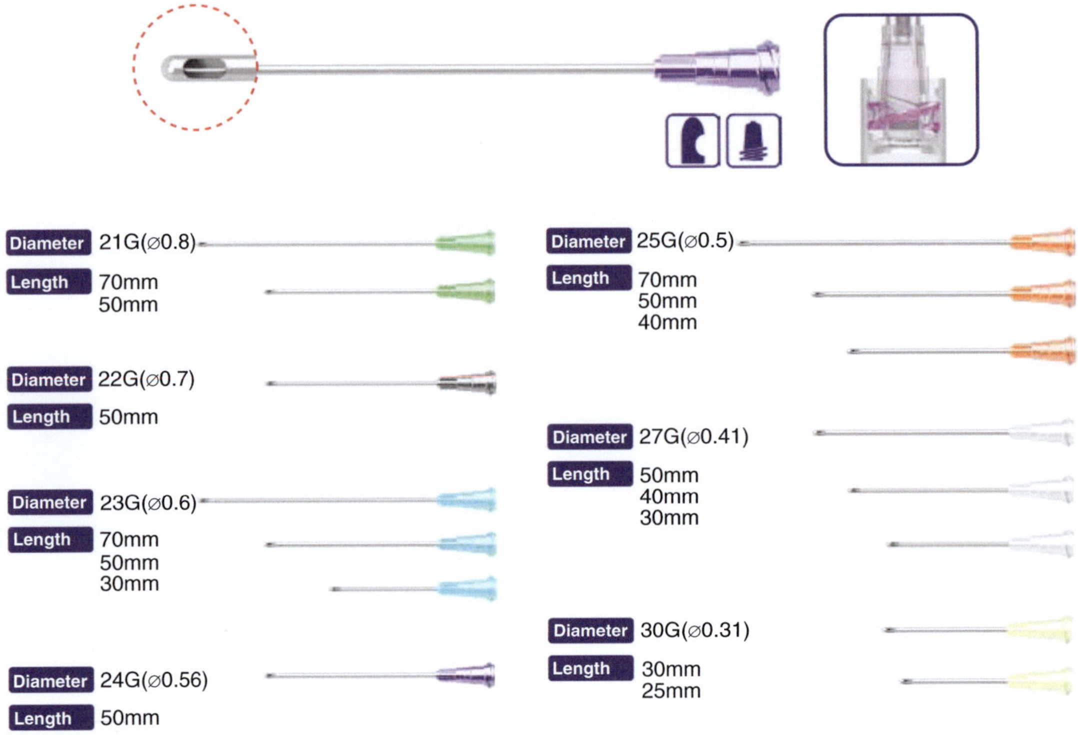

Fig. 3.5 Cannulas used for facial volumization come in a wide variety of sizes, ranging from 21G to 30G in diameter. (Courtesy of Nanum Company Co., Ltd.)

3.2 Injection Method

3.2.1 Needle vs. Cannula

Injectable fillers are still commonly referred to as "*dermal fillers*" because they had originally been developed for treating wrinkles in areas of reduced skin elasticity. Where fillers were used primarily for wrinkle treatment, needles had traditionally been the instrument of choice for delivering the filler through the stiff, rigid tissues of the dermis. However, with the evolution in the use of injectable fillers for facial volume enhancement, deep plane injection below the dermis has become the norm. When injecting the deep planes though, the use of needles carries a higher risk of traumatizing the deep-lying vessels not immediately visible from the skin surface, resulting in hematoma formation. Also, with the growing awareness over the devastating consequences of inadvertent intravascular injection of HA filler such as skin necrosis and blindness, the use of cannulas is increasingly recommended over needles for facial volumization treatments [4].

The decision whether to inject with a needle or cannula is one that should essentially rest with the injecting practitioner, as the best aesthetic outcomes are achieved by a practitioner leveraging his mastery of his most preferred technique. That said, there are certain salient advantages of using a cannula over a needle, as elaborated below. One major advantage of using a cannula over a needle lies in its significantly lower risk of penetrating a vessel, which helps to prevent bruising from unnecessary vascular damage and avoid skin necrosis and visual loss from intravascular occlusion. Accordingly, cannulas represent a much safer option when injecting into areas that are highly prone to risk of blindness such as the glabella, nose, and nasolabial folds. Incidentally, the use of a cannula may also provide the physician with better protection in the event of a litigation involving complications from intravascular filler injection.

Despite their relative inability to pierce through the vessel, it must be noted that using a cannula does not entirely preclude the possibility of a vascular complication. A cannula may be capable of perforating a weakened vessel wall, particularly when it comes to fine cannulas. Thus, extreme care should be taken when forcing a narrow-bore cannula such as a 27G or thinner through the tissue since in such case, it may behave like a needle and cut through the vessel if pushed in with too much force. Personally, I had cases where I accidentally perforated blood vessels even with a thicker 23-G cannula, which lead to in massive hematomas. In once case a female patient in her mid-70s came in for the treatment of her nasolabial folds. She had reported of having weak vessels and being prone to bruising. Even with this knowledge, however, I ended up rupturing her facial artery while advancing a 23-G cannula firmly from the lower cheek toward the nasolabial fold. Likewise, vessels trapped in the scar tissue due to a previous surgery such as fat transplant, liposuction, rhinoplasty or wounds can become highly susceptible to cannulation even with a blunt cannula. In this regard, I had a female patient in her mid-40s who presented for filler treatment in her infraorbital/anterior malar hollows with a history of a previous fat graft in the same region. Postsurgical scarring must have caused either the angular a. or a detoured branch of the facial a. to adhere to subcutaneous fat tissue. A large hematoma occurred in this patient as I forced a 23-G cannula through the tissue resistance. In both cases, a bulging hematoma appeared immediately upon the rupture of the blood vessel, leaving the patient to suffer from embarrassing bruises for several weeks thereafter.

The other benefit of using a cannula lies in its longer length which ranges between 3 and 7 cm compared with a short 0.5-in. (1.25 cm) needle. The longer reach of cannulas allows the practitioner to fill wide areas of the face from a single insertion point with greater consistency and in considerably less time. This can be of particular value when augmenting areas such as the nose and forehead prone to irregularities due to their underlying anatomy which consists of hard bone directly underlying the thin soft tissue, allowing bare minimum space for filler placement. Using a cannula also dramatically saves time when filling broad areas of the face such as the forehead. For these reasons, I almost exclusively use cannulas for augmenting the forehead apart from when only partial corrections are required.

So, what are the relevant factors for selecting the right cannula? Cannulas used for facial volumization come in a wide variety of sizes, ranging from 21G to 30G in diameter, of which 23G, 25G, 27G, and 30G are used most commonly (Fig. 3.5). Bigger, thicker cannulas are more convenient to use as they allow the product to flow more easily but can cause more discomfort to the patient while traversing through the tissues of the face. Thicker cannulas are neither ideal for performing delicate corrections that require precision and finesse. On the other hand, smaller, finer cannulas can be less painful and facilitate more detailed placement but requires greater injection pressure and takes more time to deliver the product as the material will flow more slowly. Based on these characteristics, the thicker 23-G and 25-G cannulas are more commonly used for facial volume augmentation, while the thinner 27G and 30G are utilized primarily for the refinement of static folds and wrinkles rather than for volumetric augmentation.

Meanwhile, the choice of the cannula size may also be significantly impacted by the rheology of the HA filler to the injected. Specifically, biphasic HA filler products such as Restylane® and Yvoire® require the use of cannula sizes that correspond to the particle size of the product. For example, the use of a 21-G cannula is advised for injecting large particle sized biphasic HA products such as Yvoire Contour® to minimize possible deformation of the filler particles by shear stress while they are extruded through the cannula. That notwithstanding, in my practice, I have always used a thinner 23G even for injecting these large particle products to reduce patient discomfort and pain during the movement of a thick 21G in the tissue. Nevertheless, I have observed no substantial compromise in filler longevity to date. I routinely use a 30G for injecting finer particle-sized Restylane® fillers and a 27G for Restylane® Lyft which has a relatively larger particle size. By contrast, monophasic HA fillers such as the Juvéderm®, Belotero®, and Neuramis® family of fillers allow a higher degree of freedom in terms of cannula sizes, as even the thicker, stiffer products indicated specifically for facial volume augmentation such as Juvéderm Voluma®, Belotero Volume®, and Neuramis Volume® can, in theory, be delivered via a 29-G or even a 30-G cannula. While a

25G may, therefore, be reasonably used to inject a monophasic HA filler for facial volume augmentation, I prefer to use the thicker 23G in this case. This is because while a thinner, narrower cannula has the advantage of causing less pain, it requires greater injection pressure and takes more time. Moreover, it has difficulty pushing through the resistance of the ligamentous or scar tissues during deep plane injection and tends to bend instead of properly reaching the target site.

Cannulas, however, cannot completely replace needles in all indications. For example, when treating facial wrinkles with HA filler, a sharp needle must be used for traversing through the hard dermal layer. There are times when a needle may also be used for placing volume in the subcutaneous or subdermal planes. A case in point is temples augmentation, where the use of a needle becomes the preferred option, as the blunt cannula is incapable of penetrating the thick temporal fascia covering the temporal fossa to deliver the necessary volume.

While some practitioners advocate the use of a cannula in the temples and suggest the HA filler may instead be placed in the space *between* the superficial and the deep temporal facias, locating this space with precision can be tricky and time consuming. By comparison, a direct supraperiosteal injection deep to the temporalis m. using a 21-G needle represents a much quicker and simpler approach without surface bumpiness. That being the case, the temples represent the one exception where I prefer to use a needle over a cannula in a facial volumization treatments. The needle sizes most often used for injecting HA fillers are 27G, 29G, 30G, each 1.25 cm in length. However, longer 23-G and 21-G needles can also be employed when filling deep locations spanning wide areas. Aspiration prior to filler injection is vital when injecting with a needle to confirm that it has not inadvertently entered a blood vessel. In particular, when undertaking linear threading technique, etc., where the tip of the needle constantly changes position, aspiration should be performed at each new location the needle tip is moved to before depositing the filler. Entry of the needle into the vein can be detected by aspiration prior to injection. Meanwhile, penetration of the deep temporal artery can be immediately identified by the instantaneous reflux of blood up the syringe due to the arterial pressure (Fig. 3.6).

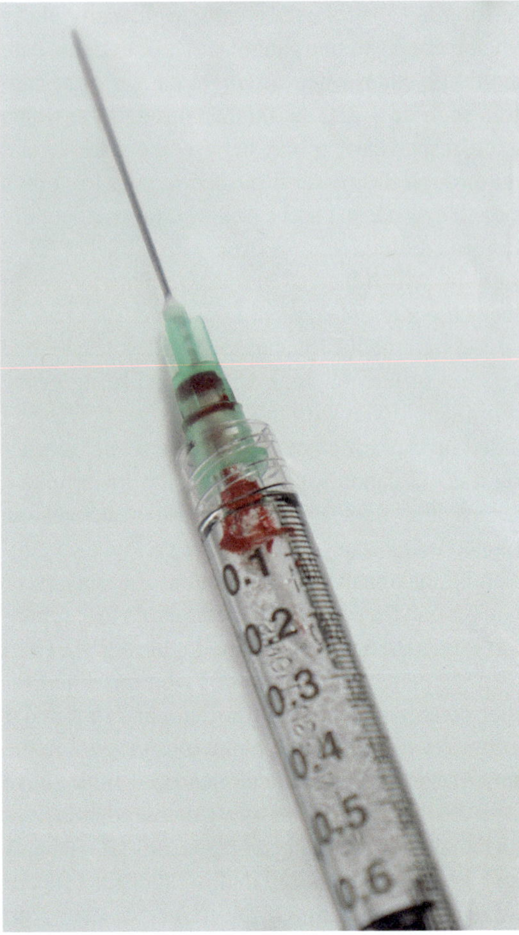

Fig. 3.6 Photo of reflux blood in the syringe by aspiration during a temple augmentation

Note, however, that a negative aspiration test does not guarantee 100% safety since finer needles in the 29-G or 30-G range do not aspirate very well in very thin vessels such as those distributed in the nasal region. According to one study in which 17 filler products and different needle sizes were used to aspirate ink reconstituted to concentrations similar to the human blood, 47% of aspiration tests showed negative results even when aspiration was performed using the needle gauge recommended by the filler manufacturer [5]. Moreover, the gauge of the needle for the positive aspiration test was found to vary according to the product [5]. At the risk of overgeneralizing, monophasic HA fillers were shown to be generally less amenable to aspiration compared with biphasic HA fillers, requiring larger bore needles to ensure adequate aspiration. It may be reasonable to assume that this is due to the rheologic property of monophasic HA fillers that tend to be sticky and viscose in nature.

Episode: Intravascular HA Filler Injection in the Nasal Area

In my practice, I have encountered five cases of vascular complications from the injection of HA filler in the nose with a needle. Fortunately, none of these events led to any disastrous consequence such as skin necrosis or blindness, for which I thank my ancestors for sending their good karma my way. In three of those cases, the vascular event went unrecognized on the day of the treatment due to lack of any noticeable symptoms. In fact it was not until the next day that mottled erythematic patches began appearing on the patients' nose, glabella, and forehead, becoming progressively larger and darker with time until they resolved spontaneously in about 1 month without medical intervention (Fig. 3.7) In the remaining two case, ischemic changes and skin blanching occurred immediately following the filler injection, to which hyaluronidase was promptly administered to dissolve the injected filler. The patient achieved full recovery within a week without any sequelae.

Three of these events represented the first three cases of intravascular filler injection I experienced since I began practicing filler rhinoplasty in 2007. Coincidentally, all three cases occurred contemporaneously within a space of 1 month and involved the use of a sharp needle and the same monophasic Juvéderm® Ultra which I had newly begun using around that time. Previously, I had exclusively used biphasic Restylane® products for injecting the nose. Preinjection aspiration was duly performed in all three cases, yet I failed to detect the inadvertent vessel entry. Given that all three cases occurred within the first month of my adopting Juvéderm® for injection in the nose, I suppose my personal lack of experience is partly to blame. More fundamentally through, the rheologic property of monophasic HA fillers not amenable to the aspiration remains a more significant cause. Needless to say, these events have since veered me away from injecting monophasic HA in the nose with a needle.

The remaining two cases involved the use of the biphasic Restylane® fillers. In one case, I had got distracted during a busy day and neglected to aspirate before injecting the filler in the nasal tip. As incredible as it may sound, I was able to spot the problem in the making as I actually witnessed the filler particle shooting up the dorsum within moments of entering the nasal tip. In the

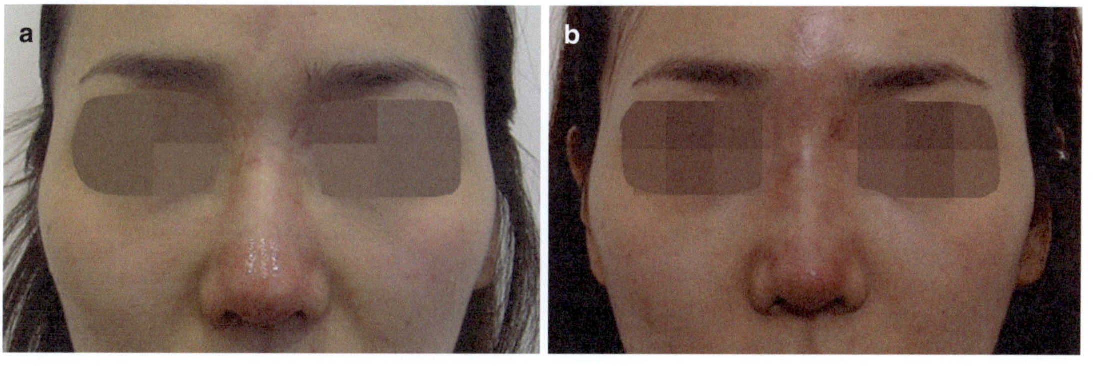

Fig. 3.7 Intravascular injection of HA fillers in the nasal area. (**a**) The next day, that mottled erythematous patches began appearing on the patients' nose, glabella, and forehead. (**b**) Mottled erythematous patches became progressively larger and darker 7 days after the injection

final case, which turned out to be the most colorful of them all, the patient had undergone two previous rhinoplasty surgeries, after which she had the implant surgically removed, which left her with a depressed dorsum for which treatment was desired. I had prior experience treating patients with similar complex histories, all of which had proven uneventful, so I proceeded with the treatment, mindful to aspirate before each injection. Despite taking utmost precaution, however, the patient showed ischemic changes in the nose shortly following the procedure to which hyaluronidase was injected immediately to have the filler reversed. The patient recovered without sequelae in a week. Ironically, however, this last case, which represented the mildest of all five complications with the quickest recovery, turned out to be the costliest, since it eventually led the clinic to pay out about 5000 USD in monetary consolation to the patient to stop her from sabotaging our business with her daily protests.

In retrospect, a common thread can be identified running through all five cases, That is, all involve the use of a needle introduced at the nasal tip. Unlike the vascular supply of the nasion located at the superior aspect of the dorsum, the vessels at the nasal tip are narrower in diameter and are distributed across different tissue layers. As such, a preinjection aspiration may not always conclusively inform whether the needle had inadvertently entered a blood vessel or not. Since then, I abandoned the use of needles for performing filler rhinoplasty and converted to using only cannulas, which spared me such problems during the past 10+ years. Sometimes it does make sense to mend the fence *even after* the horse has bolted.

3.2.2 Linear Thread Technique

This is the most commonly practiced technique for augmenting facial volume or addressing deep static lines and wrinkles with HA filler. The standard approach, referred to as the retrograde linear thread technique, consists of injecting deep beneath the fold to be corrected and depositing the product along the direction of the said fold while withdrawing the cannula/needle (Fig. 3.8). The anterograde linear thread technique is conceptually the same except that the product is deposited while the cannula/needle is being advanced forward. However, anterograde linear threading is less frequently used as it presents a relatively higher risk of intravascular occlusion.

3.2.3 Tower Technique

In this technique, the needle is inserted perpendicular to the skin down onto the periosteum to build up volume from the ground up. The product is deposited deep to the subcutaneous tissue to extend vertically from the periosteum toward the subdermal

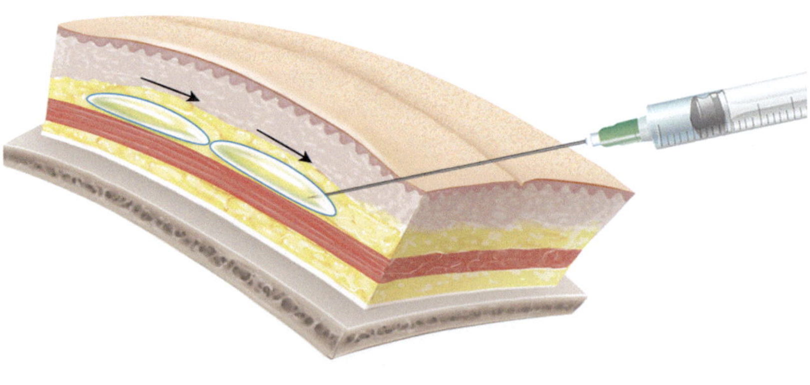

Fig. 3.8 Linear thread technique

layer in the form of a tower (Fig. 3.9) [6]. The advantage of this approach is that it avoids the risk of entering the blood vessel along its length, as the direction of the needle is perpendicular to the course of the blood vessels. Erecting HA filler towers at strategic locations also carries the advantage of reducing the amount of product needed to provide the necessary volumetric support. However, results may not be as smooth and uniform as what may be achieved with linear threading, and unevenness may be palpable when touched by hand.

3.2.4 Fern Pattern Technique (Multiple Intradermal Injection)

This technique involves multiple intradermal injections of HA filler made perpendicular to the direction of the crease or fold to be corrected along either side of said fold (Fig. 3.10). The row of fillers placed on each side of the fold resembles the shape of fern leaves with the fold itself representing the stem, hence the name fern technique (Fig. 3.11). Depositing the HA filler at a right angle to the fold produces a strong, robust dermal matrix resilient against dynamic wrinkling. While the fern technique is most frequently used for treating nasolabial folds, it is also applicable for treating the dynamic lines of the forehead and glabella. Where the same strategy is replicated for use in the wider regions of the face and body lacking skin elasticity including the arms, legs, and neck, it is referred to instead as *hydrolifting*, signifying both the lifting effect (i.e., better skin elasticity) and hydration the HA filler delivers to the skin (see Sect. 4.20). Hydrolifting provides increased elasticity to the skin, which is particularly helpful for tackling the appearance of dynamic lines in the malar, the perioral, and the cheek-areas that are not readily treatable with BoNT-A due to the risk of altering the facial expression.

The desired depth of injection for hydrolifting is at the deep dermis to minimize surface irregularities. When injecting manually using a 30-G needle, a simple test would be helpful to determine if the needle is located properly in the deep dermis. Lifting the needle upwards from under the skin, a clear silhouette of the needle should be visible if the needle is properly placed in the deep dermis (Fig. 3.12). A clear silhouette of the needle is not visible when the needle is inserted too deep into the subcutaneous layer, while a needle inserted too superficially in the

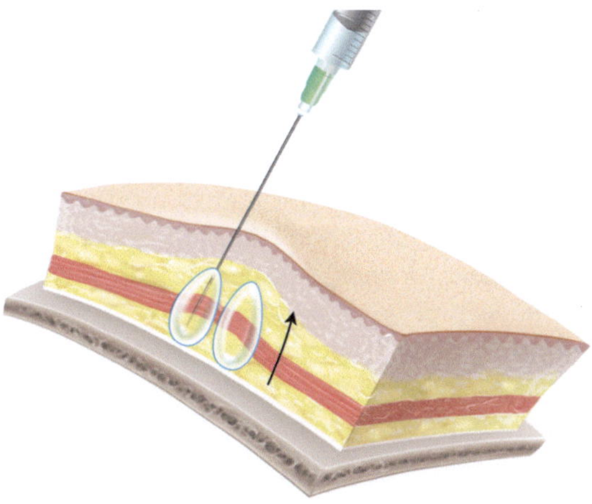

Fig. 3.9 Tower technique

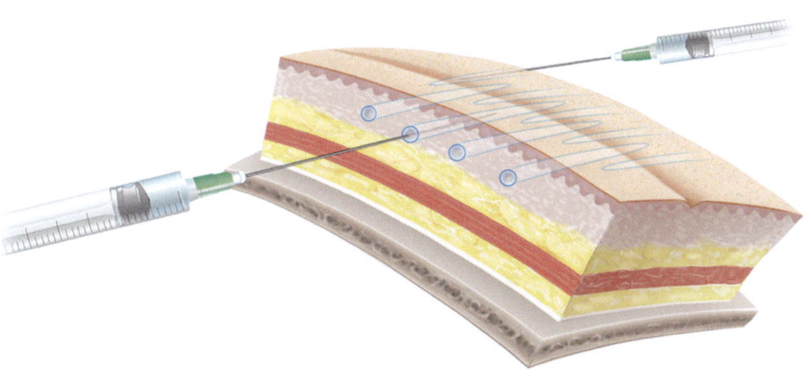

Fig. 3.10 Fern pattern technique (multiple intradermal injection)

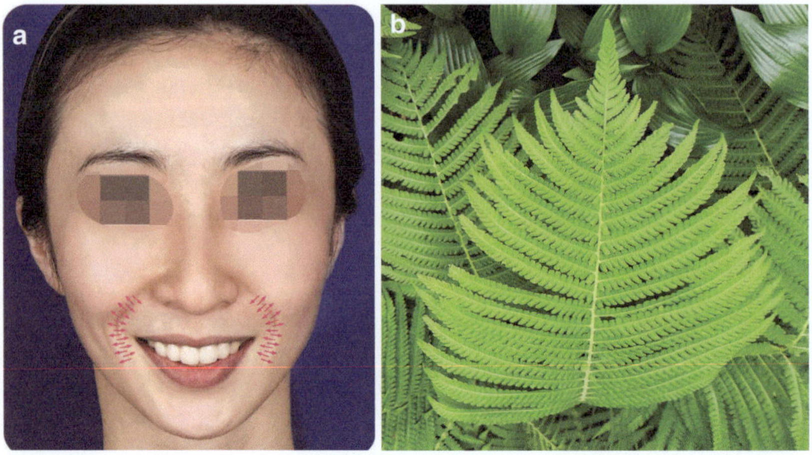

Fig. 3.11 (**a**) Fern pattern technique for the treatment of dynamic nasolabial fold. (**b**) Fern leaves

upper dermis generates a gray bluish hue of the needle visible through the skin. To prevent bumpiness in thinly skinned areas, it is advisable to perform small-volume injections targeting the deep dermis almost as if injecting the subcutaneous layer. Bented needle at a 20–30 degree angle is helpful to facilitate even injection at the dermis using linear retrograde thread technique.

3.2.5 Subcision Technique

This technique is used to release any fibrous scar tissues (i.e., acne scars) present in areas of facial volume deflation that anchor down the skin to the underlying tissue layer and deter effective HA filler placement. It is also applicable for addressing permanently etched-in grooves of the forehead, as the skin overlying the groove is also bound to the underlying tissue and has hardened like depressed scars over time. The technique involves manual severing of the scar tissue strands using the bevel of a sharp needle, to release the upper skin and create a pocket of space for filler placement (Fig. 3.13). The procedure may accompany bruising.

3.2.6 Double-Layering Technique

The double-layering technique is a technique indispensible to filler volumization, as it help to deliver both definition and volume restoration without resulting in a bulky appearance (Fig. 3.14). It requires first injecting sufficient volume in the deep plane (using the linear threading technique) before adding smaller volume in the superficial plane to build a stack of HA filler threads or HA filler towers sitting on two different tissue layers. Attempting to pump in large volumes in the deep plane alone to maximize projection will likely cause the product to instead spread laterally, leading to an unnaturally overdone appearance such as the 'Avatar nose' or the 'lion nose' often encountered after an inadequate augmentation of the nasal dorsum. In this regard, the additional injection in the superficial plane plays an important role in providing defintion and refinement to the volume restoration. Double layering is applicable to a wide range of filler indications. For treatment of deep creases, for example, the filler can be injected first in the deep subcutaneous plane to fill the groove to a substantial standard, after which superficial refinement is made either in the subdermal or dermal plane to achieve full lev-

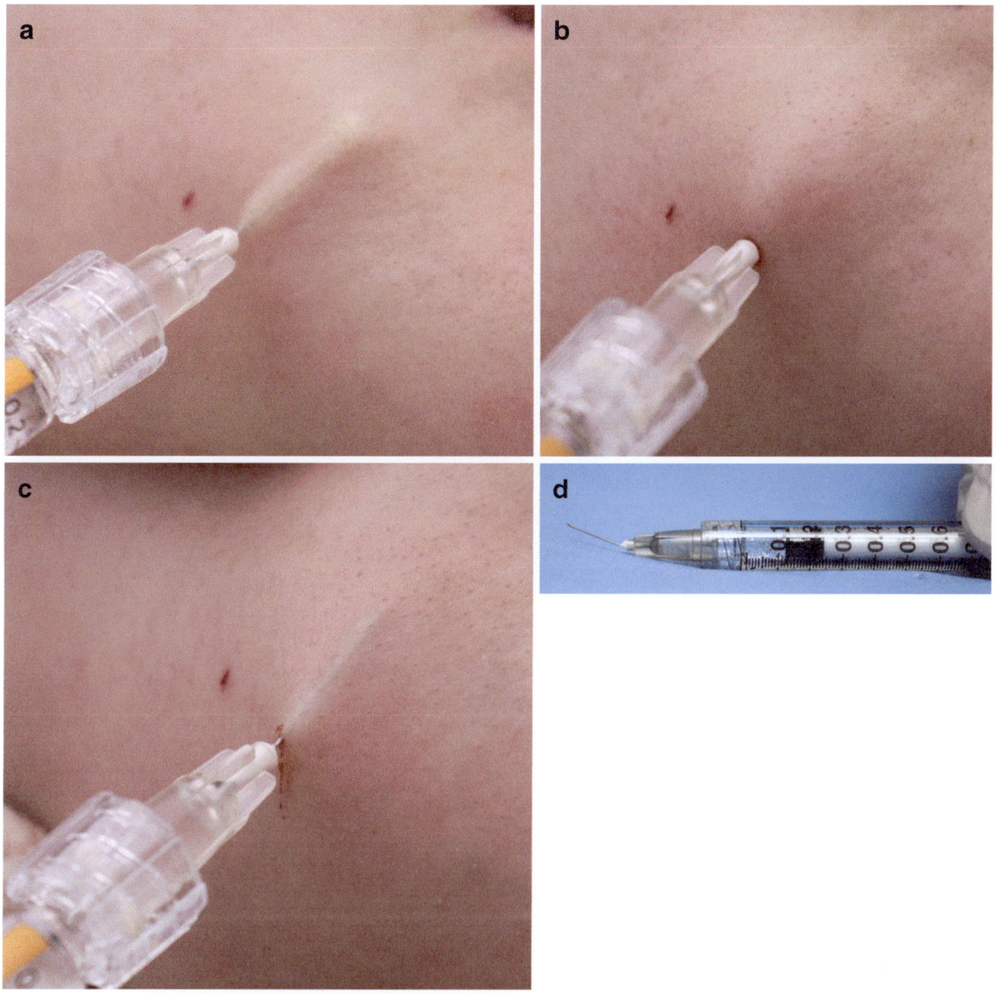

Fig. 3.12 Image of a needle inserted into the dermis depending on the depth of the injection. (**a**) Deep dermis. A clear silhouette of the needle is visible. (**b**) The subcutaneous layer. A clear silhouette of the needle is not visible. (**c**) Upper dermis. A gray bluish hue of the needle visible through the skin. (**d**) Bented needle at a 20-30 degree angle to facilitate even injection at the dermis using linear retrograde thread technique.

eling. It can also be used for addressing the infraorbital/medial malar depressions, by restoring first the deep subcutaneous volume before addressing the superficial volume in the subdermal layer for additional projection. In nasal dorsum augmentation, injecting first the deep supraperiosteal plane for the primary augmentation and subsequently in the more superficial subdermal plane allows extra elevation in nasal dorsum height without causing the filler to migrate laterally.

3.2.7 Injection Technique for Deep Static Grooves

This technique is used for addressing static grooves and creases such as the deep glabella lines and nasolabial folds. Drawing on the principle of double layering, it involves first placing a retrograde linear thread in the deep subcutaneous or supraperisoteal layer to fill the groove to a substantial standard, before completing

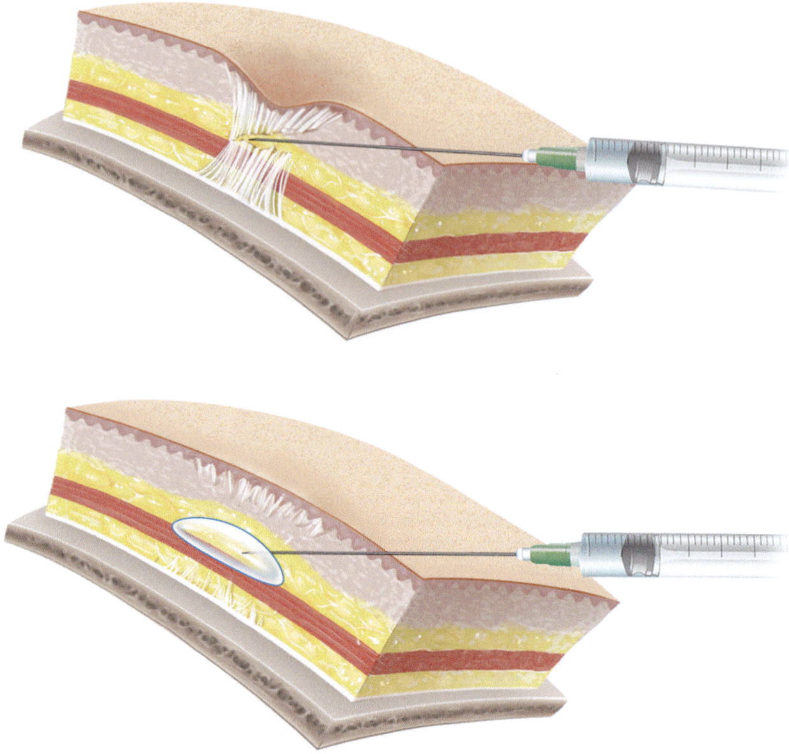

Fig. 3.13 Subcision technique

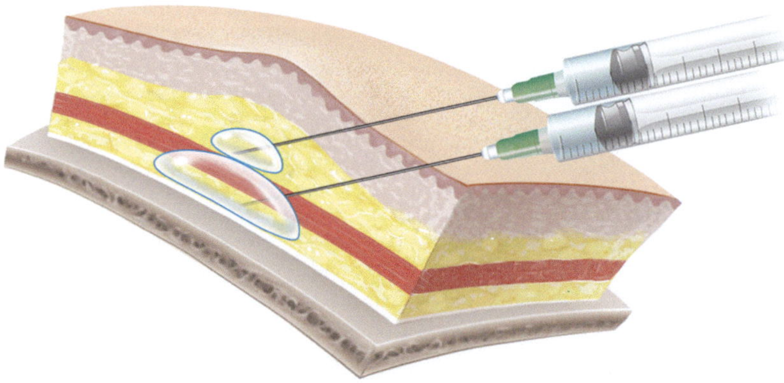

Fig. 3.14 Double-layering technique

with an intradermal or subdermal placement of a retrograde thread for full leveling. The use of a cannula is advised over a needle for deep subcutaneous or subdermal injections to avoid the risk of intravascular occlusion. A 30-G needle is more ideal for performing superficial corrections in the dermal layer. As previously noted, in the case of permanently etched-in grooves of the forehead or the glabella, the hardening of the dermis like scar tissue over time, if not the adhesion of the skin to the underlying subcutaneous tissue may prevent the injected filler from providing the necessary lift. Such limitations should be disclosed to the patient beforehand, and overcorrection should be avoided in such a case. In the alternative, the subcision method may be combined to yield more favorable results.

3.2.8 Volumizing Injection Technique

Rule 1: Double layering technique; When restoring facial volume depletion or enhancing facial features such as the nose or chin (i.e., nasal dorsum or chin augmentation), deep injection is advised to build volume from the ground up, as superficial injections just below the skin surface provide only limited volumization. Caution is required, however, when performing deep injections, as the injected volume will expand not only anteriorly or superiorly but also laterally, leading to an aesthetically displeasing bulky appearance if placed in excess amounts. For example, overfilling the nasal dorsum can widen the nose and create the appearance of the "Avatar nose," while overcorrecting the chin can result in an excessively bulky, blunt appearance of the chin. Also, filling the cheeks to perfection in patients with prominent jowls may only serve to accentuate the jowls and exacerbate the saggy appearance. In such case, the use of the double-layering technique for superficial refinements if not a slight under-correction is advised.

Rule 2: Volume matters!; It also bears noting that the primary purpose of volumizing fillers is to literally *fill out* areas of volume deficit or depletion. As such, achieving an aesthetically desirable outcome can be elusive when working with an insufficient amount of HA filler. To draw an analogy, imagine filling a balloon with water. To inflate the balloon to capacity, a certain threshold volume of water is required. If not filled enough, the balloon would remain loose and saggy rather than becoming taut and tight. The amount of water required to fill the balloon in this case depends on the size of the balloon. That is, the larger the balloon, the more water that is needed. Likewise, the more severe the volume deflation, the larger the amount of filler that is required. Otherwise, contour irregularity would continue to persist (Fig. 3.15).

Rule 3: Volumize the deepest part first; The volumizing injection technique can be applied for effective volumization of sunken areas of the face. As the first step, map out an elliptical outline of the volume-depleted area, reflecting its overall size and shape. Next, mark the longitudinal axis of the elliptical outline, and create an entry point along this longitudinal axis 1 cm lateral to the border of the ellipse. Identify the deepest point of the depression (usually located at the center of the depression) and inject volume deeply into the subcutaneous fat underlying this central point using the retrograde linear thread technique. Upon filling the central area to the desired height, repeat the same approach in the adjacent left and right areas to even out the contour (Fig. 3.16). When redirecting the cannula to fill the adjacent left and right areas, make sure to retract the cannula almost all the way out of the entry point before forming a new path different from the central path. Changing directions mid-path may lead to surface irregularities and cause most of the injected volume to end up at the center instead of the adjacent left and

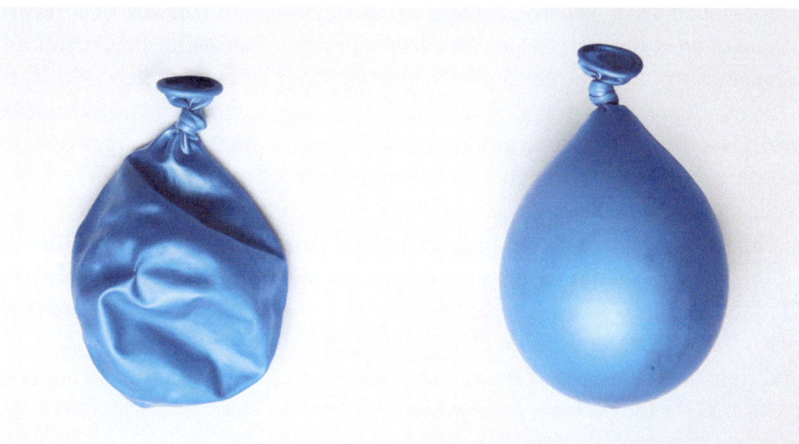

Fig. 3.15 To inflate the balloon to capacity, a certain threshold volume of water is required. If not filled enough, the balloon would remain loose and saggy

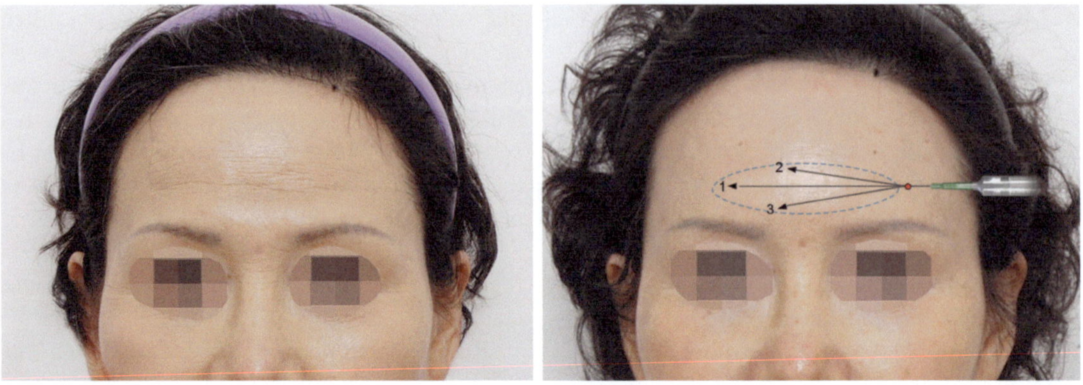

Fig. 3.16 Volumizing injection technique for correction of forehead concavity

right areas of the depression. As illustrated in Fig. 3.16, this volumizing injection technique is applicable to forehead augmentation where the aim is to fill out a concave forehead. Here, volume is injected first into the central and deepest point of the hollowness between the superciliary arch and the frontal eminence, after which additional injections are performed in areas immediately above and below the central deepest point to smoothen out the contour.

Rule 4: Regard facial depressions as simplified 3D shapes; It is vital to analyze the face from a three-dimensional perspective when assessing the target area and envisioning the desired outcome. Bear in mind that the face consists of arcs and curvatures instead of straight lines. One useful strategy for implementing a three-dimensional facial assessment is to visualize the facial depression in terms of simplified 3D shapes such as a sphere, a cone, a triangular prism, or an ellipsoid if not a water drop. Holding a mental image of a water drop when evaluating a facial depression, for example, informs that when HA filler is placed to volumize the ellipsoidal depression using the retrograde linear thread technique, smaller volumes should be dispensed at either end of the long axis plane while the bulk of the volume should be injected in the middle. On the short-axis plane, greater volume is to be placed at the center relative to the adjacent left and right aspects so that a smooth fluid curvature is formed on the surface. Meanwhile, the fan of columns deposited along the transverse plane (using the fanning technique) should consist of short columns outermost at the left and right border of the waterdrop or ellipsoid and progressively longer columns toward the middle (Fig. 3.17). For the relevant volumization technique pertaining to each facial region, see the respective sections.

Rule 5: Leverage the effect of visual illusions (Fig. 3.18): While it is impossible to remove protrusions in facial contour using injectable fillers, it is possible to visually diminish or deemphasize their relative prominence by padding volume in the adjacent areas. This approach can be leveraged to obscure a prominent lateral zygoma by filling the relative hollows in the posterior cheek or temples (Fig. 1.4). By the same token, filling in the nasolabial folds and anterior cheeks and giving anterior projection to the chin can balance out the appearance of a protruded mouth. Meanwhile, as facial proportionality is defined by the ratio between the width and height of the face, a wide or round face can be made to appear slimmer and longer by adding vertical length to the chin (Fig. 1.5).

3.2.9 The Role of the Nondominant Hand

The role of the nondominant hand is often overlooked during filler procedures since the actual injection is performed with the dominant hand.

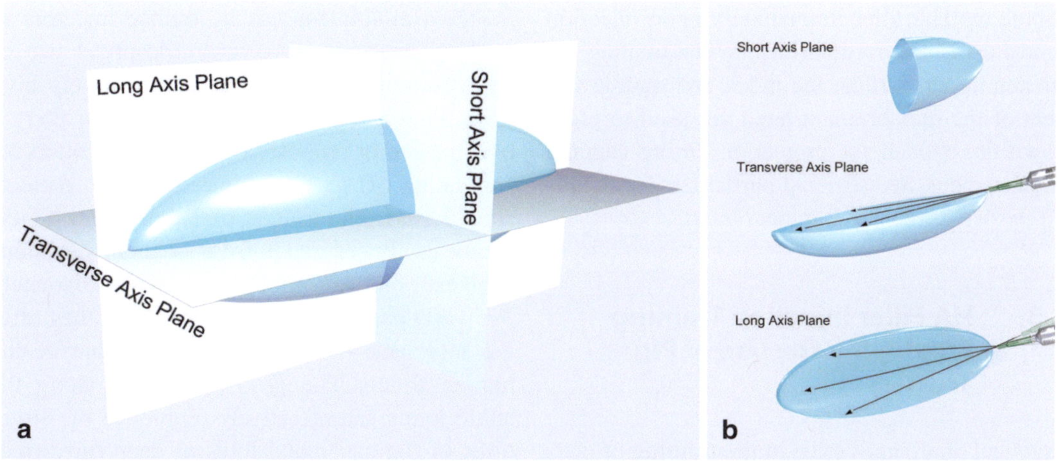

Fig. 3.17 Three-dimensional perspective for volumization. (**a**) A mental image of a ellipsoid water drop when filling a facial depression. (**b**) Smaller volumes should be dispensed at either end of the long axis plane while the bulk of the volume should be injected in the middle. On the short-axis plane, greater volume is to be placed at the center relative to the adjacent left and right aspects so that a smooth fluid curvature is formed on the surface. Meanwhile, the fan of threads deposited along the transverse plane (using the fanning technique) should consist of short outermost threads at the left and right border of the waterdrop or ellipsoid and progressively longer threads toward the middle

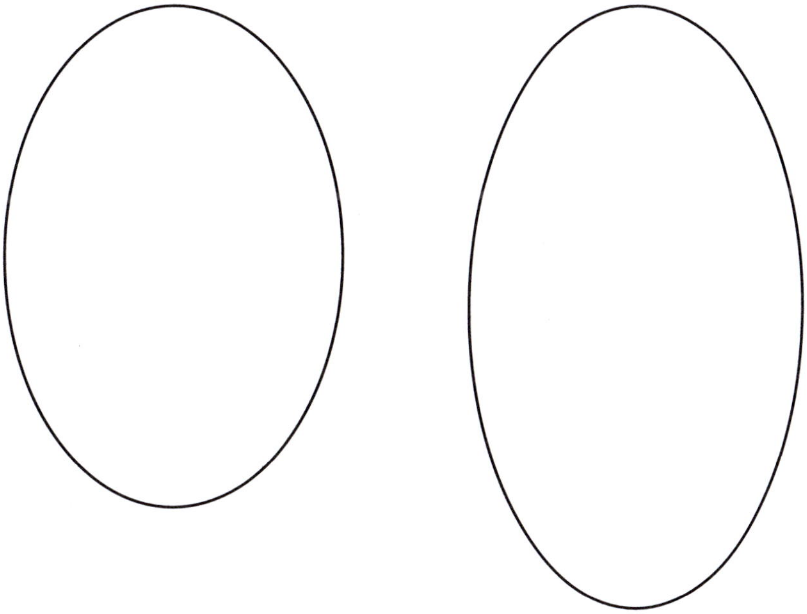

Fig. 3.18 Leverage visual illusion

However, the nondominant hand plays just as important a function as the dominant hand during the filler injection in the following respects. First, the nondominant hand is engaged to pull the skin opposite to the direction of the needle or cannula to facilitate its insertion and traction under the skin. Also, during nasal dorsum augmentation, the thumb and index finger of the nondominant hand is used to pinch the sidewalls of the nasal dorsum to prevent widening of the nose. During forehead augmentation, the nondominant hand must be used to constantly mold and evenly distribute the HA filler immediately upon injection to avoid surface irregularities. When treating the sunken upper eyelids, the index and middle fingers of the nondominant hand are used to press down the eyeball for protection during cannula advancement. See regional particulars for details on the use of the nondominant hand.

3.3 HA Filler Injection Training Employing the Use of Pig Trotters

Practical challenges exist in the training of novice injectors on HA filler injection techniques. First, HA filler procedures are performed primarily by physicians in private practice rather than by tertiary medical institutions such as university hospitals specializing in training medical residents. Further, unlike surgical procedures where the patient is typically placed under general anesthesia, HA filler procedures are undertaken with the patient alert and fully conscious, which limits the opportunity for the teaching of procedural skills, let alone the attendance by trainees during the procedure. Under the circumstances, it is absolutely out of the question for trainees go anywhere near an actual live patient in-clinic for a practice session. This being the case, beginning practitioners have little choice but to take what techniques they have managed to glean from watching live courses or have learned over-the-shoulder from advanced injectors and to try them out first on their dearest and nearest (i.e., usually family members) before going out on a limb to work with actual patients. Due to the absence of systematic training, trials and errors are inevitable during this process, subjecting injectors to various technical issues and adverse events which, in turn, erode patient satisfaction and confidence.

In this regard, Allergan is known to have developed facial injection dummies, which it makes available for use by trainee injectors in training courses. However, widespread use of such dummies is limited by the relatively high price point and lack of reusability. As an alternative, the author proposes the use of pig trotters for simulating HA filler injection on patients (Fig. 3.19a). The trotters of 1-month-old piglets can be easily ordered in from local butcher shops at an extremely affordable price of approximately 3–5 USD per cut. More than anything, they offer the look and feel quite similar to that of the human tissue. The grooves formed along the ankle joints can effectively reproduce the structures of the nasolabial folds or deep furrows of the forehead or glabella in a human face (Fig. 3.19b). In addition, the curvatures present on the calf provide an excellent platform for practicing facial volumization with HA (Fig. 3.19c). As the first step, the areas requiring volume enhancement is marked out. Next, HA is injected into center of the marked-out area (where volume deficit is usually the greatest) using the retrograde linear thread technique. Upon filling the central area to the desired height, the same approach is repeated in the adjacent areas to even out the contour (see Sect. 3.2.8). Furthermore, the skin of the pig's trotters can be used by trainee injectors to familiarize themselves with the intradermal injection, fern pattern technique, and hydrolifting technique (or multiple intradermal injection of HA filler) (Fig. 3.19d).

HA fillers past their expiry date or without cross-linking may be obtained from filler manufacturers upon request or purchase and used for training purposes. Mixing a small amount of blue dye with the HA filler can help establish the depth of the injected HA filler after injection upon dissction of the treated area. To mix the HA filler with the blue dye, it is recommended to connect the syringes holding HA filler and blue dye onto a three-way or a "transfer" and pump the liquid back and forth in a piston movement at least 20 times.

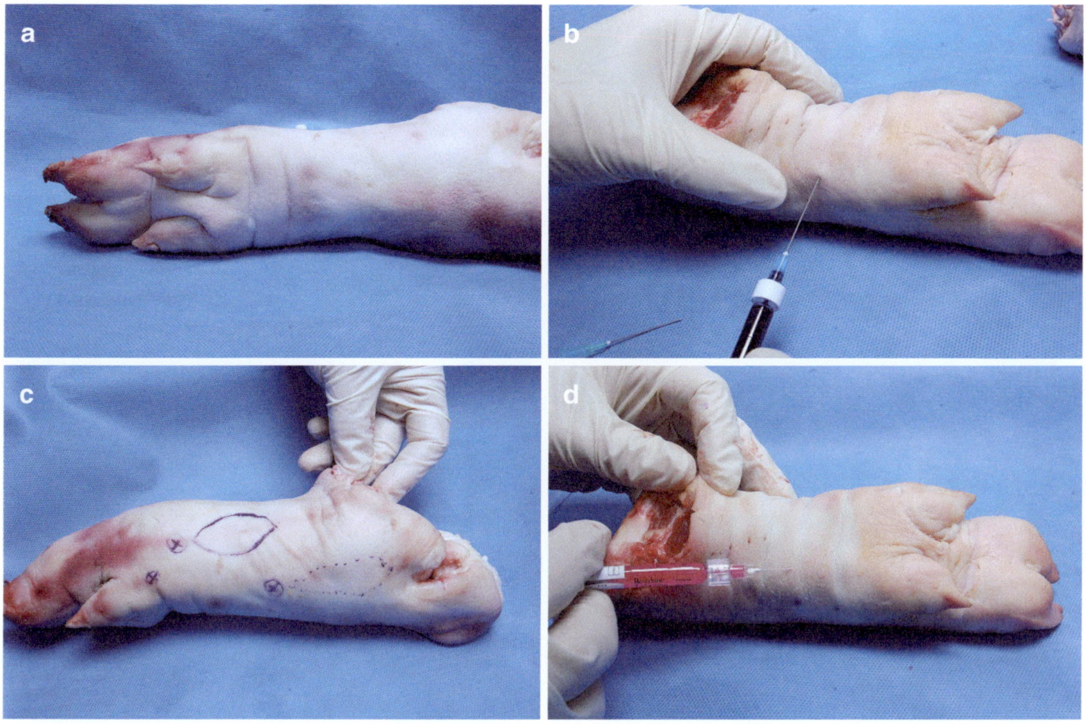

Fig. 3.19 The use of pig trotters for HA filler injection training. (**a**) The trotter of 1-*month-old piglets*. (**b**) The grooves formed along the ankle joints can effectively reproduce the structures of the nasolabial folds or deep furrows of the forehead or glabella in a human face. (**c**) The curvatures present on the calf provide an excellent platform for practicing facial volumization with HA. (**d**) The skin of the pig's trotters can be used by trainee injectors to familiarize themselves with the intradermal injection

References

1. Seo KK. Botulinum toxin for Asians. Singapore: Springer Nature Ltd.; 2017. p. 175–6.
2. Kim HJ, Seo KK, Lee HK, Kim JS. Clinical anatomy of face for botulinum toxin and filler injection. Berlin: Springer; 2016. p. 28–31.
3. Heuss LT, Inauen W. The dawning of a new sedative: propofol in gastrointestinal endoscopy. Digestion. 2004;69(1):20–6.
4. Kim HJ, Seo KK, Lee HK, Kim JS. Clinical anatomy of face for botulinum toxin and filler injection. Berlin: Springer; 2016. p. 169–73.
5. Casabona G. Blood aspiration test for cosmetic fillers to prevent accidental intravascular injection in the face. Dermatol Surg. 2015;41(7):841–7.
6. Sattler G. Tower technique of filler injection. In: Carruthers J, Carruthers A, editors. Soft tissue augmentation. Philadelphia: Elsevier; 2018. p. 175–83.

4 Regional Particulars

4.1 Forehead Augmentation

Difficulty Level: C, Effectiveness: A, Complications: C

> *Summary 1*: 23-G Cannula is used for injection. Monophasic HA filler with high lifting capacity and high cohesivity is recommended.

> *Summary 2*: Fillers should be placed at the supraperiosteal layer under the frontalis m.

> *Summary 3*: The relevant injection volume is 2–6 mL for forehead concavity correction and 3–10 mL for forehead sloping correction.

> *Summary 4*: Pre-injection of botulinum toxin is highly advised prior to forehead augmentation in order to avoid irregularites caused by the movement of the frontalis and corrugator supercilii muscles. To ensure overall facial balance, concurrent augmentation of the temples and the nose should also be considered.

The purpose of forehead augmentation is primarily two-fold: to correct forehead concavity and to address forehead sloping. Correction of forehead concavity aims to smoothen the contour of a concave or scalloped forehead by filling the hollowness between the superciliary arch and the frontal eminence (Fig. 4.1). In comparison, the latter indication aims to rebalance a backward sloping forehead on the lateral view by projecting it slightly forward (Fig. 4.2).

Forehead concavity or a sunken forehead can be caused either by the congenital bossing of the frontal bone or by the progressive depletion of frontal fat due to aging or weight loss, which serves to reveal the underlying protrusions and depressions of the frontal bone structure [1]. Deep forehead concavity accentuates the prominence of the superior orbital ridge, a trait commonly associated with a strong masculine image. Therefore, forehead augmentation for a smooth convexity is a commonly requested indication among young female patients to create a softer, more feminine facial appearance. Revolumizing a concave forehead also holds significant value for older patients, as it helps to recreate the smooth youthful facial contour lost to facial deflation and descent with age, In brief, forehead augmentation serves not only as a beautification tool in young patients in their 20s and 30s but also as a rejuvenation tool in older patients in their fourth decade and above.

HA filler placed in the forehead is reasonably expected to last between 5 and 10 years. The

K. K. Seo, *Facial Volumization with Fillers*, https://doi.org/10.1007/978-981-33-6212-3_4

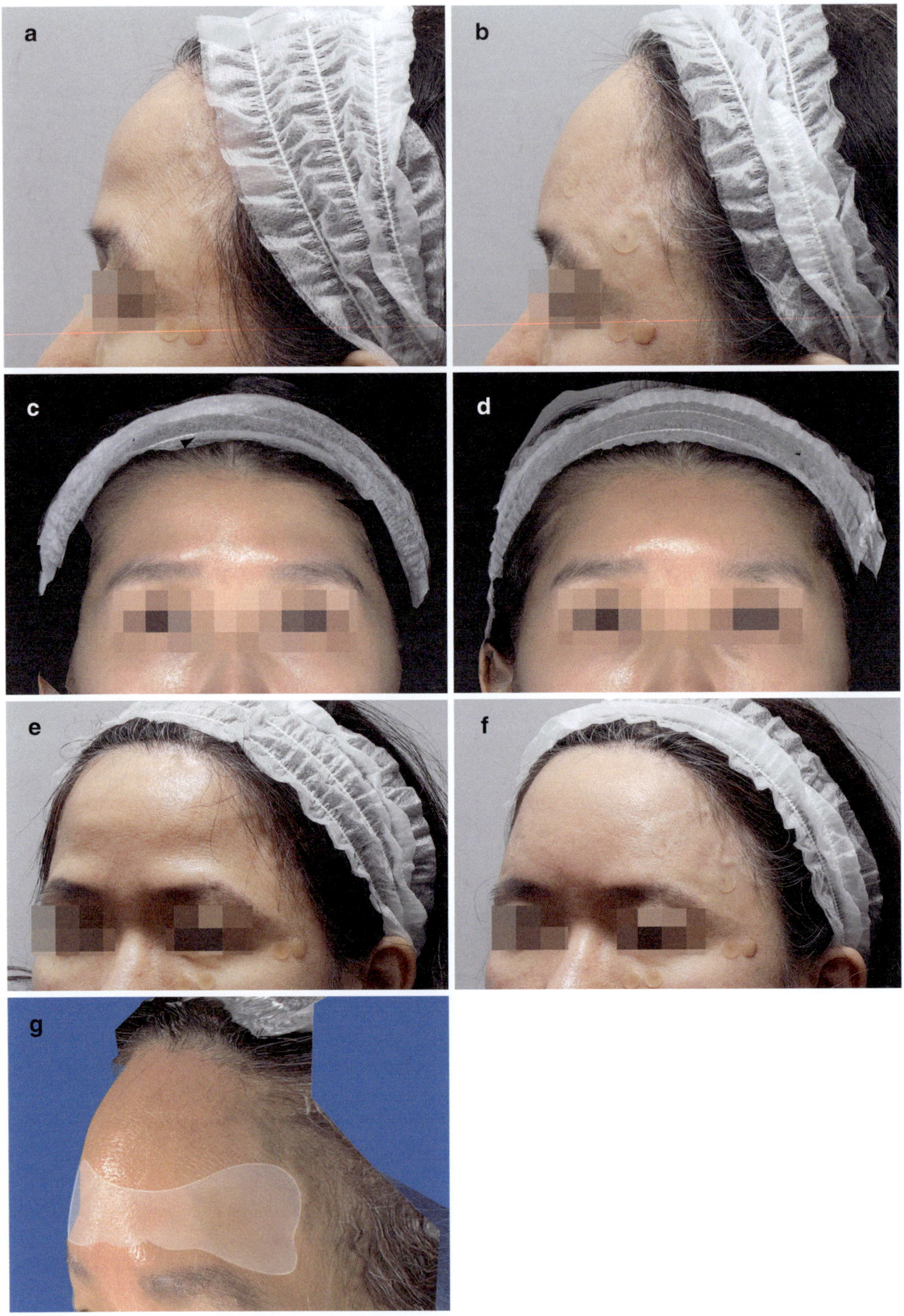

Fig. 4.1 Correction of forehead concavity ((**a**, **c**, **e**) before, (**b**, **d**, **f**) after, (**g**) Superimposed image of forehead before and after augmentation clearly domonstrates the smoothened forehead concavity as well as the appropriate location of the volume restoration

forehead, together with the nose and pretarsal roll, represents an area where the duration of the deposited HA filler tends to be the longest. Presumably, this may be correlated with the specific technique employed for the placement, that is, injection of boluses, which better protects the HA filler against enzymatic biodegradation by hyaluronidase. On the other hand, the limited space available for HA filler placement in the forehead, which consists of hard bone immediately underlying the thin soft tissue, means that even when HA filler is delivered evenly in the target area, subsequent contractions of the frontalis muscle may cause the HA filler to migrate and collect elsewhere, leading to the appearance of lumpiness in the forehead. To

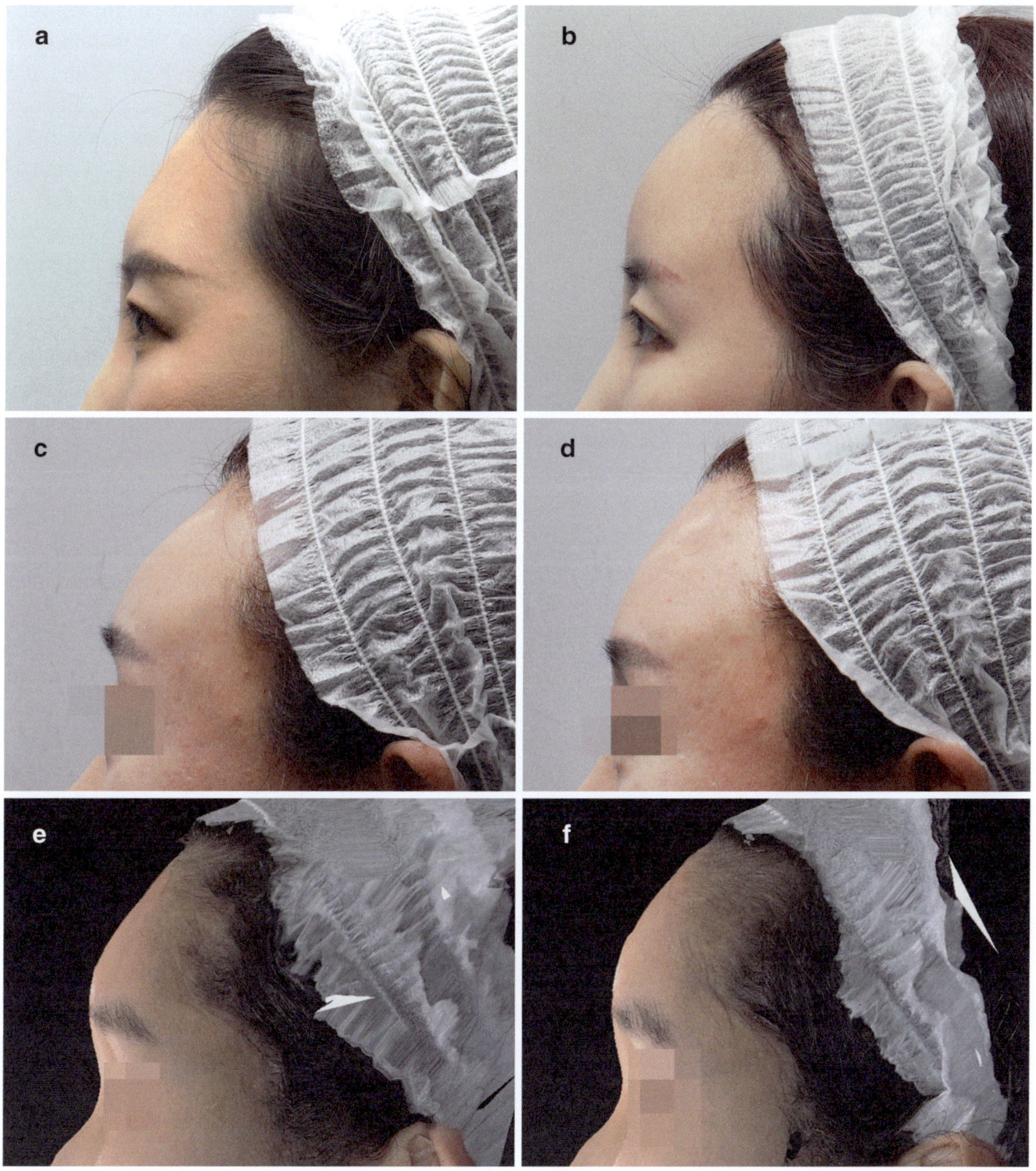

Fig. 4.2 Correction of forehead sloping ((**a**, **c**, **e**) before, (**b**, **d**, **f**) after, (**g**) Superimposed image of forehead before and after augmentation clearly domonstrates the improved sloping of forehead)

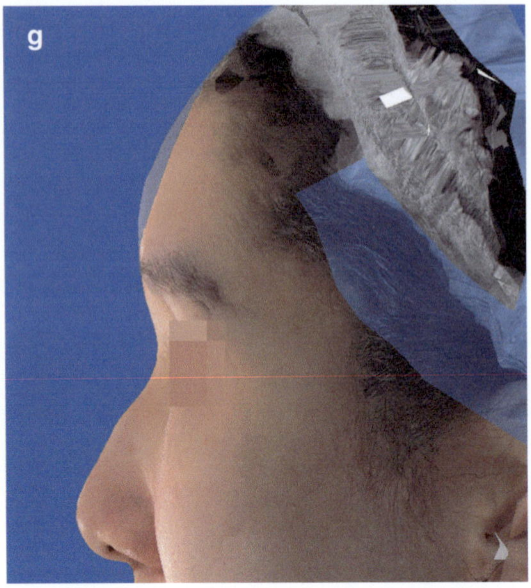

Fig. 4.2 (continued)

avoid such occurrence, preinjection of BoNT-A in the frontalis and glabella 1–2 week(s) prior to forehead augmentation is strongly recommended. Optimum maintenance treatment for forehead augmentation should preferably consist of follow-up BoNT-A injections repeated at regular intervals rather than any periodic top-up of volume with HA filler. That said, results can be well maintained without adjuvant BoNT-A injections in patients who rarely animate the frontalis muscle for conveying facial expressions.

4.1.1 Anatomical Considerations

The soft tissue layers of the forehead from the outer to inner consist of the skin—subcutaneous layer—frontalis m. and galea aponeurosis—loose connective tissue—periosteum [1]. Caution should be taken when creating the entry points with a needle to avoid perforating the vessels, which in turn may bring about surplus volume change in the depressed area due to bruising. This would disturb the appropriate placement of filler for forehead augmentation. The relevant vessels at risk include the sentinel v. and the superficial temporal a. located lateral to the orbital rim as well as the supratrochlear a. and supraorbital a. located near the glabellar region [2]. Since all these vessels run between the frontalis m. and skin, the filler should be placed at the supraperiosteal layer under the frontalis m. for the purpose of avoiding intravascular filler injection (Fig. 4.3) [3]. Moreover, placing the filler under the frontalis muscle is also helpful for preventing irregularities caused by the frontalis muscle movement.

4.1.2 Pretreatment Assessment

Pretreatment considerations include, among others, the location and severity of the frontal concavity, the gradient of the forehead slope, the patient's gender, dermal thickness, prominence of the relevant mimetic muscles such as the frontalis m., and corrugator supercilii m., presence of any blepharoptosis or eyelid hooding, as well as such subjective factors as the patient's expectation concerning the desired posttreatment volume and contour improvement.

Location-wise, forehead concavity can be present in the central forehead region and/or the left and right lateral forehead above the eyebrows. Whether to confine treatment to either the central or lateral forehead depressions only or to treat both aspects in tandem ultimately depends on the location and the severity of the relevant frontal hollowing. Note that in the case of pronounced lateral forehead depressions, indentations can extend as far out as the hairline from above the eyebrows.

The severity of frontal hollowness also becomes a key pretreatment consideration since it dictates the amount of volume to be placed. The severity of forehead concavity can be graded based on a five-point scale, scored as follows. 0 = an overall round convex forehead devoid of concavities, projecting slightly forward when viewed in profile, 1 = a flat forehead extending from the frontal eminence to the supraorbital ridge without any intervening depressions, 2 = presence of mild depression between the frontal eminence and the supraorbital ridge, 3 = presence of moderate depression in the said region, and 4 = presence of severe depression in the said region, representing frontal bossing in its severest form (Fig. 4.4).

Concerning gender considerations, unlike in female patients, full correction or leveling of forehead concavity is not advised in men since

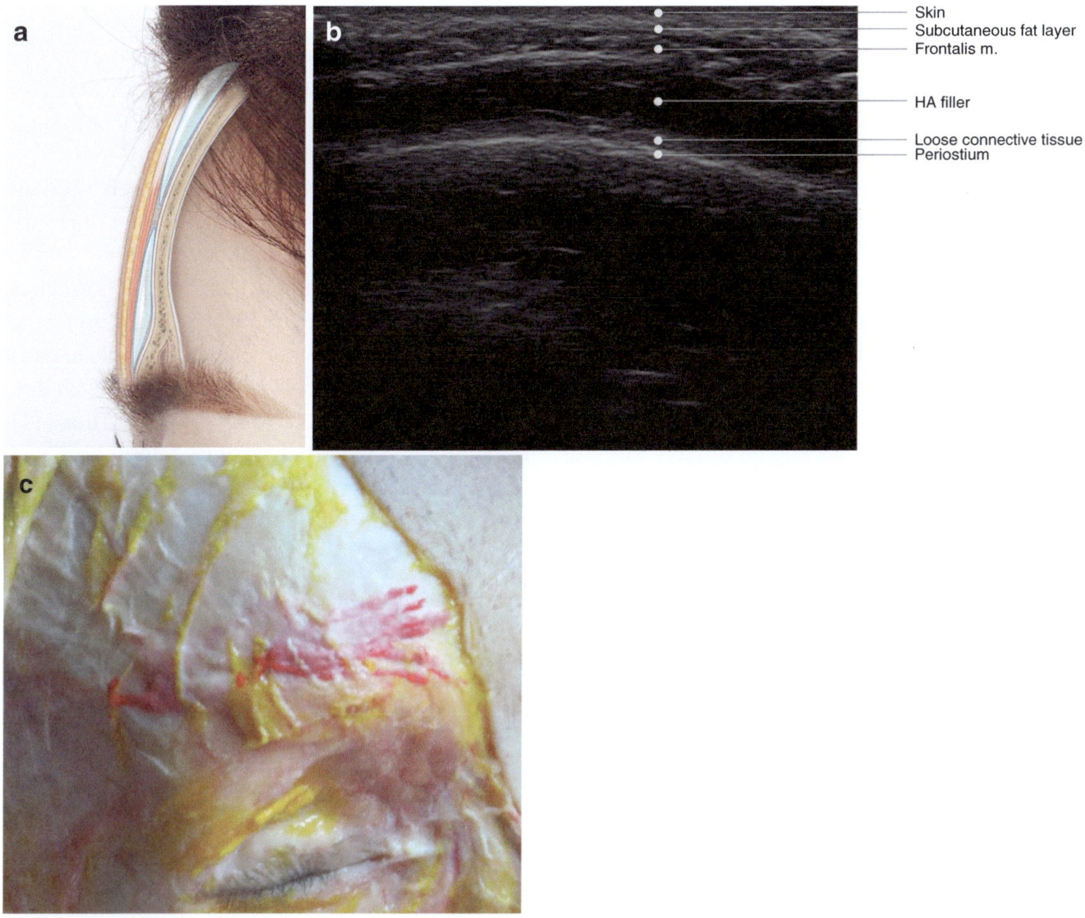

Fig. 4.3 Depth of injection for forehead augmentation. (**a**) Fillers should be placed at the supraperiosteal layer under the frontalis m. for the purpose of avoiding intravascular injection. (**b**) Sonography image displaying the evenly placed HA filler at the supraperiosteal layer. (**c**) Proper placement of HA under the frontalis muscle on the cadaveric forehead (courtesy of Pf. Kim Hee-Jin)

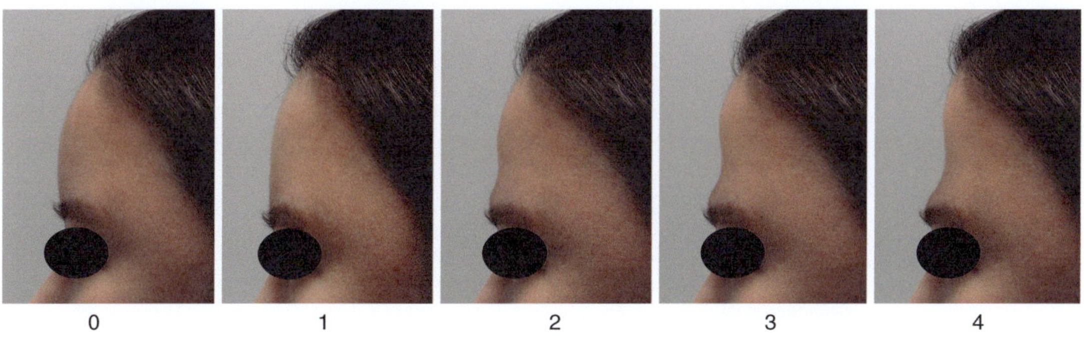

Fig. 4.4 The scale for grading the severity of forehead concavity. *0*: an overall round convex forehead, *1*: a flat forehead, *2*: mild forehead concavity, *3*: moderate forehead concavity, *4*: severe forehead concavity

the appearance of a mildly rugged forehead with slightly prominent superciliary arches is considered a desired masculinizing trait. Accordingly, a reduced dose just enough to ameliorate the severity of the frontal irregularity is advised in the male forehead, though actual volumes may vary based on the patient's subjective preference and the desired forehead shape.

Meanwhile, the slant of the forehead describes the degree to which the frontal bone slopes backwards from the superciliary arch up to the hairline. Forehead slant or sloping can be graded according to the inclination, with 0 = slight protrusion of the forehead (on profile) anterior to a line connecting the hairline and the superciliary arch, 1 = a straight forehead profile, with the superciliary arch falling vertically from the hairline, 2 = mild sloping of the forehead, 3 = moderate sloping, and 4 = severe sloping (Fig. 4.5) [4]. Asians are known to have more of a backward-sloping forehead compared with Caucasians [5].

4.1.3 Injection Technique for Forehead Concavity and Forehead Sloping (Table 4.1)

The use of a 23-G cannula is advised to avoid bruising and inadvertent intravascular injection of filler. The relevant cannula entry points differ in location depending on whether the correction is for forehead concavity or forehead sloping. As regards frontal concavities, medial forehead entry points are created 1.5–2 cm superior to each eyebrow along the respective midpupillary lines [1]. Meanwhile, the left and right lateral forehead entry points are made 1 cm above the eyebrow along a vertical line drawn 1 cm lateral to each

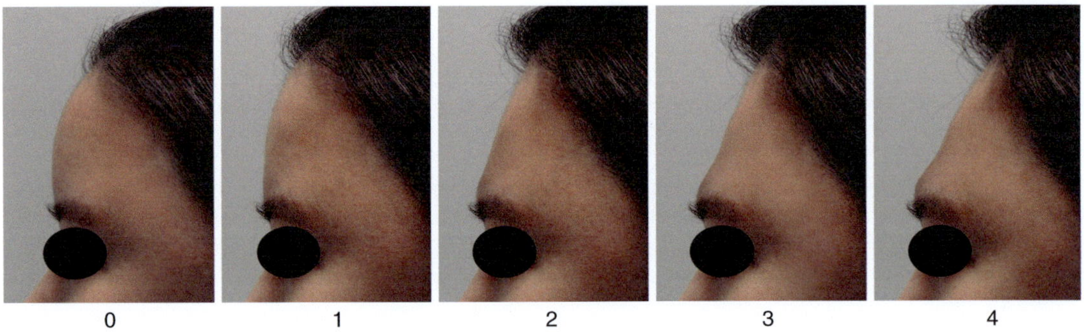

Fig. 4.5 The scale for grading the severity of forehead sloping. 0: an overall round convex forehead, *1*: a flat forehead, *2*: a mildly sloping forehead, *3*: a moderately sloping forehead, *4*: a severely sloping forehead

Table 4.1 Summary of forehead augmentation injection technique

Item	Contents
Needle vs. Cannula	23-G 5-cm Cannula
Choice of HA filler	Monophasic HA filler with high lifting capacity
Amount of HA filler	2–6 mL for correction of forehead concavity 3–10 mL for correction of forehead sloping
Depth of injection	Supraperiosteal layer
Entry point for cannula	For forehead concavity, medial forehead entry points are created 1.5–2 cm superior to each eyebrow along the respective midpupillary lines. Meanwhile, left and right lateral forehead entry points are made 1 cm above the eyebrow along a vertical line drawn 1 cm lateral to each lateral canthus For forehead sloping, entry points are created 1–2 cm inferior to the hairline along each lateral limbus line, while the left and right lateral entry points are made 2–4 cm superior to each eyebrow along the respective lateral canthal lines
Target area	Correction of forehead concavity aims to fill the hollowness between the superciliary arch and the frontal eminence Correction of sloping forehead aims to volumize upper part of forehead under the hairline
Anesthetics	Supraorbital and supratrochlear nerve blocks

lateral canthus and (Fig. 4.6). Note that the precise location of cannula access points may also vary according to the actual size and extent of the frontal depression.

As regards forehead sloping, since the main target of augmentation is the upper forehead region extending to the hairline, medial forehead entry points are made 1–2 cm inferior to the hairline along each lateral limbus line, while the left and right lateral entry points are made 2–4 cm superior to each eyebrow along the respective lateral canthal lines (Fig. 4.6). In either case, the relevant plane of injection is the supraperiosteal layer deep to the frontalis m (Fig. 4.3).

For the treatment of forehead concavity, insert a 23-G cannula through the medial entry point on the left mid pupillary line, and first fill the deepest (middle) part of the central forehead concavity. The cannula should be inserted deeply down to the periosteum and advanced practically scraping the surface of the periosteum. Once reaching the right medial entry point, deposit the HA filler

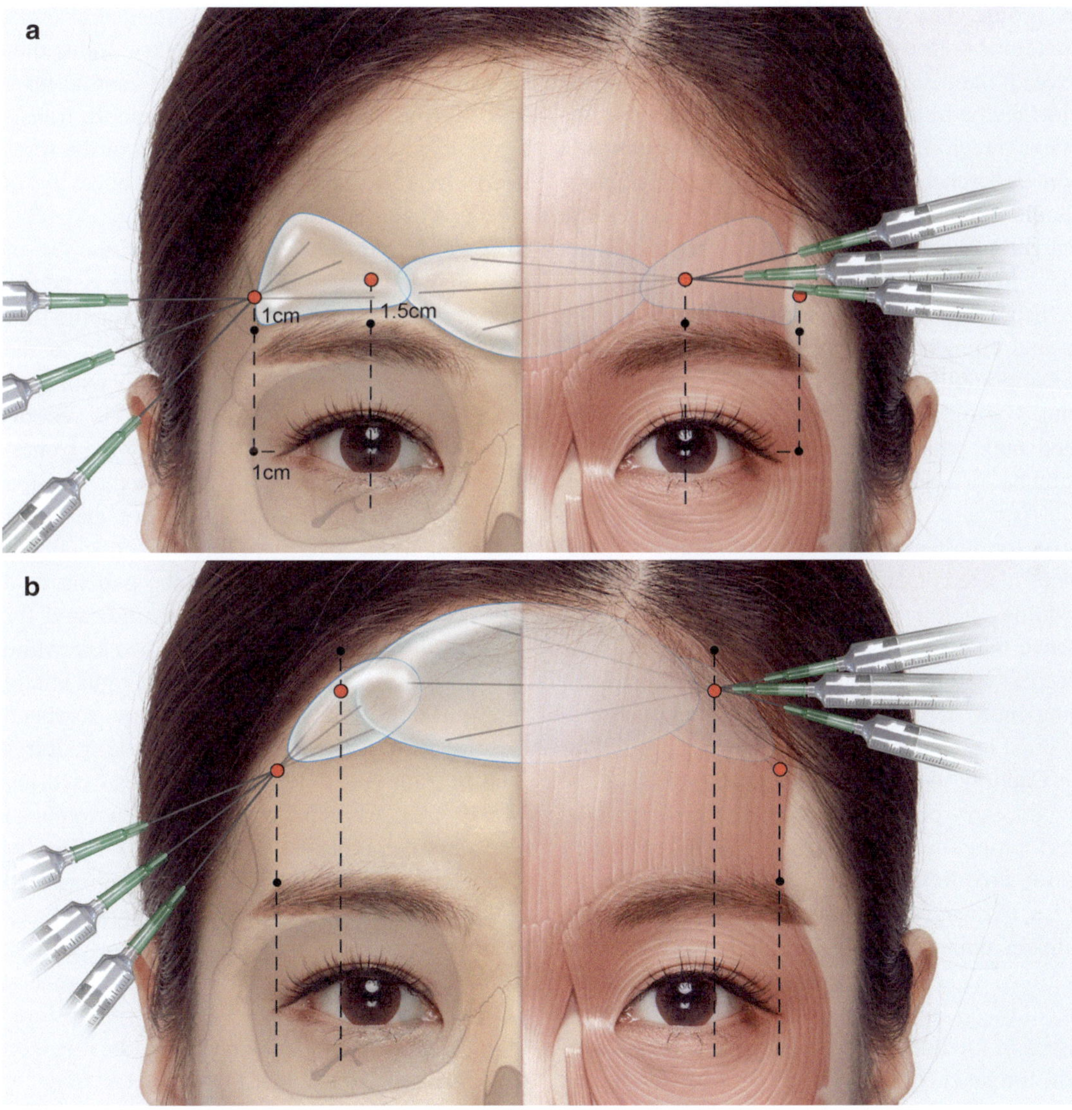

Fig. 4.6 (**a**) Injection technique for forehead concavity, (**b**) Injection technique for forehead sloping

supraperiosteally while withdrawing the cannula. Fill to the desired height maintaining constant injection pressure to avoid unwanted contour irregularities (Fig. 4.6).

Once the desired volume is achieved, repeat the same technique in areas located immediately above and below the deepest part (middle part) of the central forehead concavity, extending up to the frontal eminence superiorly and down to the glabella inferiorly (Fig. 3.16). In case a mildly convex forehead is desired, augment the middle part of central forehead concavity to project slightly beyond the frontal eminence from the profile view. Where instead a smooth straight contour is preferred, the relevant areas should not exceed the frontal eminence from the profile view but be treated just enough to blend with the glabella region. Note, however, that even where a convex forehead is desired, the forehead contour should flow as a smooth arc from above the patient's own frontal eminence on the profile view. In other words, care should be taken to not to disproportionately augment the area below the frontal eminence to such extent that it appears unharmonious with the rest of the foreheard contour. The right medial entry point should be created only where necessary for treating a wide forehead or a large central depression. Meanwhile, the right and left lateral entry points should be used for addressing the lateral forehead depressions located on either side of the forehead. Here, volume should be injected starting from just above the eyebrows where the depression is the deepest before tapering off towards the frontal eminence, with progressively lower volumes applied in the upper aspect.

Caution should be taken when creating the lateral entry points with a 21-G needle to avoid perforating the sentinel vein or the frontal branch of the superficial temporal artery running nearby. Also, to create a smooth gradation from the most sunken point of the forehead toward adjacent regions, make sure to taper the injection volume accordingly, applying progressively lower volumes in the upper and lower aspects of the central forehead concavity and reduced volumes in the upper/lateral aspects of the lateral depressions. On the other hand, as regards forehead sloping, insert a 23 G cannula through an medial entry point at the upper forehead created along the left lateral limbus line, and proceed first to fill the upper central forehead near the hairline to the desired height, before proceeding towards the cannula entry point in the same manner. Once the desired volume is achieved in the area close to the central portion of the hairline, repeat the same technique in the area located immediately below, extending down to the frontal eminence inferiorly in amounts adequate for projecting the slanted forehead with progressively lower volumes applied in the lower aspect. Next, repeat the same process on the contralateral side of the forehead slope using the opposite medial entry point. Finally, using the lateral entry points created along the right and left lateral canthal lines place further volume to ensure a smooth transition to the lateral and inferior aspect of the forehead slope to achieve a smooth convexity in forehead contour.

Regarding the choice of HA filler, the use of soft, malleable monophasic HA filler is generally advised for the augmentation, given the limited space available for filler placement in the forehead. Also, monophasic HA filler with high lifting capacity and high cohesivity is recommended considering the movement of the frontalis muscle in the area. As regards the desired dose, while actual injection volumes may vary according to the severity of forehead concavity as well as the volume desired by the patient, as a general rule of thumb, 1–3 mL is indicated for treating the central forehead hollowness while 1–2 mL is required for the left and right lateral forehead concavities. A mildly hollow forehead (scoring 2 on forehead concavity scale) requires 2–3 mL, a moderately hollow forehead (scoring 3) 4–5 mL, while a severely sunken forehead (scoring 4) requires 6 mL or more of HA filler for forehead augmentation. With respect to forehead sloping, 3–5 mL of HA filler is required for augmenting a grade 2 forehead, 6–8 mL for grade 3, and 10 mL or more for a grade 4 forehead primarily in the upper-mid portion of the forehead. The nondominant hand should be engaged to constantly mold the injected HA filler to smoothness. The use of 4 × 4 gauze molding would be helpful to even out the forehead surface after forehead filler injection (Fig. 4.7).

Anesthesia: Supraorbital and supratrochlear nerve blocks are required to minimize the pain and discomfort during the supraperiosteal placement of HA fillers in the forehead (Fig. 3.4). Upon applying the nerve block, massage and wait for approximately 20 mins for the volume of the injected local anesthetic to subside. Preinjection of dental lidocaine intradermally in the cannula entry points may provide further comfort. The patient should be made to understand in advance that while the anesthesia helps to numbs any significant pain during treatment, they may still feel an odd sensation of the cannula scraping against their periosteum; and that in case the cannula were to hit a sensory nerve, they may experience a sharp tingling sensation radiating cephalically and a weird feeling of hair on the vertex suddenly being tugged backwards.

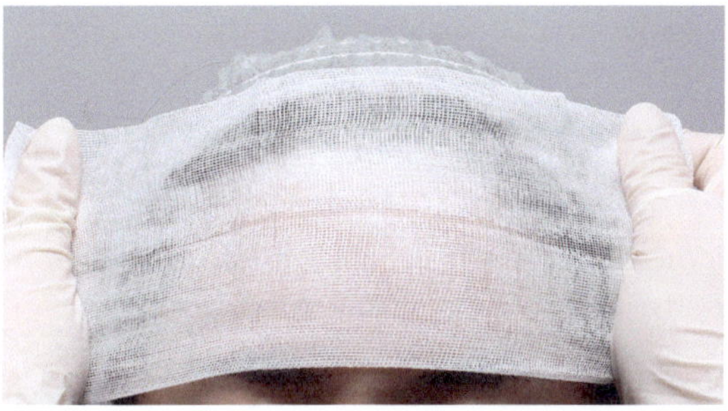

Fig. 4.7 The 4 X 4 gauze molding would be helpful to even out the forehead surface after forehead filler injection

4.1.4 Combination Treatment

Pre-injection of botulinum toxin (BoNT-A) injection is highly advised prior to the filler injection in the forehead to avoid irregularities caused by the frontalis and corrugator supercilii muscle movement. For the same reason, a follow-up injection of botulinum toxin repeated every 3–6 months would be helpful for the optimum maintanance of results especially in patients with unconscious expression habit on the glabella and forehead area. It would be necessary to make two additional BoNT-A injections (0.5–1 U) above the eyebrows, on the midpupillary line and along the lateral canthal line respectively, in patients displaying active corrugator muscle movement above the eyebrows when frowning (Fig. 4.8) [6].

For the purpose of ensuring optimum facial balance, temple augmentation should be

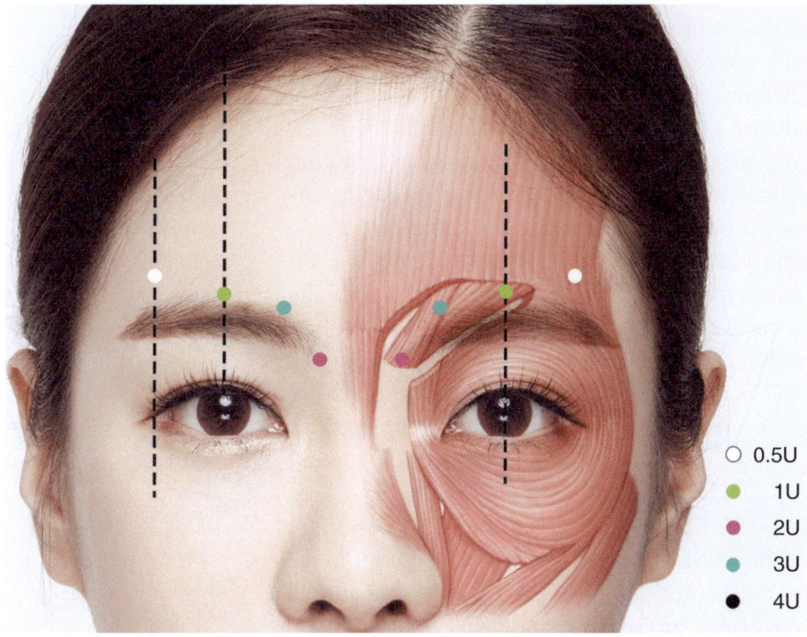

Fig. 4.8 Injection points of BoNT-A in patients with an active corrugator muscle movement above the eyebrows

concomitantly performed in patients with temple depressions. In the same context, concurrent nose augmentation would be required in patients with a low-set nasal dorsum.

4.1.5 Complications

The most frequent and aesthetically displeasing adverse event following forehead augmentation is contour irregularity. The limited space available in the forehead between the frontal bone and skin means the implanted HA filler, unless placed evenly with meticulous care, is prone to irregularity and clumping. In this respect, the use of a cannula rather than a needle is advised, since its longer length allows filling of more areas from a single access point with less trauma, creating a smoother and more even result. Meanwhile, the noninjecting hand must be used to constantly mold and evenly distribute the HA filler immediately postinjection to remove any irregularities. Where irregularities are present due to a previous fat graft procedure, the injection of HA would sometimes aggrevate such irregularities due to the scar tissues under the skin.

By the same token, a hyperactive frontalis or corrugator m. can also result in the appearance of dimpling or hollowing in the treated area, as the pronounced movement of these muscles may cause volume to shift from its implanted location. As such, BoNT-A injection is highly advised prior to filler injection in the forehead. And also, Care should be taken not to overfill the central forehead, as it may create an odd localized protrusion resembling the bump on a dolphin's forehead. More importantly do not overfill the lateral part of the forehead, which also results in awkward bumpiness.

Necrosis due to intravascular injection of filler may occur in the forehead when injections are performed with needles. Other complications include a sharp tingling sensation radiating cephalically when the skin around the brow area is touched, which may arise either as a side effect of the nerve block or from a partial compromise to the sensory nerves caused by the cannula movement during the treatment.

Episode: Forehead Augmentation Nightmare

I refer to two nightmarish cases involving forehead fillers dating back to the early 2000s when I had just started practicing forehead augmentation. The first case involved an aspirant Korean idol trainee in his early 20s who presented with harsh frontal bossing and bulging brow ridges which gave the face a distinctly gorilla-like appearance.

Those were still early days when fillers were used predominantly in the forehead for addressing horizontal lines and creases, and augmenting a sunken forehead was a novel indication. Personally, I hardly had any prior experience performing forehead volumization at the time. Upon starting the procedure, I was instantly struck by the seemingly inordinate amount of filler the patient's forehead appeared to be consuming, even though the angularity in the forehead contour seemed to persist regardless of the volumes being pumped in. I struggled laboriously for more than 40–50 min to smoothen the contour irregularity, to no avail.

On reflection, I realize that the problem did not lie in placing *too much* volume but rather the lack thereof. If I felt the 3–4 mL I was injecting was a worryingly large amount, it in fact fell far short of the 6–10 mL advised for patients with such a severely sunken forehead. Moreover, long disposable cannulas had yet to be introduced at the time, and it was tricky to achieve uniformity using a 1.25 cm needle to inject multiple areas across the vast frontal area. Fortunately, with the subsequent introduction of cannulas, I came to handle even the most severely depressed foreheads with a flourish in under 10 mins.

The young male patient had since gone on to become a fairly renowned celebrity who, to this day, sports a hairstyle covering up his forehead. I feel bad for the young man each time I see him on TV but, understandably, he was never to return to my clinic.

The other case involved a young male patient who manifested a severe horizontal depression across the forehead like a deep furrow. In this case, while the indentation seemingly diasppeared immediately following treatment, for some inexplicable reason it would invariably reappear in about a week. Three to four rounds of touch-ups were provided, though to no avail, and the problem ultimately went unresolved.

In hindsight, I now realize that the patient may have been the type that relies heavily on the use of forehead muscles to lift the upper eyelid, in which case, the frequent movement of the frontalis m. tends to displace the filler from the deposited location. Prior injection of BoNT-A in the forehead and glabella to relax and minimize the muscle movement can help to avoid such adverse events.

4.2 Temple Augmentation

Difficulty Level: A, Effectiveness: A, Complications: B

Summary 1: Inject HA filler directly onto the periosteum deep to the temporalis m. using a 21-gauge sharp needle and the bolus injection technique without withdrawing the needle.

Summary 2: Care should be taken to avoid the rich vasculature of the temple region to prevent bruising and embolization. Preinjection aspiration is a prerequisite when injecting with a needle.

Summary 3: To achieve the ideal oval face shape by rounding out the zygomatic prominence, HA filler should be injected in the lateral part of the temporal fossa. To diminish the prominence of the orbital rim, volume should be placed at the medial and superior aspects of the temporal fossa.

Recessed temples may either be a congenital feature or caused by the loss of temporal volume with aging or weight loss. Concavity in the temples creates a relative prominence of the adjacent zygomatic and supraciliary arches, skeletonizing the facial contour and giving the face a severe, austere, and aged appearance. In this regard, temple enhancement serves not only to ovalize the face by obscuring the prominence of the lateral zygoma but also helps to create a softer, more rested appearance by smoothening out the perceived protrusion of the orbital rim (Fig. 1.4 and Fig. 4.9).

4.2.1 Anatomical Considerations

The temporal fossa is delineated superiorly by the superior temporal line, inferiorly by the zygomatic arch, medially by the superciliary arch and the frontal process of zygoma, and laterally by the temporal peak or the hairline down to the sideburns. The soft tissue layers of the temporal fossa from the outer to inner consist of the skin—subcutaneous layer—superficial temporal fascia —superficial layer of deep temporal fascia-temporal fat pad—deep layer of deep temporal fascia-temporal extension of the buccal fat pad-temporalis m.-temporal bone [1]. The temporal area is rich in blood vessels, and vigilance must therefore be taken to avoid extensive bruising from vessel injury or embolization from intravascular filler injection. The relevant vessels at risk include, among others, the sentinel v. located lateral to the orbital rim, the superficial temporal a. and v., the middle temporal v., and the deep temporal a. and v. (Fig. 4.10).

The sentinel v. is present lateral to the eyes and the brow, and is visible with the naked eye. Careful observation is thus required during injection to avoid the rupture of this vein since it

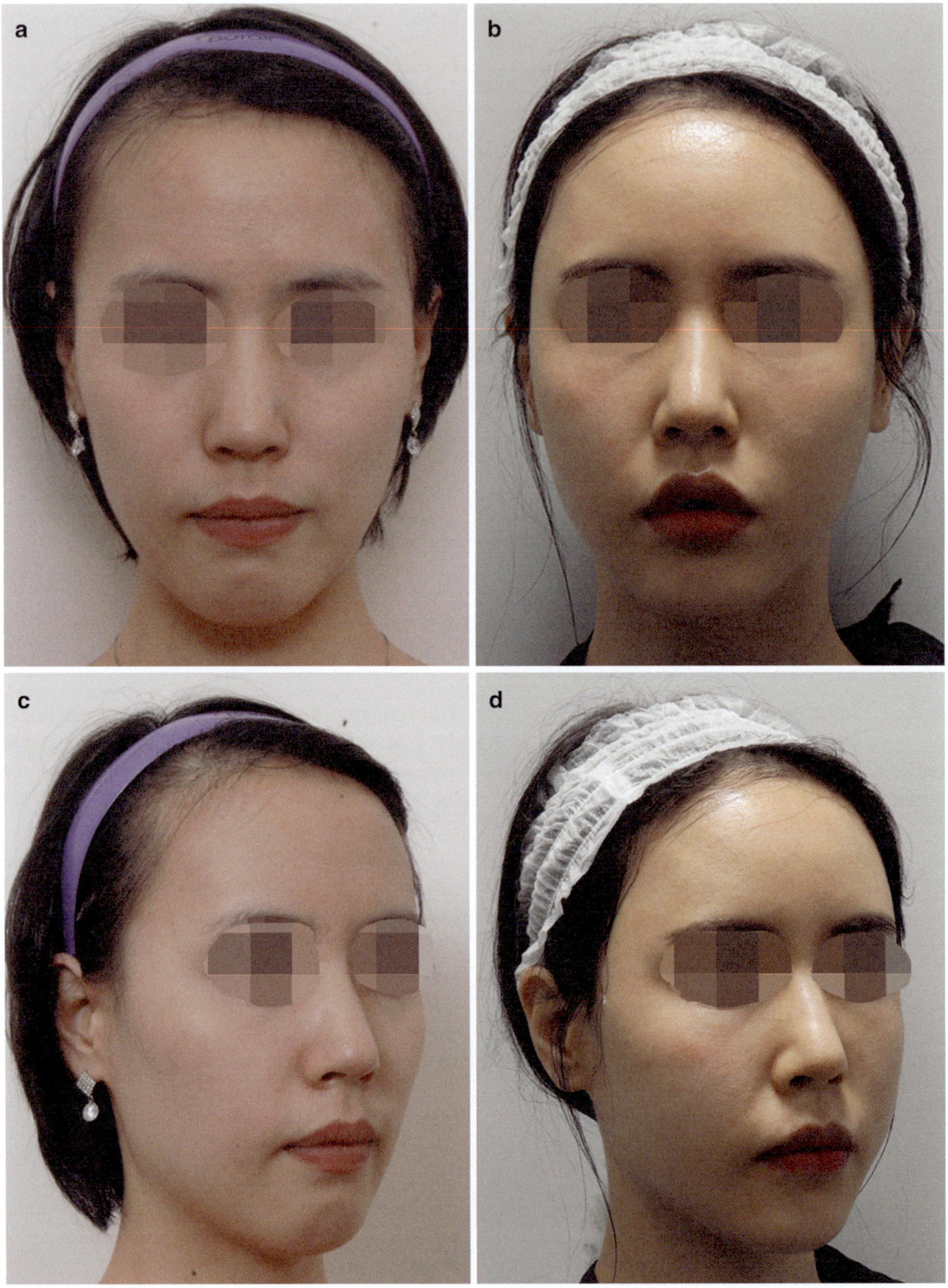

Fig. 4.9 (**a**, **c**, **e**, **g**) Before and (**b**, **d**, **f**, **h**) after temple augmentation

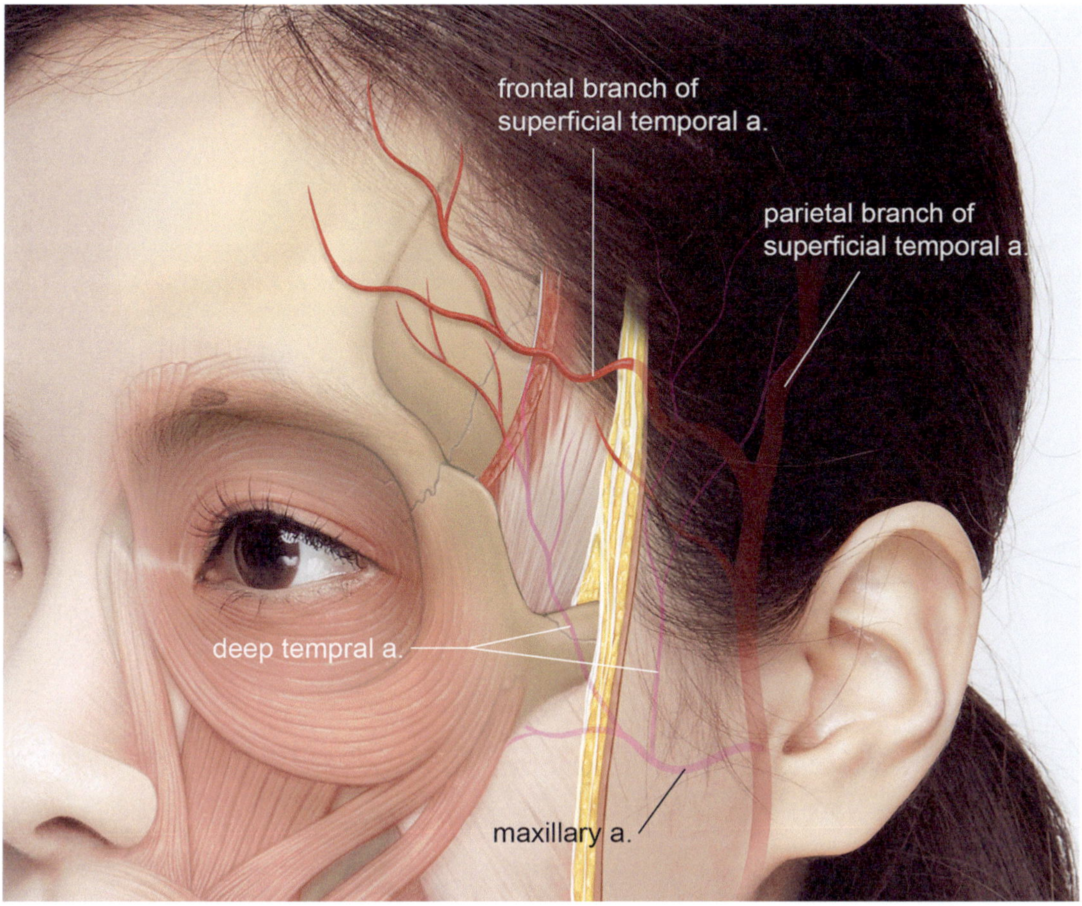

Fig. 4.10 Arterial distribution in the temple

can lead to severe bruising. The superficial temporal a. runs between the superficial and the deep temporal fascia and bifurcates into the frontal branch and the parietal branch at a point 37 mm superior and 18 mm medial to the tragus [7].The frontal branch of the superficial temporal a. courses obliquely in a superomedial direction toward a point located 2 cm superior to the eyebrow on a vertical line drawn from the lateral canthus (Fig. 4.11). The middle temporal v. as a branch of the superficial temporal v. is situated deep to the deep temporal facia and runs anterior to the ear toward the orbital rim, approximately 2 cm or one fingerbreadth above and parallel to the superior margin of the zygomatic arch (Fig. 4.12). The deep temporal a. branching from the maxillary a. gives off multiple small branches, which within the substance of the temporalis m., ascend superficially toward the muscle surface (Fig. 4.10).

To sum up, from a clinical standpoint, the relevant vessels to avoid during temple augmentation are the sentinel v. when filling the medial aspect of the temporal fossa, the middle temporal v. when treating the inferior aspect, the deep temporal a. when treating the deeper aspect, and the superficial temporal a. when filling the superior aspect of the temple. While the sentinel v. is easily observed by the naked eye, the others are deep structures hidden from view. Make sure to perform slow injections of HA filler down into the periosteum to avoid inadvertently entering these structures. Aspiration before each injection must be performed as a matter of course to minimize the risk of intravascular filler injection despite taking such precautions (Fig. 3.6).

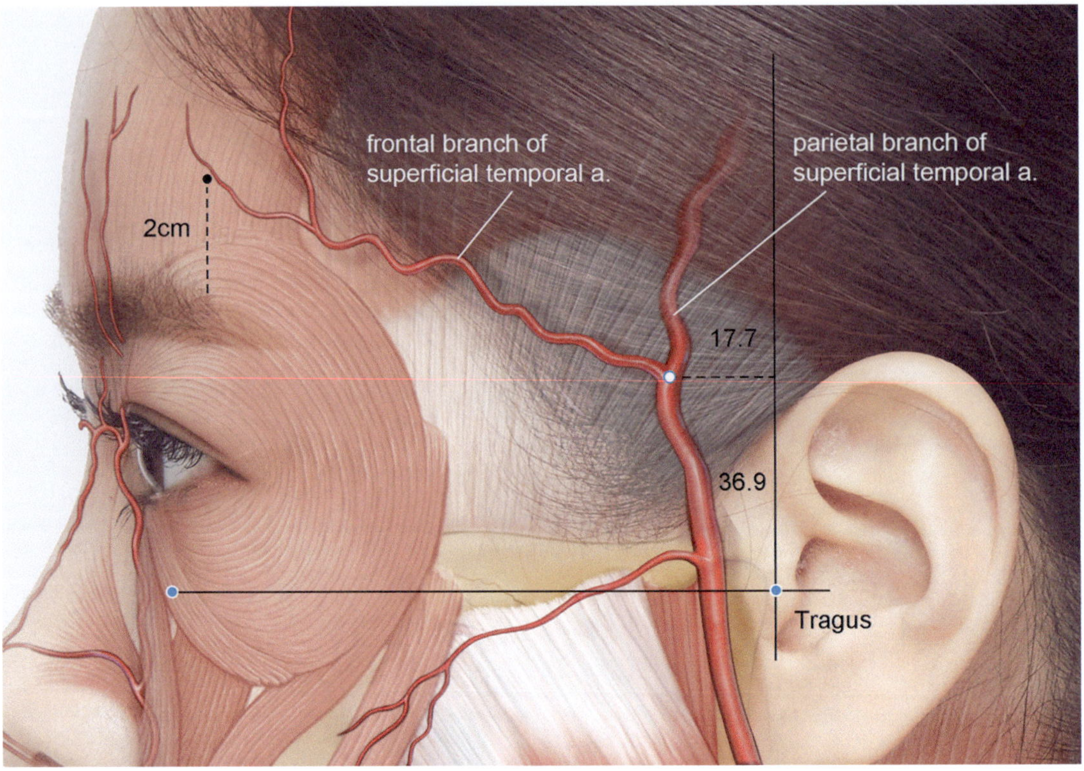

Fig. 4.11 The superficial temporal a

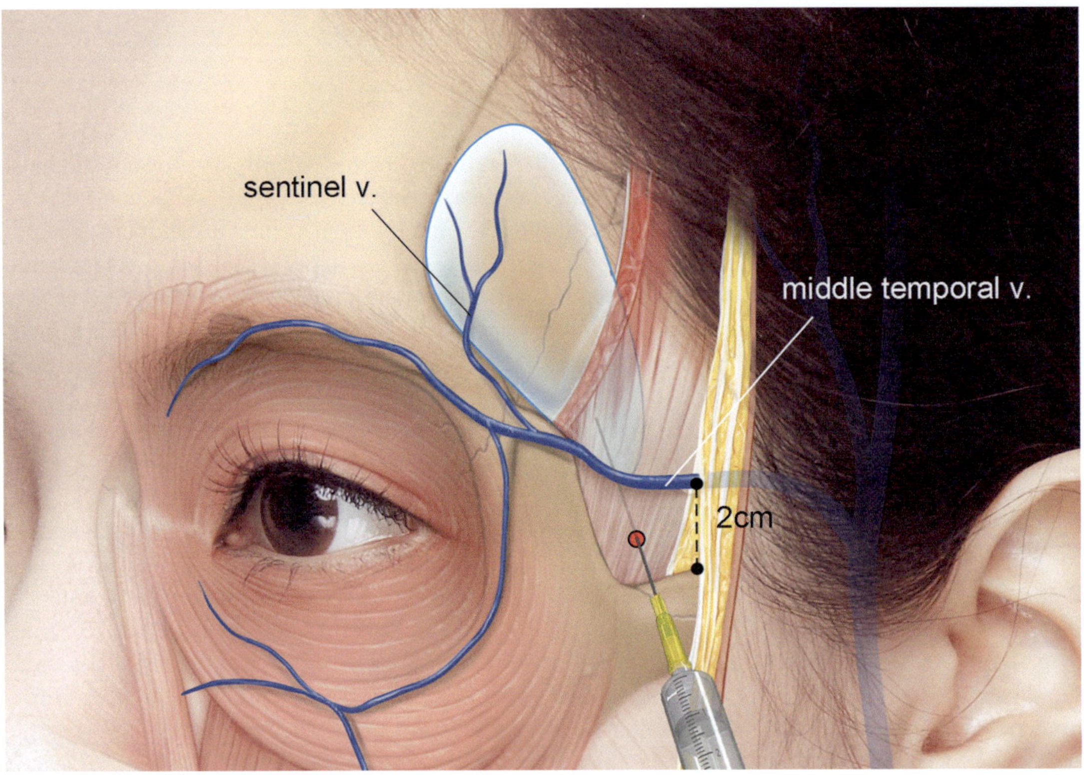

Fig. 4.12 The middle temporal v

4.2.2 Pretreatment Assessment

It is first necessary to assess where and to what extent volume is lacking within the temporal fossa. Additionally, the patient's subjective aesthetic goal for the treatment must be established during consultation since the actual site and volume of injection varies depending on the respective indication. Confirm with the patient whether the aim is to achieve an oval face shape by balancing out the prominent zygoma, or to create a softer impression by smoothening the harsh transition to the orbital rim. Significantly, ethnic differences in facial aesthetic standards must be taken into consideration. For example, full rounded temples are considered an auspicious and favorable attribute among Chinese women since, according to the traditional Chinese physiognomy, it is believed to bring them a perfect husband. Accordingly, when treating a Chinese female patient, full leveling or convexity across the entire temporal fossa is advised. On the other hand, subtle concavity in the temples is considered a desired trait among Caucasians, as it highlights the malar eminence and completes the Ogee curve regarded as essential to facial attractiveness in Caucasians (Fig. 4.13). By the same token, temporal hollowing in men requires less recontouring than in females since a slight angularity in facial contour can be a masculinizing trait that lends more strength and charisma to the face.

4.2.3 Injection Technique (Table 4.2)

As previously noted, the relevant area of injection within the temporal fossa differs according to the specific indication. To ovalize the face by deemphasizing the prominence of the lateral zygoma, HA filler is placed in the lateral part of the temporal fossa. To soften and blend the prominence of the orbital rim, volume should be directed toward the medial and superior aspects of the temporal fossa. The medial and superior temporal fossa are also targeted when temple enhancement is undertaken in conjunction with forehead augmentation to smoothen the transition between the relevant structures.

Significantly, the temple region represents the one area where the author prefers to use needles when performing volumization with HA filler.

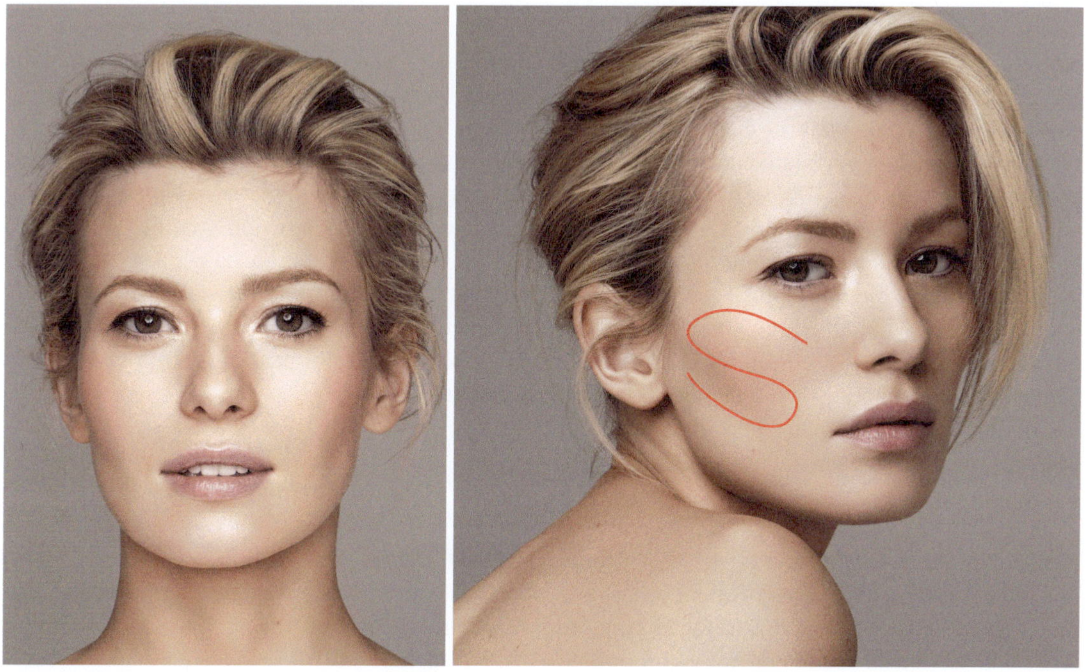

Fig. 4.13 Ogee curve (Photo: Courtesy of Galderma)

Table 4.2 Summary of temple augmentation injection technique

Item	Contents
Needle vs. Cannula	21-G needle (Aspiration is prerequisite prior to injection)
HA filler	Monophasic or biphasic with high lifting capacity
Amount of HA filler	1–4 mL per side
Depth of injection	Supraperiosteal or deep muscular level
Entry point for needle	Medial part: 1 cm behind the frontal process of the zygoma and 1 cm above the zygomatic arch Lateral part: 3 cm behind the frontal process of the zygoma and 1 cm above the zygomatic arch. Additional entry point for lateral part: 2.5 cm behind the frontal process of the zygoma and 1 cm above the zygomatic arch if necessary
Target area	Medial part of the temporal depression for smoothening the orbital rim contour Lateral part for the oval face line
Anesthetics	Topical anesthetics

This is because the blunt tipped cannula is not capable of piercing through the thick membrane of the underlying superficial and deep temporal facias. On the other hand, deep injection right onto the periosteum using a sharp needle allows for a quick and easy correction of volume deficiency without leaving any surface irregularities. For this reason, the procedure can be performed even by novice injectors subject to following certain precautions. Standard precautions include choosing the needle entry points with care to avoid bruising, aspirating before each injection, and pressing down the treatment area hard for 3 mins. post procedure to prevent the incidence of hematoma formation. A 21-G long needle is used for injecting the temple. The location and direction of needle entry and advancement vary depending on the relevant indication.

Specifically, to soften the transition with the orbital rim, the needle should be inserted deeply at a point 1 cm posterior to the frontal process of the zygoma and 1 cm superior to the zygomatic arch, and advanced superomedially through to the medial and superior parts of the temporal fossa (Fig. 4.14a). To achieve an oval facial shape by offsetting the prominent zygoma, the needle is inserted deeply through the entry point created 3 cm behind the frontal process of the zygoma and 1 cm above the zygomatic arch and guided superolaterally to fill the deficiency in the lateral aspect of the temporal fossa (Fig. 4.14b). Where additional volume correction is desired immediately superior to the zygomatic arch, an entry point is created 2.5 cm behind the frontal process of the zygoma and 1 cm above the zygomatic arch for making deep injection in the posterior direction (Fig. 4.14c).

The needle should be introduced tangentially to the skin at a 30°–45° angle with a downward-facing bevel until it reaches the bone. Once the needle tip touches the bone, aspirate before depositing a full 1 mL of HA filler right on the bone without withdrawing the needle (Fig. 4.14d). Unlike the retrograde threading technique typically employed in volumizing HA filler treatments where the substance is deposited while the instrument is being withdrawn, here, a full 1 mL bolus is dispensed into the point of the most significant volume depletion. The bolus of HA filler diffuses evenly to adjacent areas in a smooth fluid manner which the author postulates is most probably due to the tight cover, or resistance, provided by the overlying structures of the temporalis m. or the deep temporal facia. Where 1 mL falls short of achieving the intended result, additional volume may be placed in or around the injection site. Any odd lumps or bumps from the injected HA filler can easily be massaged and blended in.

Concerning the injection volume, 1–2 mL of HA filler is usually dispensed per site, depending on the indication. While 1–4 mL is generally injected per side, as much as 5–6 mL may be deposited per side in patients with a severe temporal recess.

4.2.4 Complications

4.2.4.1 Bruising

Vessel injury during temple augmentation can result in extensive bruising. Caution should be exercised therefore to avoid the sentinel v. observable by the naked eye and running in proximity to

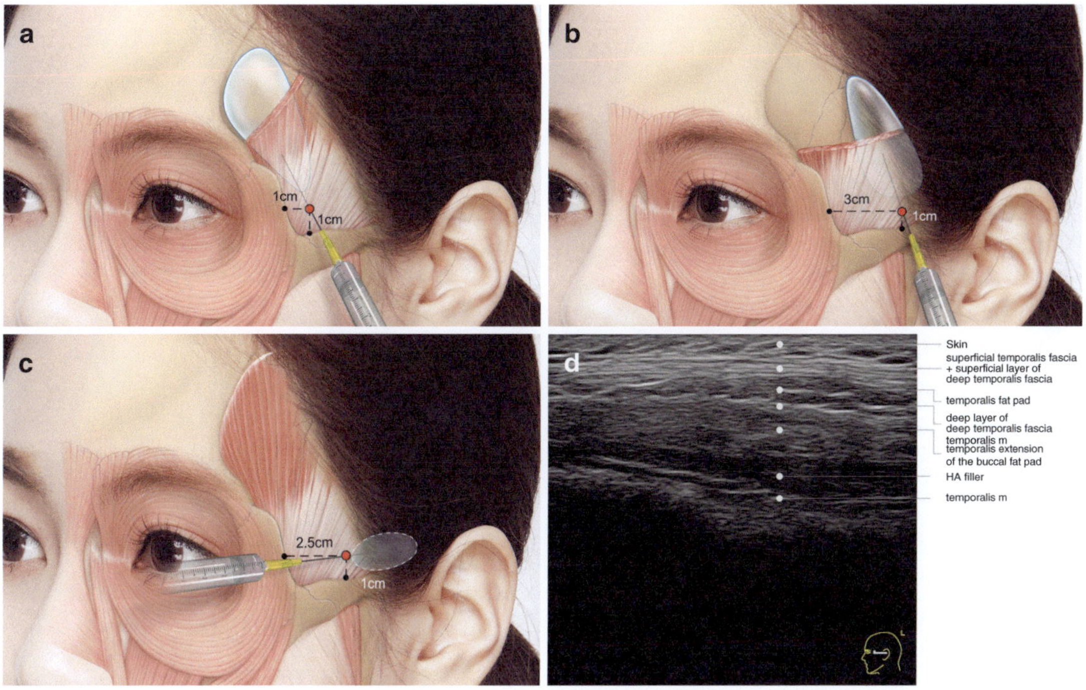

Fig. 4.14 Injection technique for temple augmentation. (**a**) Medial aspect of temple depression. (**b**) Lateral aspect of temple depression. (**c**) Inferolateral aspect of temple depression. (**d**) Proper placement of HA filler for temple augmentation as demonstrated by sonography

the orbital rim. Regarding the deeper lying vessels not immediately visible to the eye including the superficial temporal a. and v. and the middle temporal vein, an educated guess has to be taken regarding their possible pathways. Note, however, that individual variations exist in the course of these blood vessels and that deep structures such as temporal a. may be at risk during the deep periosteal injection. Therefore, compression of the treatment area for at least 3 min is required following treatment to prevent any unexpected hematoma formation, Failure to do so may cause the patient to experience immediate bulging at the temporal fossa or lumpiness under the zygomatic arch on the following day as a result of the hematoma trickling downwards through temporal extension of the buccal fat pad (Fig. 4.15). However, this should not be too much of a concern since the hematoma typically resolves spontaneously in approximately 1–2 week.

4.2.4.2 Embolism

Given its extensive vascularity, the temple area is susceptible to vascular embolism following treatment with HA fillers or Sculptra [8]. In this regard, the author's preferred method of delivering HA filler supraperiosteally via direct needle injection avoids the danger of severe vascular injury apart from the potential risk to the deep temporal a. and v. In each case, however, entry of the needle in the vessel is easily detectable. Penetration of the deep temporal artery can be immediately identified by the instantaneous reflux of blood up the syringe due to the arterial pressure (Fig. 3.6). Meanwhile, entry of the needle into the vein can be detected by aspiration prior to injection. Withdrawal of blood upon aspiration requires the needle to be removed and bleeding to be controlled with firm pressure for 5 mins before the procedure can be resumed.

4.2.4.3 Headache

Headache may occur for 1–2 days following treatment. Where persistent pain continues for more than 1–2 weeks, it is best to dissolve the HA filler with hyaluronidase. In my practice, I have observed only two cases involving persistent headaches following temple augmentation out of

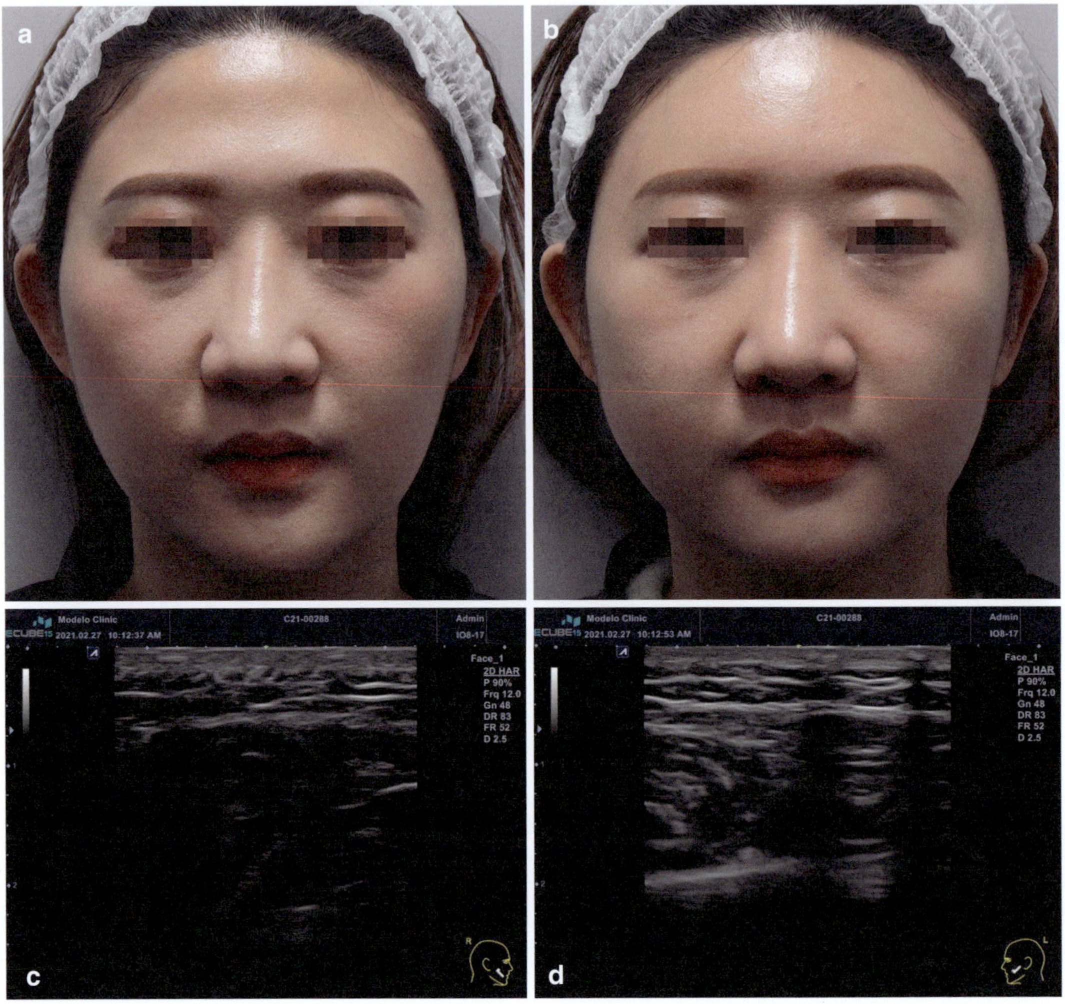

Fig. 4.15 Swelling developed at right buccal cheek 2 days after temporal volumization with HA filler. (**a**) Before (**b**) 2 days after injection (**c**) Sonography of right cheek clearly establishes the presence of hematoma, hypoechoic mass under the subcutaneous fat layer. (**d**) Sonography of normal cheek (left)

the hundreds of cases performed. The fact that symptoms resolved spontaneously upon dissolution of the HA filler suggests causation with HA filler placement.

4.2.4.4 Irregularity

The author's preferred approach of placing volume deep to the muscle avoids the risk of surface contour irregularities as the taut overlying structures bear down on the injected HA filler and even out its distribution. In contrast, superficial injections into the subcutaneous fatty layer or beneath the superficial temporal facia may result in the appearance of lumpiness, which must be dissolved away with hyaluronidase.

Tips: Use of needles and appropriate level of the injection for temple augmentation

While the author generally prefers the use of a cannula in performing volumizing HA filler treatments to minimize the risk of bruising and embolization, temple augmentation represents the one exception to the rule. In the case HA filler is placed superficially into the subcutaneous fatty layer, the thin skin overlying the temples is prone to resulting in product visibility, that is, the appearance of visible lumps and unevenness, and product palpability where the material tends to retrude and sink in when pressed down with the hand. In the alternative, some practitioners suggest that strategic placement of HA filler in the space between the superficial temporal fascia and the deep temporal fascia can achieve a more uniform distribution of HA filler while requiring less product than placements made deep to the muscle. In this approach, it is advised to pinch and lift the overlying skin away from the underlying muscle to pave the way for cannula advancement toward the proposed target space, as the superficial temporal fascia is attached to the skin while the deep temporal fascia has adhered to the muscle. However, it is not necessarily a straightforward matter to determine whether the right plane has been injected. Plus, the risk of visible irregularities and product palpability still exists though to a lesser degree than subcutaneous injections.

On the other hand, deep supraperiosteal injection using a 21-G long needle directly on bone allows for a quick and easy correction of recessed temples without the risk of surface irregularity thanks to the tight cover provided by the overlying structures of the temporalis m. or the deep temporal facia (Fig. 4.14d). The procedure is simple enough that it can be performed even by novice injectors. To the extent that the needle is used for the injection, however, aspiration prior to injection is a prerequisite.

4.3 Deep Glabella Furrow

Difficulty Level: B Effectiveness: A Complications: C

Summary 1: Caution must be taken to avoid the supratrochlear a. and supraorbital a. lying close to the glabella furrows, as inadvertent intravascular injection of HA filler into these arteries may result in devastating consequences of skin necrosis and blindness.

Summary 2: A glabellar "spread test" may be performed to assess the extent to which satisfactory improvement may be produced.

Summary 3: A 27-G × 3-cm cannula is used to inject HA filler deeply into the subcutaneous fat layer above the periosteum (i.e., the supraperiosteal layer) as well as superficially in the subdermal layer. A 30-G needle should be used exclusively for intradermal injections. Biphasic HA fillers with medium-sized particles or monophasic HA fillers with moderate viscoelasticity are acceptable for use.

Summary 4: The adjunct use of BoNT-A is required to relax the corrugator m. as the underlying cause giving rise to the appearance of dynamic glabella lines.

Loss of skin elasticity with age and repeated wrinkling in the glabella complex over time leads to the development of deep static glabella furrows engraved in the form of number 11 (hence the name "11 lines") or the Chinese character for "stream" (川). Unlike Caucasians who routinely mobilize the muscles of the forehead and glabella for communucating a broad range of thoughts and feelings, Asians tend to associate glabella lines primarily with negative sentiments such as frustration and anger, as these lines are considered to be formed principally by frowning and scowling. For this reason, correction of glabella lines represents the most popular indication for BoNT-A treatment in Koreans [6]. However, while the appearance of dynamic glabella lines may be reversed with BoNT-A injections, removal of deep static glabella furrows requires filling in with HA filler (Fig. 4.16).

4.3.1 Anatomical Considerations

The supratrochlear a. and supraorbital a. arising from the ophthalmic a. are located in the glabella

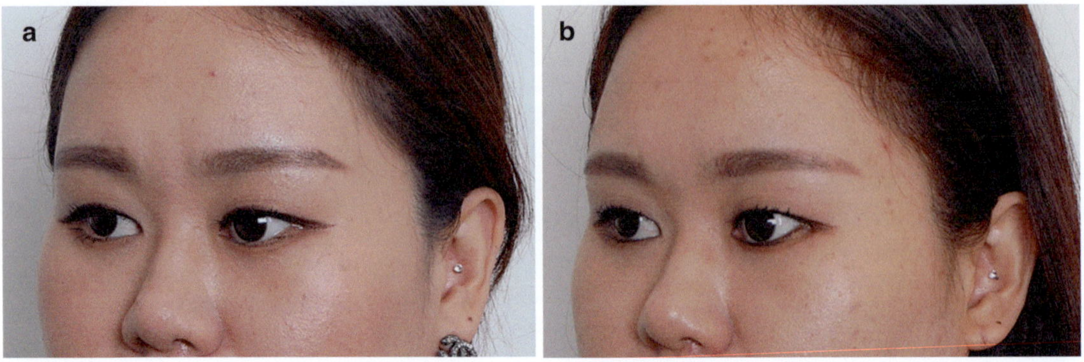

Fig. 4.16 Deep glabella furrows. (**a**) Before and (**b**) after injection of HA filler

complex. The supratrochlear a. arises near the medial canthus of the eye, while the supraorbital a. emerges from the supraorbital foramen or notch, and exits the orbit by piercing the orbital septum before ascending superiorly to the forehead where it courses between the frontalis m. and skin (Fig. 4.17) [7]. The supratrochlear a. not only lies relatively closer to the glabella furrows compared with the supraorbital artery but also runs superficially close to the skin surface. Consequently, the supratrochlear a. is at a greater risk of inadvertent intravascular filler injection during the HA treatment of the glabella which may result in subsequent necrosis of the skin or loss of vision. That said, injecting within the 18–22 mm area between the supratrochlear arteries is believed to be relatively safe because the supratrochlear artery usually runs 9–11 mm lateral to the midline of the glabella [8]. However, it is important to note that there are many variations in their branching pattern.

Though extremely rare, BoNT-A or local anesthetic agents targeted at the glabella area may accidentally be injected into the supratrochlear a., due to the proximity of the supratrochlear a.to the relevant injection points. When this occurs, the inadvertently injected BonT-A or nerve block can actually be observed shooting up toward the forehead through the supratrochlear a. coursing superficially beneath the skin surface. Supposing the injected material consisted of HA fillers, the occlusion of the supratrochlear a. in such case would lead to the devastating complication of necrosis of the forehead skin. Significantly, given that HA filler for glabellar rhytide correction is injected retrograde to the direction of the blood flow of the supratrochlear a., the resulting back-flow of the filler embolus into the ophthalmic a. would most likely lead to the disastrous complication of visual loss (see Sect. 5.1.4). Significantly, Beleznay et al. found the glabella to be the most commonly implicated site of filler-related blindness [9]. To avoid such dire consequences, the use of a cannula should be preferred to the needle for HA filler injections in the glabella, apart from when addressing surface wrinkles in the dermis, in which case, a needle should be used.

4.3.2 Pretreatment Assessment

To define the relevant treatment area, determine first whether the furrows are configured in the form of number 11 or the Chinese character for stream (川) fanning out over a wider territory. It must also be decided whether the patient requires volume restoration of the deep furrows only or additional refinement of static lines ingrained on the skin surface like scratch marks. This is because HA fillers are suitable primarily for filling in deep grooves or depressions, rather than addressing skin surface changes. Permanently etched-in glabella lines on the skin surface are typically associated with textural changes on the skin surface, as well as the adhesion of the skin overlying these lines to the scar-like fibrous tissue lying below. As such, superficial etched-in lines on the skin surface are generally not amenable to treatment with HA filler alone (Fig. 4.18).

Consideration must also be given to any concurrent central forehead depressions above the glabella region or any horizontal indentations or depressions in the nasion located below. Undercorrection is advised in patients with a prominent

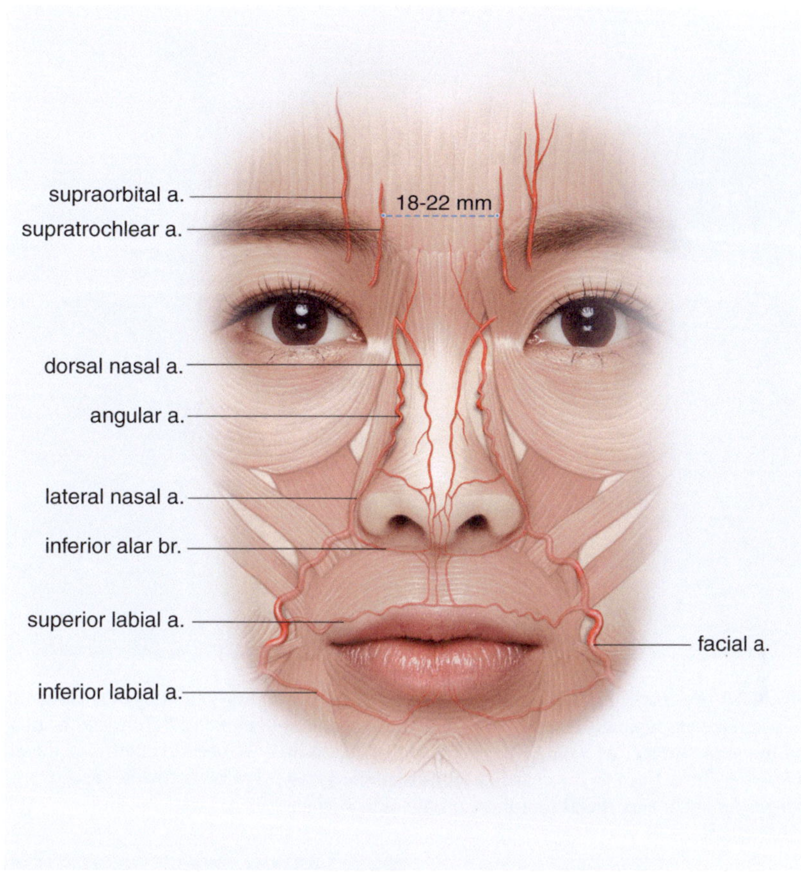

Fig. 4.17 Vascular patterns of the nose and glabellar region

superciliary arch, as full leveling of the glabella furrows in these individuals serves to highlight the left and right superciliary ridges above the medial canthus. A glabella "spread test" can be used to determine the spreadability of the furrow and the extent to which a satisfactory improvement may be produced (Fig. 4.18).

4.3.3 Injection Technique (Table 4.3)

A biphasic HA filler with medium-sized particles or a monophasic HA filler with moderate viscoelasticity is recommended for treating the glabella region. For deep glabella furrows, a 27-G × 3-cm cannula is used to deliver the HA filler in the deep subcutaneous plane above the periosteum (supraperiosteal layer) via the retrograde linear threading technique and subsequently in the subdermal layer to complete the

Table 4.3 Summary of glabella furrow injection technique

Item	Contents
Needle vs. Cannula	27-G 3-cm cannula for the deep layer 30-G needle for the intradermal layer
HA filler	Biphasic HA filler with intermediate particle size or monophasic HA filler with moderate viscoelasticity
Amount of HA filler	0.3–1 mL
Depth of injection	Supraperiosteal layer and deep subcutaneous layer Intradermal layer for superficial correction
Entry point for cannula	0.5–1 cm above each furrow
Target area	Deep glabellar furrows rather than the fine lines etched on the skin surface
Anesthetics	Topical anesthetics
Nondominant hand	Hold the forehead skin upward

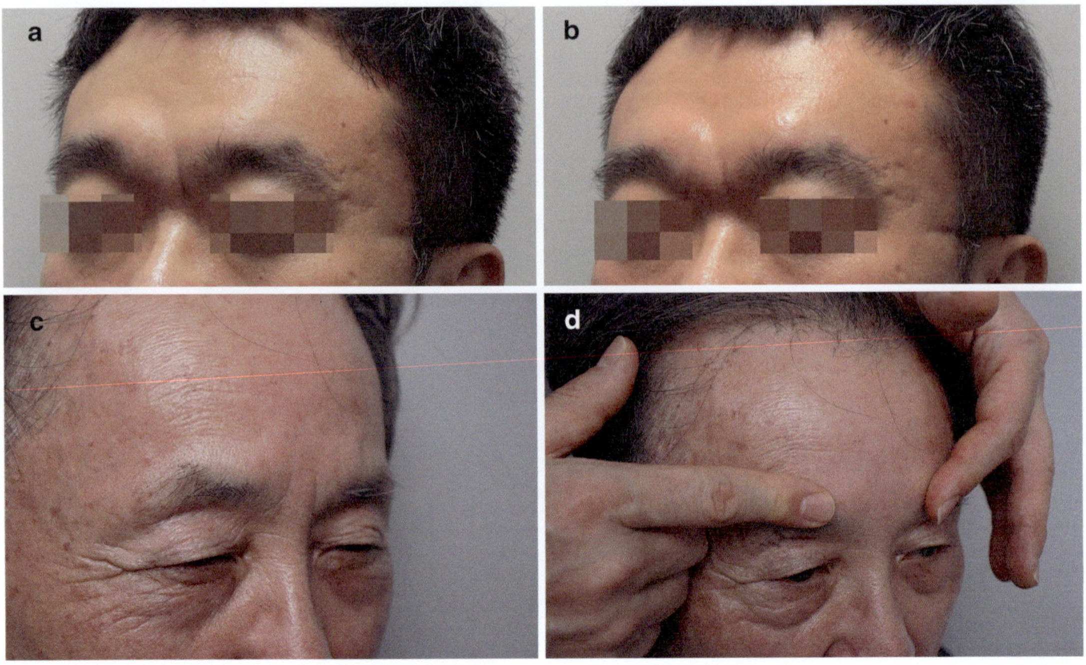

Fig. 4.18 Permanently etched-in glabella lines on the skin surface are typically associated with textural changes on the skin surface, as well as the adhesion of the skin overlying these lines to the scar-like fibrous tissue lying below. As such, superficial fine lines on the skin surface are generally not amenable to treatment with HA filler alone (**a** before and **b** after). A glabella "spread test" can be used to determine the efficacy of filler injection for the galbella furrow (**c**, **d**)

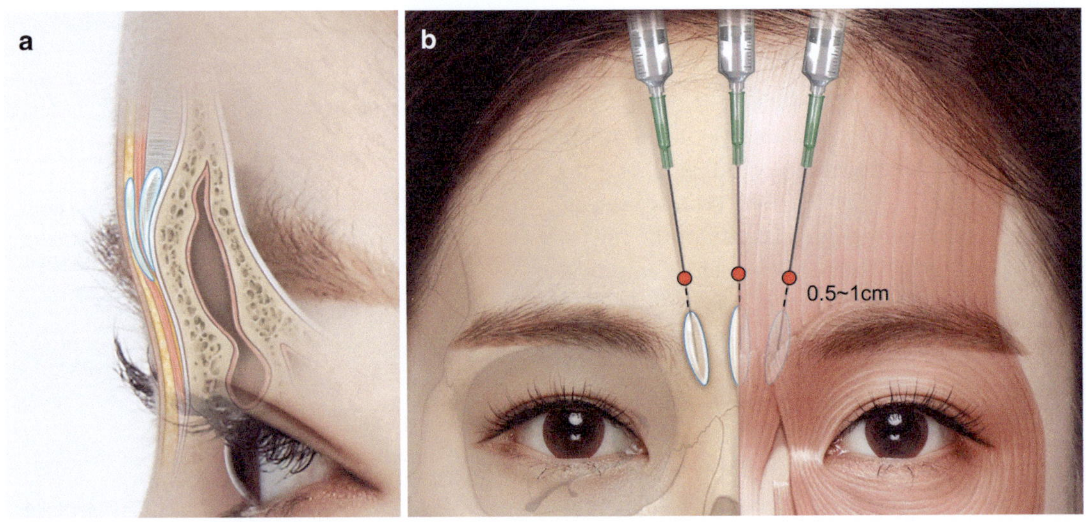

Fig. 4.19 Injection technique for deep glabella furrows. (**a**) HA filler placed in the deep subcutaneous plane above the periosteum and subsequently in the subdermal layer. (**b**) The cannula entry point

procedure (Fig. 4.18). A 30-G needle may be used for superficial correction of residual surface wrinkles in the dermal layer. To prevent inadvertent intravascular filler injection, the procedure should be performed exclusively using a cannula. The needle may be used only for performing superficial corrections in the intradermal layer. The cannula entry point is created 0.5–1 cm above each furrow as it extends superiorly toward the forehead (Fig. 4.19). The injection volume usually ranges from 0.3 to 1 mL depending on the depth or severity of the groove.

The use of topical anesthetic cream is sufficient for local numbing. The nondominant hand is used to stretch the forehead skin superiorly during the injection. HA filler treatment of glabella furrows should preferably be combined with the BoNT-A injection to the corrugator m., the contraction of which triggers the appearance of glabella furrows in the first place. In the absence of adjunct BoNT-A injections, the frequent movement of the corrugator muscles may displace the HA filler from its originally deposited location, leading to the recurrence of glabella grooves or the migration of HA filler to noninjected areas. Where concavities are concurrently present in the central forehead, volume should also be added in the sunken forehead to allow a smooth transition down to the glabella. Likewise, in patients presenting with a congenitally low nasion or horizontal indentation traversing under the glabella, it is advisable to restore volume in these areas simultaneously.

4.3.4 Complications

Irregularities: Full leveling of the glabella furrows in patients with a pronounced superciliary arch or a sunken central forehead may accentuate the prominence of the superciliary arch. Meanwhile, treatment of glabella furrows with HA fillers alone without the combined use of BoNT-A may cause migration and aggregation of the injected HA filler due to surrounding muscle contractions, resulting in contour irregularities.

Skin necrosis and blindness are also potential complications (see Sect. 5.1.4).

4.4 Sunken Eyes Volumization

Difficulty Level: C, Effectiveness: A, Complications: B

> *Summary 1*: Treatment is performed with a 27-G 5-cm cannula. The target plane of injection is the preseptal layer.

> *Summary 2*: The cannula entry point is created 0.3 mm lateral to the bony orbital rim at the level of the lash line or the tarsal fold. Insert the cannula at a 20°–30° angle to the horizontal and coronal plane, and advance along the margin of the orbital rim toward the superomedial direction. Place product below the bony orbital roof while withdrawing the cannula.

> *Summary 3*: Aim for a moderate undercorrection of 50–70% improvement with the eyes open to prevent the appearance of bulges when the eyes are closed.

> *Summary 4*: Identify the presence of any eyelid ptosis or hooding as the underlying cause of sunken eyes. Refer the patient for surgery where conditions are severe.

Hollowness in the upper eyelid is one of the key indicators of an aging face. Sunken eyes, also referred to as sunken upper eyelids, sunken superior sulcus, or upper eyelid hollowing, can occur due to a multitude of factors. It can be caused by a congenitally prominent orbital bony framework typically found in Caucasians or can be associated with an underlying eyelid ptosis or a severe dermatochalasis, in which case, the patient may seek to compensate for their weak levator m. by contracting the frontalis muscle to open the eye. Supraorbital hollowing may also appear due to the loss of septal fat volume with aging or weight loss. Though rare, septal fat loss may also occur due to its aggressive removal during an upper eyelid blepharoplasty. In Caucasians who tend to have a narrow distance between the eyes and the brow, the appearance of deep-set eyes is often innately created by a combination of congenital factors including the relatively protruded bony orbit and the direct insertion of the levator palpebral superioris m. into the dermis. By contrast, in Asians with a wide distance between the eyes and the brow, the levator m. attaches to the tarsus rather than the skin, causing the septal fat to descend and sit on the eyelid and contributing to

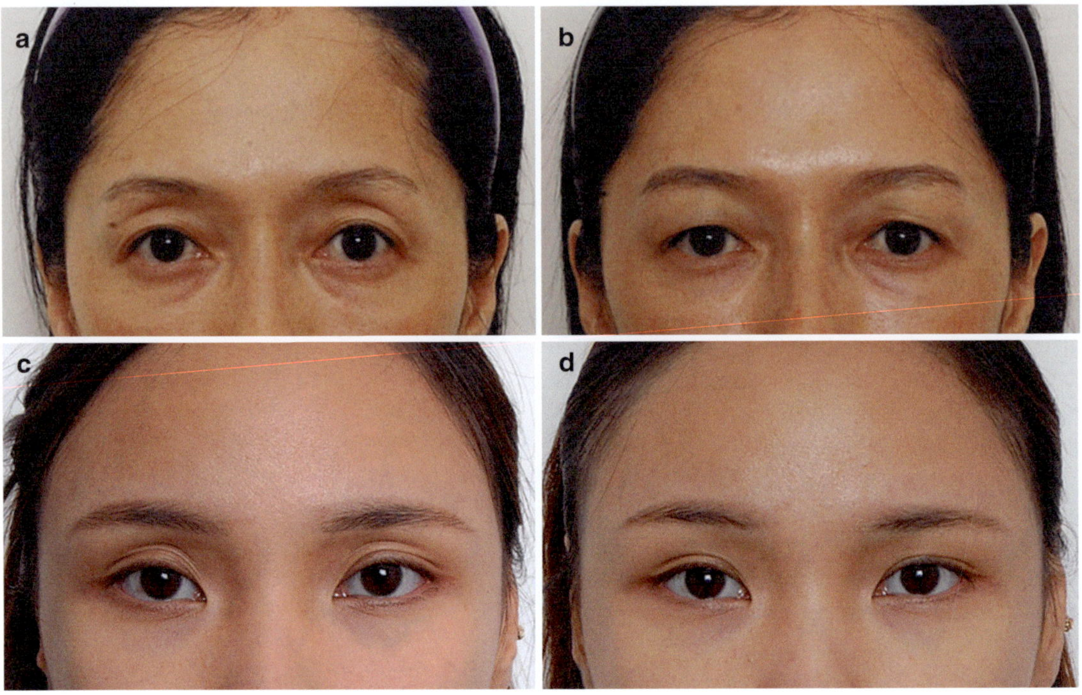

Fig. 4.20 (**a**, **c**) Before and (**b**, **d**) after sunken eye volumization

an innate fullness in the eyelid. For this reason, hollowness in the upper eyelid in Asians tends to impart an overaged appearance (Fig. 4.20).

The relevant solution to upper eyelid hollowness varies according to the underlying cause of the problem. Where the sunken appearance is traceable to an underlying eyelid ptosis or dermatochalasis, surgical corrections such as a ptosis surgery or blepharoplasty can provide the definitive solution by obviating the need for compensatory frontalis m. contraction for retracting the eyelid upwards. Such improvements can be mimicked, to a certain degree, by use of BoNT-A for relaxing the frontalis m. in patients with eyelid ptosis (Fig. 4.21). On the other hand, where the supraorbital hollowing is caused by the loss of septal fat, correction is provided by replacing the lost volume via surgical septal fat repositioning, fat grafting, or HA filler placement. It bears noting that sunken eye augmentation is a technically challenging procedure requiring extreme precision and finesse in technique, as the molding after the injection is almost impossible due to the soft characteristics of eyeball. Moreover, the fine skin overlying the upper eyelid tends to easily reveal any filler imperfections, while the bumpiness further increases when the eye is open and closed.

4.4.1 Anatomical Considerations

From the outer to inner, the upper eyelid is layered as follows: the skin—subcutaneous fat—orbicularis oculi m—preseptal fat—orbital septum—septal fat or intraorbital fat (Fig. 4.22) The fat tissues of the upper eyelid consist of the subcutaneous fat underlying the skin, the preseptal fat present anterior to the orbital septum, and the septal fat, also known as the retroseptal fat or the intraorbital fat lying behind the septum. While the septal fat constitutes the bulk of the upper lid volume, volume replacement with HA is directed primarily at the preseptal space since the cannula cannot easily penetrate and reach behind the rigid orbital septum.

4.4.2 Pretreatment Assessment

Assess the eyes for any underlying conditions such as eyelid ptosis or hooding (dermatochalasis)

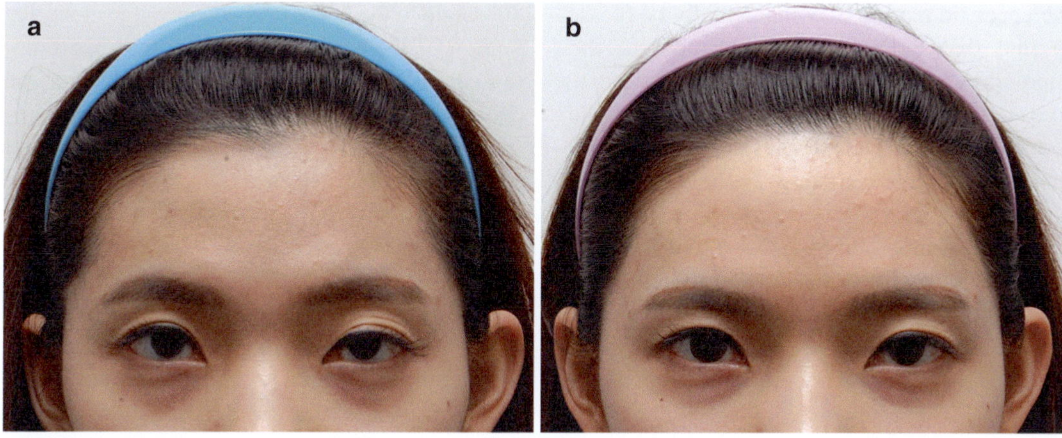

Fig. 4.21 Botulinum toxin injection for relaxing the frontalis m. in a 26-year-old patient with eyelid ptosis may improve the sunken eye. (**a**) Before and (**b**) after injection

Fig. 4.22 Depth of injection for sunken eye volumization

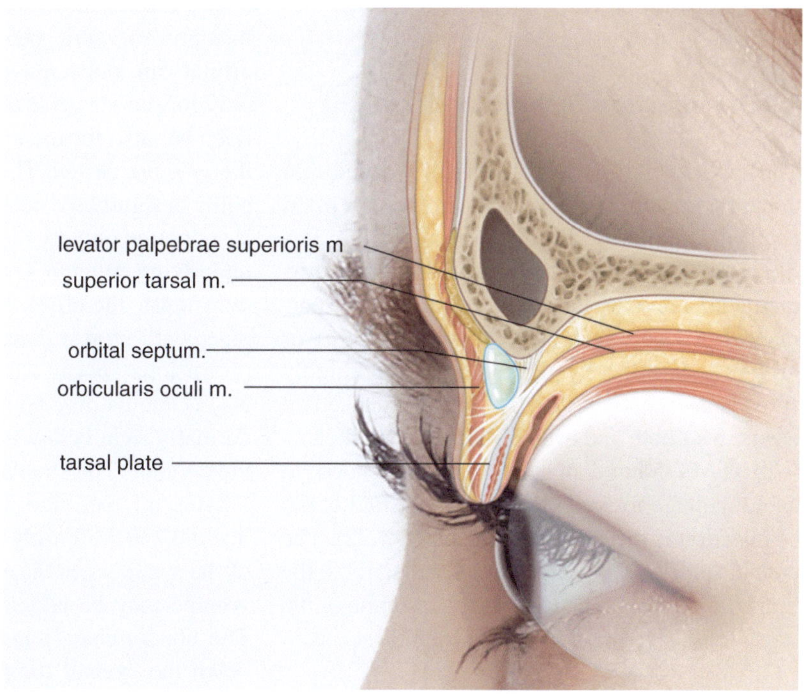

which may give rise to the sunken appearance. Where conditions are severe, the patient should be advised to undergo a definitive surgery instead. While ptosis per se does not constitute a contraindication for sunken eye correction with HA, patients with droopy eyelids may occasionally complain of perceived heaviness when opening the eyes following treatment. In a vast majority of cases, however, patients tend to express greater comfort with which they can roll up their eyelids post-treatment. It can be conjectured that this is due to the lubrication and hydration provided by the HA filler placed between the septum and the orbicularis oculi m.

Regarding patient selection, patients in their late 50s and above presenting with severely hooded eyelids are not ideal candidates as the procedure may serve to exacerbate the redundancy of the eyelid skin, reducing, if not eliminating, the visibility of the pretarsal crease as a result. On the other hand, patients with eyelid ptosis manifesting an abnormally low position of the upper lid margin may incidentally be pleased to find that the volume replacement to their supraorbital hollows has helped to restore the folds to the normal height. Finally, the procedure is not suitable for patients presenting with exophthalmoses, as it may cause the bulging appearance of the eyes to become more pronounced.

It is also important to assess the precise location, that is, medial or lateral, and severity of the volume loss in the upper eyelid. Note that less is best when volumizing this area, and that the treatment should aim for a moderate under-correction, or a 50–70% improvement in the hollowness with the eyes open, as even severe hollowness is inconspicuous when the eyes are closed. Full correction with the eyes open may thus result in bulging of the lids when the eyes are closed.

4.4.3 Injection Technique (Table 4.4)

The upper eyelid is a delicate area of reduced skin thickness, where volume replacement can often result in lumpiness. Accordingly, reversible HA fillers are the ideal choice for injecting this unforgiving area and are more preferable to other permanent products such as collagen stimulators or fat grafts. Specifically, the use of soft and highly spreadable monophasic HA filler is advised to ensure a smooth and even distribution of filler.

A 27-G 5-cm cannula is recommended to avoid damage to the eyeballs. The desired depth of injection is the preseptal layer (Fig. 4.22). The cannula entry point is created 0.3 cm lateral to the bony orbital rim at the level of the lash line or the tarsal fold (Fig. 4.23). Insert the cannula at a 20°–30° angle to the horizontal and advance along the margin of the orbital rim toward the superomedial direction. More importantly, advance the cannul at a 20°–30° angle posteriorly at the coronal plane before touching the bony orbital roof. Place the material below the orbital roof while withdrawing the cannula. As noted above, the relevant injection plane is in the preseptal layer superficial to the septum, as penetrating the tough, rigid orbital septum with a cannula is extremely difficult and painful even if it were possible. Where hollowness is the severest in the medial aspect of the upper eyelid, most of the volume should be located in the medial hollows, followed by HA filler delivered under constant pressure along the orbital rim margin using the retrograde linear thread technique. Finish the injection 0.5 cm before reaching the lateral orbital rim and remove the cannula. Check not only for the presence of lumps when the eyes are open but also for the appearance of bulges when the eyes are closed. The upper eyelid is not amenable to significant postinjection molding since it is supported only by the soft eyeball with no hard underlying structures to push against. The procedure must, therefore, be undertaken in the first place with utmost precision and caution. In case protrusions appear when the eyes are closed, a 30-G cannula may be used to add HA filler subdermally right below the protrusion to smoothen the contour. The standard amount of HA filler is 0.2–0.5 mL per side. It is advisable to initially inject 0.2–0.3 mL only and check for any bulging of the eyelid when the eyes are closed. Additional volume may be added as needed subsequently. The nondominant hand should be used to press down the eyeball for protection during cannula advancement. Apart from the slight discomfort felt when the eyeball is pushed downward, there is hardly any pain during HA filler injection. Concerning anesthesia, a local anesthetic applied at the cannula entry point should suffice.

Table 4.4 Summary of sunken eye augmentation technique

Item	Contents
Needle vs. Cannula	27-G 4-cm
HA filler	Monophasic HA filler
Amount of HA filler	0.2–0.5 mL per side
Depth of injection	Preseptal layer
Entry point for cannula	0.3 cm lateral to the bony orbital rim
Target area	Sunken upper lid sulcus
Anesthetics	Local anesthetics at the entry point
Nondominant hand	Press the eyeball downward

4.4.4 Complications

Irregularities: The skin overlying the upper eyelid is thin and prone to developing lumpiness when injected with HA fillers. Hence, aiming for

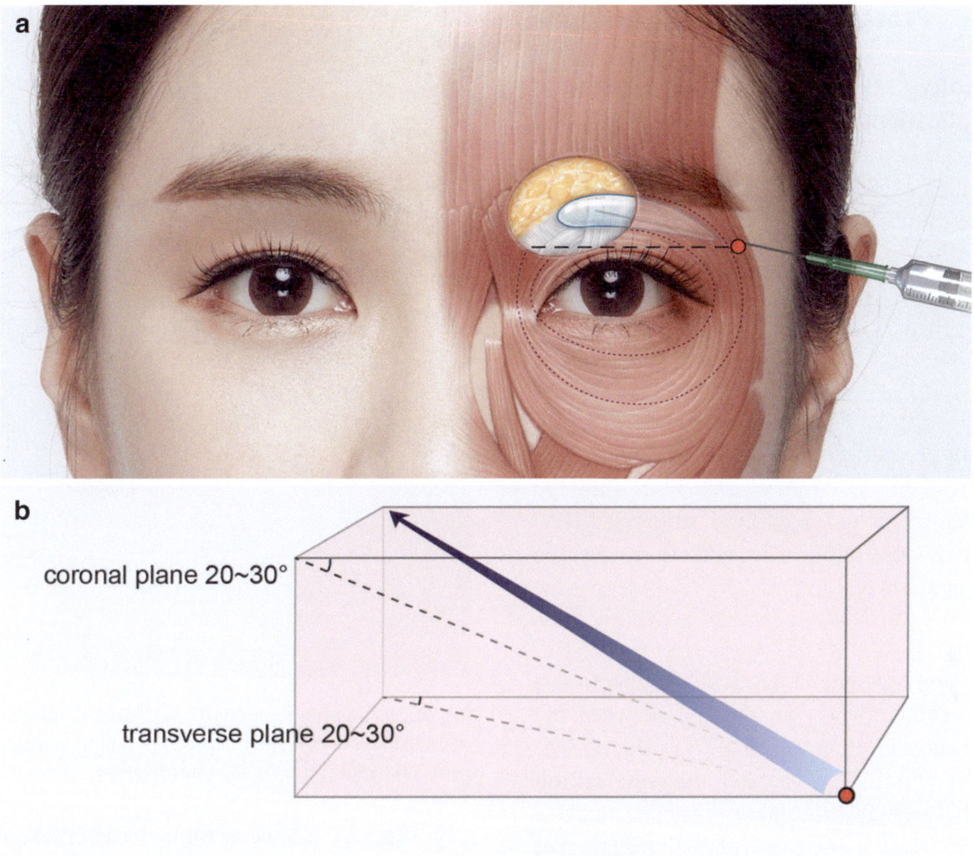

Fig. 4.23 The entry point and the direction fo the cannula for sunken eye volumization (**a**) Insert the cannula at a 20°–30° angle to the horizontal toward the superomedial direction. (**b**) advance the cannul at a 20°–30° angle posteriorly from the coronal plane before touching the bony orbital roof

full correction with the eyes open can lead to the appearance of lumps when the eyes are closed (Fig. 4.24). Contour irregularities from HA injection cannot be massaged in easily and should rather be dissolved away.

Bruising: Care should be taken to avoid damaging the sentinel v. or the superior palpebral v. running in close proximity to the periorbital area. Preinjection of dental lidocaine containing epinephrine at the cannula entry point is advised to reduce vascular injury.

Heaviness in the eyelid: Heaviness in the eyelid is an occasional occurrence in patients with eyelid ptosis.

Narrowing or elimination of supratarsal crease: Narrowing or elimination of the supratarsal crease is an occasional occurrence in patients in their late 40s and above presenting with eyelid hooding or dermatochalasis.

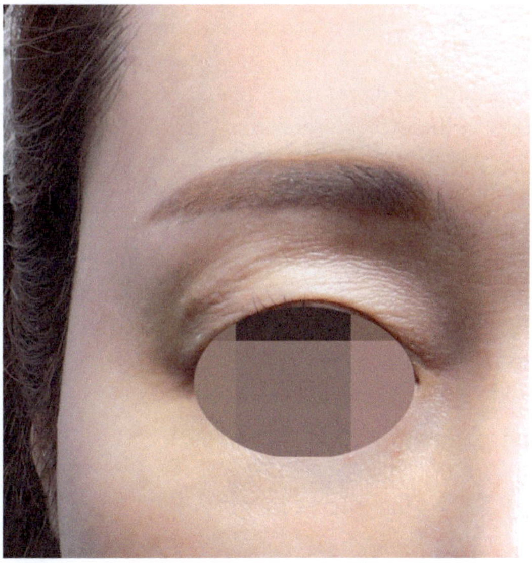

Fig. 4.24 Irregularity of the upper eyelid following HA injection for the sunken eye

4.5 Pretarsal Roll Augmentation

Difficulty Level: C, Effectiveness: A, Complications: B

Summary 1: Pretarsal roll, or the hypertrophy of the pretarsal aspect of the orbicularis oculi muscle at the lower eyelid, represents one of the salient elements that culminate in the ideal "Korean look."

Summary 2: The use of a 30-G 3 cm cannula is advised to prevent bruising and unwanted injection of HA filler into the inferior medial palpebral artery (IMPA) which runs along the eyelash under the orbicularis oculi m.

Summary 3: The target depth of injection is the subdermal layer, that is, between the dermis and the pretarsal part of the orbicularis oculi m. The shape of the pretarsal roll should ideally resemble a banana, narrow in the medial one-third, and slightly thicker in the lateral aspect.

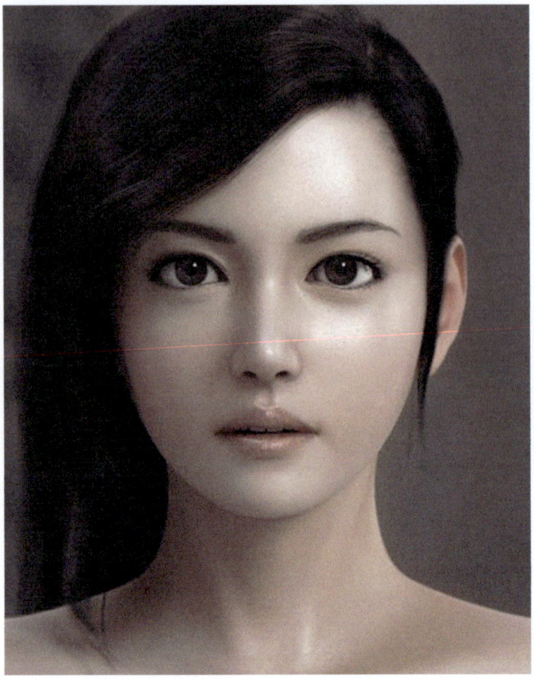

Fig. 4.25 Cyborg embodying the "Korean look" featuring a the small oval egg-shaped face, plump cheeks, large eyes, pretarsal roll and a tall narrow nose

Pretarsal roll, or the hypertrophy of the pretarsal aspect of the orbicularis oculi muscle at the lower eyelid, is a long "*roll*" formed along the length of the lower tarsal plate upon the contraction of the orbicularis oculi while smiling. Since the pretarsal roll generally becomes more pronounced upon smiling, the presence of pretarsal fullness at rest naturally imparts a soft, friendly, and smiley impression. The visual effect of the pretarsal roll on the lower eyelid is equivalent to that of supratarsal crease on the upper eyelid in terms of making the eyes appear larger overall by adding an extra frame around the eye fissure. For this reason, it is often dubbed "supratarsal crease *for the lower lid*." Volumizing the pretarsal roll also has the incidental effect of reducing the exposure of the lower white sclera in those with a scleral show, diminishing the negative, scary image associated with it.

From the Caucasian viewpoint, however, the pretarsal roll may be considered a factor that causes the relatively small palpebral aperture in Asians to appear even smaller upon smiling. In this regard, a BoNT-A indication had previously been proposed for the removal of pretarsal roll in Asians [10]. However, the result was deemed aesthetically undesirable from the Korean aesthetic standard, and there are no doctors in Korea currently performing this indication to the best of my knowledge. On the contrary, the pretarsal roll represents one of the salient elements, together with the small oval egg-shaped face, plump cheeks, large eyes, and a tall narrow nose that culminate in the ideal "Korean look" (Fig. 4.25). Accordingly, volumizing the pretarsal roll with HA fillers continues to be a popular indication among many Koreans (Fig. 1.25 and Fig. 4.26).

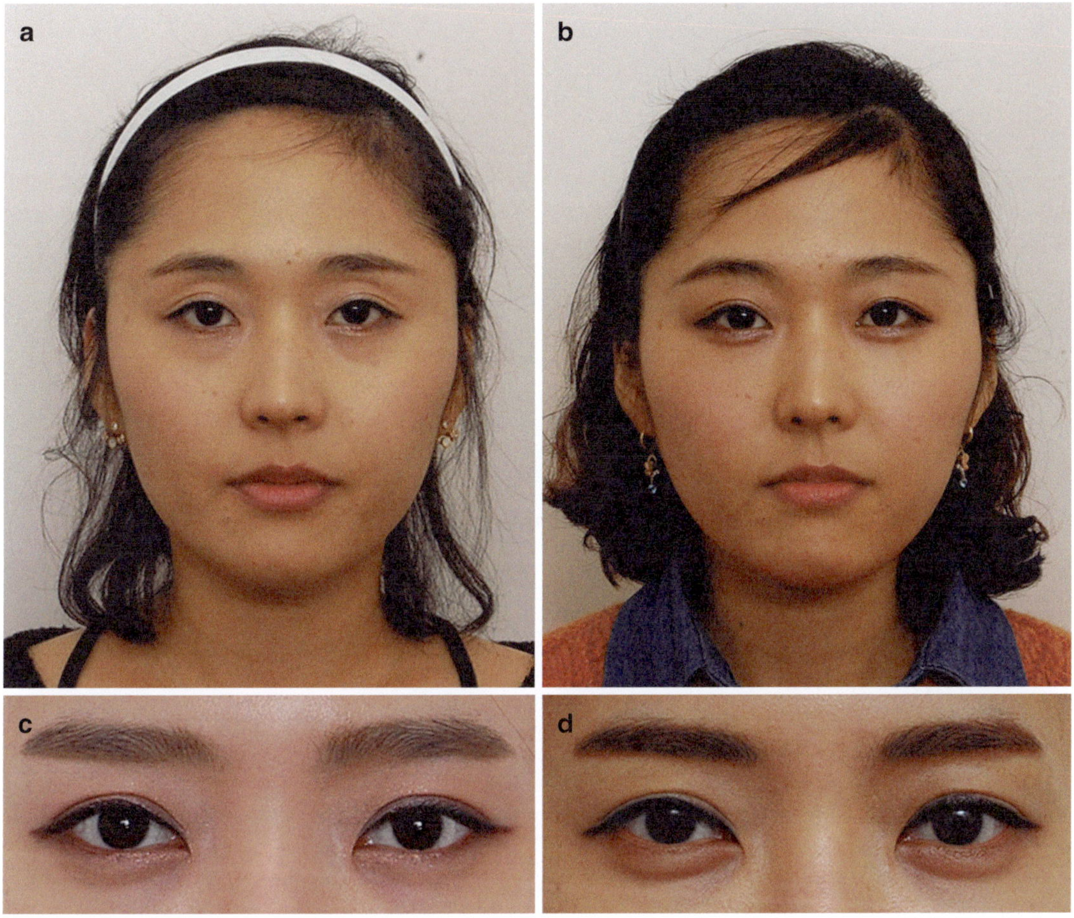

Fig. 4.26 (**a**, **c**) Before and (**b**, **d**) after volumizing the pretarsal roll with HA filler combined with the volumization of sunken eyes and infraorbital hollows

4.5.1 Anatomical Considerations

The anatomical layers of the lower eyelid from the outer to inner consist of the skin—subdermal layer—orbicularis oculi m.—tarsal plate—mucosa. At the pretarsal roll, the inferior medial palpebral artery (IMPA), a branch of the ophthalmic a. runs along the eyelash between the tarsal plate and orbicularis oculi m. (Fig. 4.27) [7]. This arterial branch supplies the tarsal plate of the lower eyelids and has a diameter of approx. 1 mm at the medial canthus. For this reason, injecting too deep near the tarsal plate using a needle may cause intravascular injection of filler directly through the ophthalmic a. [11].

4.5.2 Pretreatment Assessment

Prior to treatment, due consideration must be given to the patient's age, skin elasticity, the width and height of the eyes, the thickness of tarsal plate (i.e., size of the pretarsal roll), presence or absence of lower eyebag, as well as any history of a previous lower blepharoplasty. Age should be checked for the same reason as the patient's skin elasticity; patients in their fifth decade and above and, for that matter, patients below the age of 50 but demonstrating skin laxity are at a greater risk for developing contour irregularity or an overly thickened pretarsal roll.

The thickness of the patient's own tarsal plate informs the potential shape and size of the

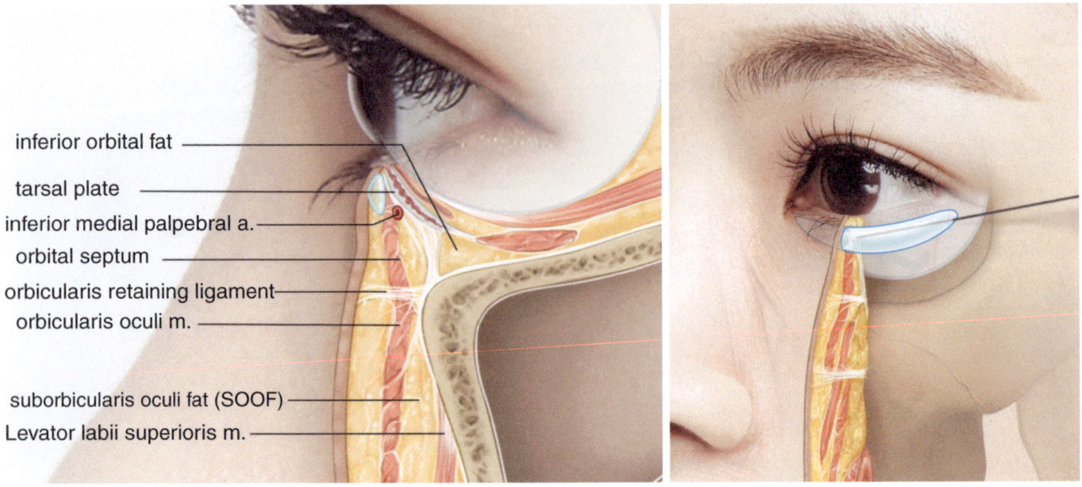

Fig. 4.27 Depth of injection for pretarsal roll augmentation

pretarsal roll to be obtained posttreatment, which can be assessed by instructing the patient to smile to trigger the contraction of orbicularis oculi m. or by manually pushing the patient's tarsal plate upwards with a finger. The patient should be advised, however, that the actual thickness of the pretarsal roll created with HA is greater than what is spontaneously generated by the contraction of the orbicularis oculi m. during smiling. Whereas the pretarsal fullness from orbicularis oculi contraction manifests in the form of a narrow roll under the lower lash line protruding forwards upon a smile, the pretarsal roll created with HA is subject to pressure from multiple directions which causes the deposited volume to diffuse omnidirectionally, that is, expanding not only anteriorly but also inferiorly, resulting in greater thickness.

Next, assessment should also be made of the width and height of the eyes, or more technically, the horizontal length and vertical height of the eye aperture. An overly thick pretarsal roll relative to the size of the eye aperture can appear disproportionate and out of balance. Note that pronounced pretarsal fullness on eyes with short width of eye aperture creates a particularly odd, worm-like appearance. The appropriate thickness of the pretarsal roll relative to the width and height of the eye aperture, based on measurements taken of ten Korean female celebrities with natural-looking pretarsal rolls including Tae-Hee Kim, was found to be within 30% of the eye width and 65% of the height (Fig. 4.28).

The presence of lower eye bags must also be identified as any incorrect positioning of the HA filler below the lower tarsal plate can exacerbate the puffy appearance of the lower eyelid area. To prevent such occurrence, the HA filler should be placed as close to the lower lash line as possible to create a sharp distinction from the infraorbital fat located inferior to the pretarsal roll. Alternatively, surgical removal of the eye bags might be a more viable option where the lower eye bags is such that it obscures the appearance of the patient's own pretarsal roll.

Note that pretarsal roll augmentation is relatively contraindicated in patients with a history of lower eyelid blepharoplasty or trichiasis surgery (Fig. 4.29). Scar tissue adhesions formed in the lower eyelash from such procedures limit the space for HA filler placement along the lash line and result in lumpiness even if the HA filler is placed slightly inferior to the lash line.

That notwithstanding, pretarsal roll augmentation may still be attempted despite such history where the patient so desires, considering the visibly softer appearance it helps to foster. Besides, reversing the HA filler is a straightforward matter if the outcome turns out to be unfavorable. In the author's experience, one-third of the patients in

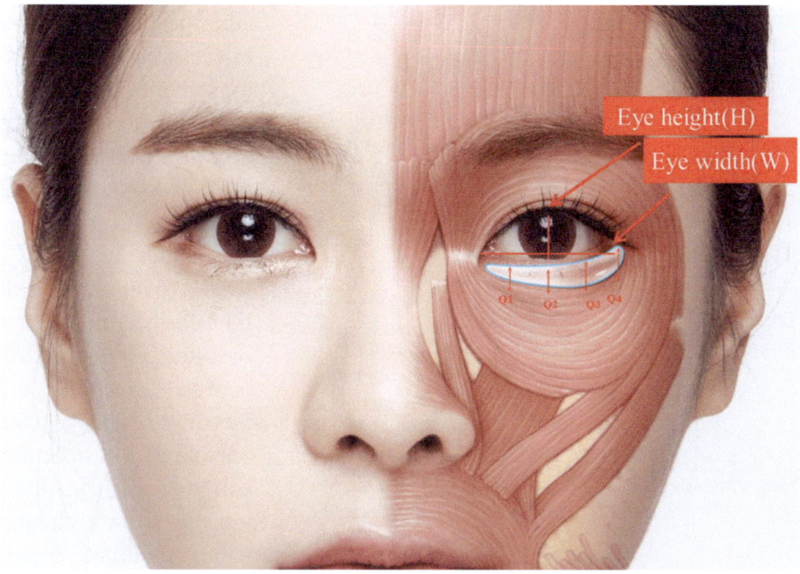

Fig. 4.28 Attractive thickness of a pretarsal roll relative to the width and height of the eye aperture, based on measurements taken of ten Korean female celebrities with natural-looking pretarsal rolls including Tae-Hee Kim, Young-Ae Lee, Hye-Kyo Song, etc, was found to be within 30% of the eye width and 65% of the height

Proportion to the width of eye aperture(%)				Proportion to the height of eye aperture(%)			
Q1	Q2	Q3	Q4	Q1	Q2	Q3	Q4
19	24	24	27	51	63	64	72

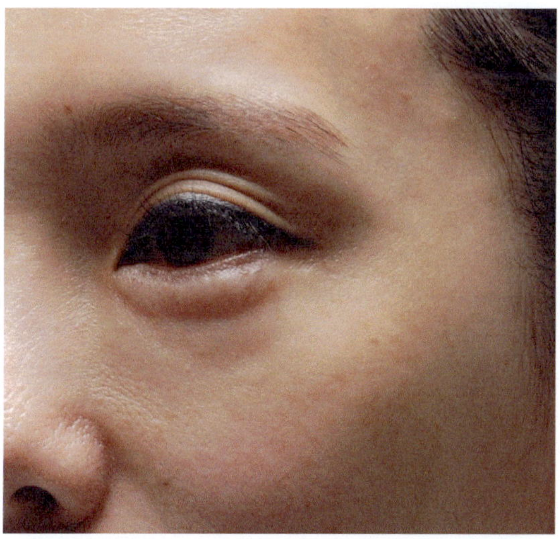

Fig. 4.29 Irregularity in pretarsal roll augmentation in a 45-year-old woman with scar tissue adhesions formed in the lower eyelash due to a history of lower eyelid blepharoplasty

such case eventually chose to have the HA filler dissolved, while the remaining two-thirds opted to retain the pretarsal fullness. In this respect, patients with a previous medial or lateral canthoplasty must also be forewarned of potentially suboptimal outcomes in their previously operated sites.

4.5.3 Injection Technique (Table 4.5)

To avoid the Tyndall effect, it is preferable to use a biphasic HA filler, given its lower water retention property, while keeping the injection volume to the minimum. The use of a 30-G 3cm cannula is advised to prevent bruising and unwanted injection of HA filler into the inferior medial palpebral artery (IMPA). The entry point for cannula insertion is made 0.5 cm inferolateral to the

Table 4.5 Summary of pretarsal roll augmentation injection technique

Item	Contents
Needle vs. Cannula	30-G 3-cm cannula
HA filler	Biphasic HA filler with intermediate particle size
Amount of HA filler	0.1–0.3 mL per side
Depth of injection	Subdermal layer
Entry point for cannula	0.5 cm inferolateral to the lateral canthus
Target area	Pretarsal roll
Anesthetics	Epi-lidocaine injection in the cannula entry points or an infraorbital nerve block Application of local eye drop with alcaine
Nondominant hand	Press and bend the cannul tip during the advancement of the cannula and press the lower border of pretarsal roll upward during injection

lateral canthus (Fig. 4.30). On occasion, an additional entry point may be created midway along the pretarsal roll in eyes with significant horizontal length. The target depth of injection is the subdermal layer, that is, between the dermis and the orbicularis oculi m., to avoid hitting the IMPA running deep to the orbicularis oculi m. (Fig. 4.28). The shape of the pretarsal roll should ideally resemble that of a banana, narrow in the medial one-third, and slightly thicker in the lateral aspect. This is achieved by depositing the HA filler in a retrograde manner starting with tiny amount of filler from near the medial canthus immediately below the lower eyelash to run parallel to the lower lash line, while excercising particular care to inject with precision and constant pressure to avoid lumpiness or an overly thick appearance.

The pretarsal region is a soft, delicate region not readily amenable to substantial postinjection molding. As such, the use of HA fillers is advised given their reversibility in case of any contingencies. Also, the use of biphasic HA is preferred over the more hydrophilic monophasic HA, to minimize the risk of the Tyndall effect or swelling from excessive water retention. The adequate injection volume is 0.1–0.3 mL per side, subject to individual variations in the desired volume. Anesthesia consists primarily of epi-lidocaine injection in the cannula entry points, as the use of topical anesthetic ointment is not readily applicable in the periorbital region. An infraorbital nerve block may be considered in patients with low pain tolerance. Alcaine® eye drop (i.e. a local anesthetic eye drop) can be used prior to injection in case bleeding occurs from the rupture of the IMPA, to numb the mucosal part of the lower eyelid before cotton tips are applied to control the bleeding. Once the IMPA is ruptured by a needle or even a cannula, it is difficult to control the bleeding simply by compressing the site from the outside as the structure is supported only by the soft eyeball. In such case, compression with cotton tips from both sides of the lower eyelid can better facilitate bleeding control. During the advancement of the cannula, the second finger of the non-dominant hand should be engaged to slightly press and bend the cannula tip at the medial one third of the pretarsal roll in order to facilitate the movement of the straight cannula through the convexly curved pretarsal roll. During the injection, the second and third fingers of the nondominant hand should be engaged to press the lower border of pretarsal roll upwards in order to avoid an overly thick pretarsal roll from the spreading down of the deposited HA filler during injection.

4.5.4 Complications

Complications relating to pretarsal roll volumization consist largely of aesthetic concerns arising from poor placement such as lumpiness (Fig. 4.31), sub-optimal shape, an overly thick appearance, and other complications such as the Tyndall effect and vascular compromise including bruising and intravascular injection, among others. As mentioned, rupture of the IMPA may occur even with the use of a cannula. Failure to control the bleeding immediately and properly in such event may lead to severe bruising that can spread even into the white sclera, resulting in an unsightly bloodshot appearance for up to one month. Therefore, timely detection of the rupture is of essence, as is its adequate management consisting

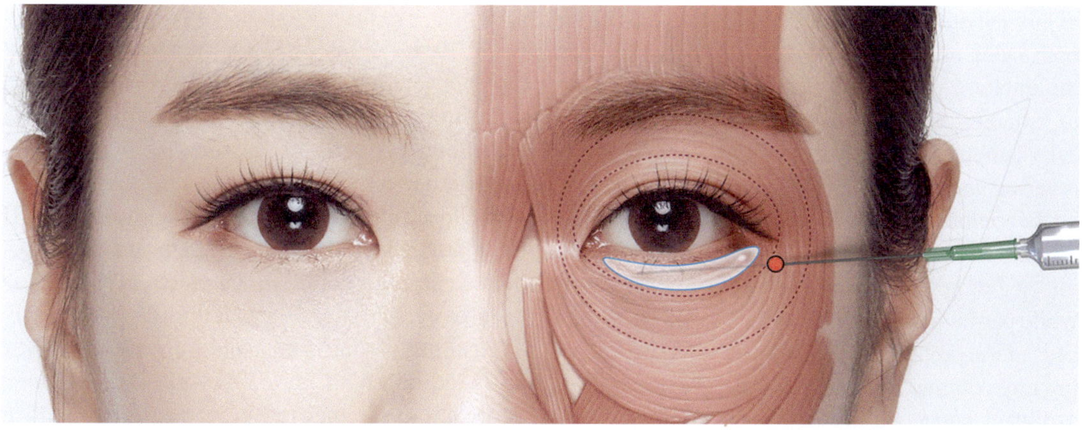

Fig. 4.30 Appropriate shape of the pretarsal roll and cannula entry point for pretarsal roll augmentation

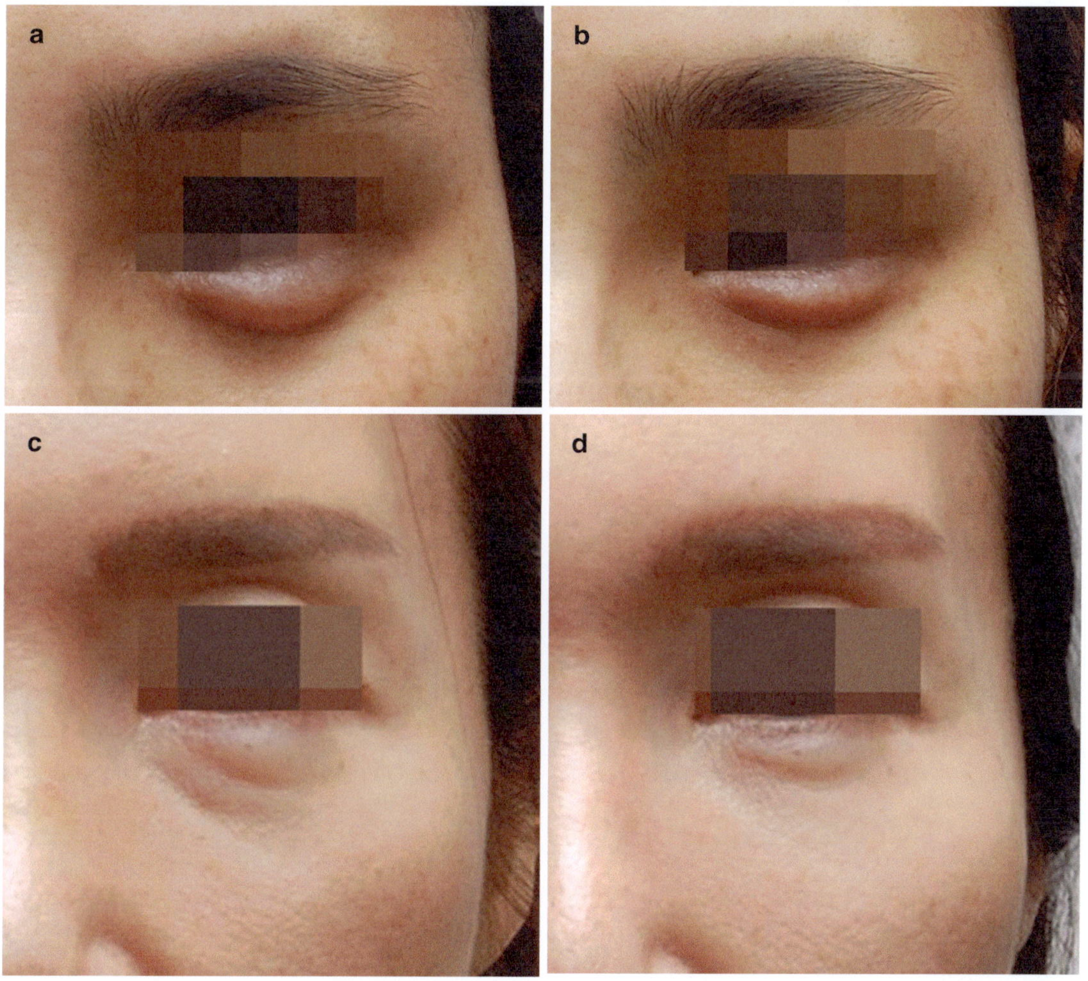

Fig. 4.31 (**a**) An overfilled pretarsal roll. (**b**) After partial reduction by hyaluronidase injection. (**c**) Disfiguring lumpiness after pretarsal roll augmentation. (**d**) After partial reduction by hyaluronidase injection

of immediate compression with cotton tips from both sides of the lower eyelid. Considering that the duration of pretarsal roll augmentation tends to extend for more than 5 years, any aethetically suboptimal placement of HA fillers are best reversed and reapplied.

To completely dissolve the misplaced HA filler, 0.5–1 mL of hyaluronidase (150 U/mL) is to be injected directly at the center of the pretarsal roll, while partial dissolution to reduce localized thickness of the pretarsal roll can be achieved by injecting tiny volumes of hyaluronidase (0.1–0.2 mL) at a diluted concentration of 30–50 U/mL slightly inferior to the overly thickened portion.

4.6 Inferior Orbital Hollow, Tear Trough, and Palpebromalar Groove

Difficulty Level: C, Effectiveness: A, Complications: C

Summary 1: Inferior orbital hollowness consists of three components: the tear trough in the medial aspect, the central infraorbital hollow in the central aspect, and the palpebromalar groove in the lateral aspect.

Summary 2: For superficial volume correction, HA is injected in the subdermal layer with a 30-G × 3-cm cannula. For deep volume correction, volume is placed in the submuscular layer with a 27-G or 30-G × 3-cm cannula. The use of fine biphasic HA fillers is advised for injecting the infraorbital area.

Summary 3: In patients displaying hypertrophy of the medial band of the orbicularis oculi m., the adjunctive use of BoNT-A is advised at two to three spots (1.5–2 U per spot) along the medial band. In patients manifesting anterior malar depression, concurrent volume restoration is advised in the anterior malar region.

Under-eye discoloration, colloquially referred to as "dark circles," is a multifactorial problem, the four leading causes of which include ethnic skin tones (pigmentation), visibility of the bluish vasculature underlying the skin, skin wrinkling, and the appearance of shadows on the skin surface. Specifically, Fitzpatrick skin phototypes III to IV are genetically more predisposed to periorbital hyperpigmentation, which tends to become progressively more pronounced with age. Congenitally robust vasculature under the eyes or the dilation of blood vessels due to sleep deprivation or menstruation can also induce infraorbital darkening. Wrinkling of the infraorbital skin due either to aging or to chronic dermatitis such as atopic dermatitis or allergic dermatitis may also cause darkening of the skin under the eyes. The discoloration may also be caused by congenital or progressive shadowing under the eyes due to the hollowing of the infraorbital region or the herniation of the suborbital fat (a.k.a. eye bags) or sagging of the lower eyelid. Of the aforementioned factors, correction of under-eye shadows represents the simplest and most straightforward solution to the appearance of dark circles. While surgery is required for treating lower eyebags or lower eyelid sagging, volume deficit in the infraorbital area can be addressed with HA fillers for immediate rejuvenation of the dark circles.

Infraorbital hollowness consists of three parts depending on the location, namely the tear trough on the medial aspect, the central infraorbital hollow on the central aspect, and the palpebromalar groove on the lateral aspect (Fig. 4.32) [12]. The tear trough is formed at the medial 1/2 of the infraorbital hollowness, where the thin skin of the periorbital region meets the thicker skin of the malar region. The palpebromalar groove represents the lateral 1/2 of the infraorbital hollowness resembling the indentation marks left after wearing goggles. The central infraorbital hollow is located outside the bounds of these two regions, inferior to the pretarsal roll or the inferior tarsus. The tear trough and the central infraorbital hollow can be a congenital feature, found commonly in young people as well, while the palpebromalar groove tends to be more prevalent among older patients presenting with malar mounds and infraorbital fat herniation (Fig. 4.33).

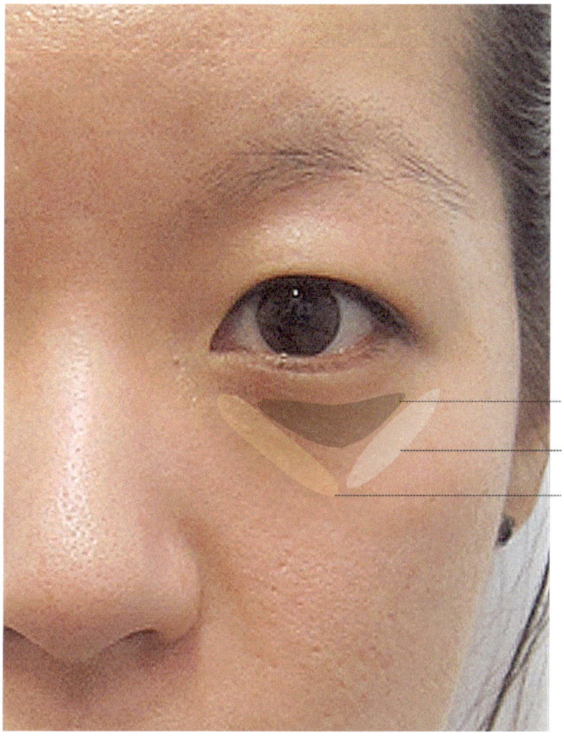

Fig. 4.32 Infraorbital hollowness consists of three parts depending on the location, namely the tear trough on the medial aspect, the central infraorbital hollow on the central aspect, and the palpebromalar groove on the lateral aspect

4.6.1 Anatomical Considerations

The tear trough commences at the medial canthus and extends inferolaterally along the orbital rim to converge with the palpebromalar groove at the midpoint of the orbital rim. A sagittal section of the infraorbital region shows that the relevant layers from the superficial to the deep consist of the skin—subdermal layer—orbicularis oculi m.—preseptal fat layer—orbital septum—inferior orbital fat (Fig. 4.34) [13]. The location of the tear trough is also consistent with that of the orbital retaining ligament (ORL), which spans the orbital bone and inserts into the orbicularis oculi m. The clinical photo in Fig. 4.35 well illustrates the location of the ORL represented in white in the picture due to the vasoconstriction induced by diffusion of the epinephrine mixed with lidocaine injected in the cannula entry point (Fig. 4.35). The ORL tethers the orbicularis oculi m. down to the bone, and it is this firm attachment that prevents any downward sagging of the infraorbital fat. Instead, the infraorbital fat herniates forward along the perimeter of the ORL. It remains unclear, however, as to whether the ORL inserts all the way up to the skin.

Meanwhile, the palpebromalar groove runs inferomedially from the lateral canthus parallel to the orbital rim and meets the tear trough in the middle of the inferior orbital rim. It also lies lateral to the arcus marginalis of the orbital rim. While the palpebromalar groove can be a congenital condition, it is more often associated with the aging-related protrusion of malar festoons and lower eye bags. The use of a cannula is advised for injecting these periorbital regions to avoid hitting the inferior palpebral v. and the angular a. running in the area.

4.6.2 Pretreatment Assessment

Start by assessing the severity and the position of the infraorbital hollowness, that is, the tear trough, the central infraorbital hollow or the palpebromalar groove. While in a vast majority of cases depression is visible only in the tear trough region, checks should nonetheless be made for

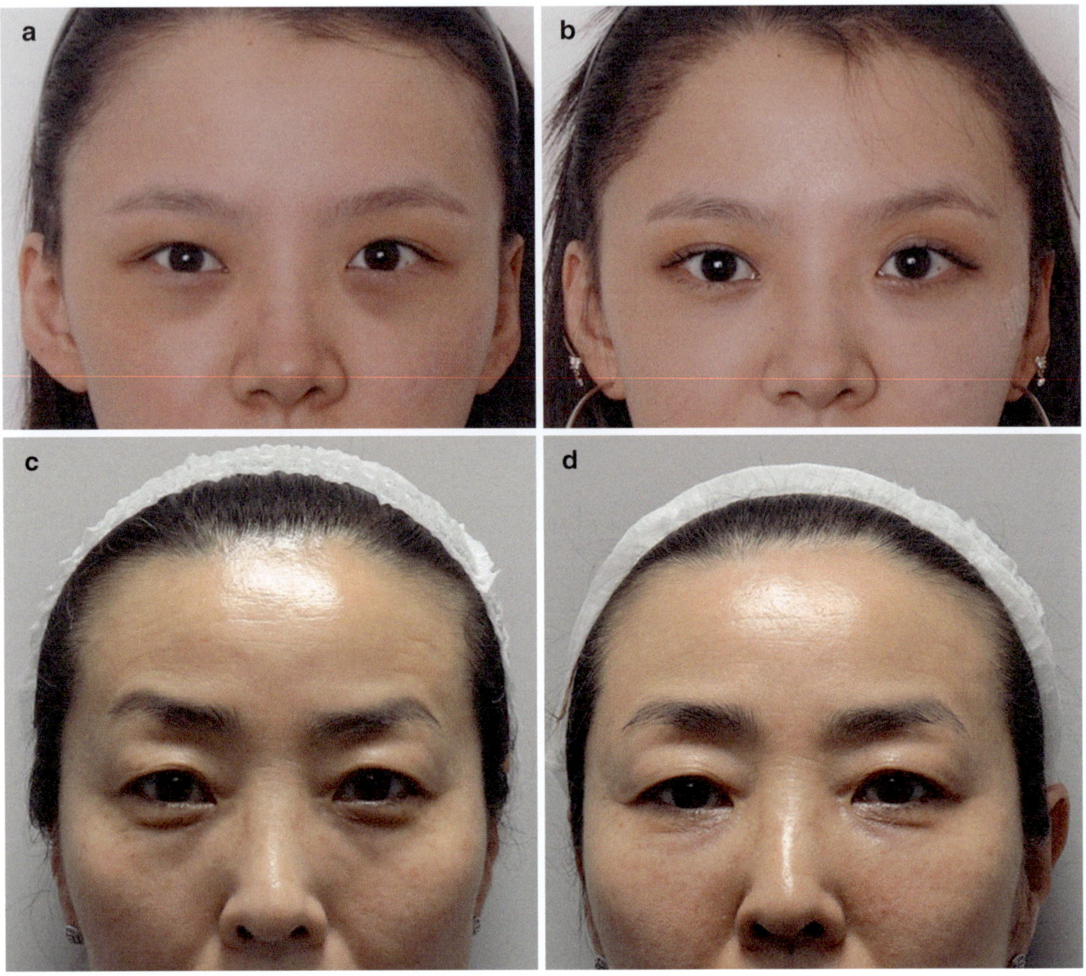

Fig. 4.33 (**a**) Before and (**b**) after tear trough volumization in a 28-year-old female. (**c**) Before and (**d**) after volumization of the tear trough, palpebromalar groove, and anterior malar depression in a 48-year-old female

any concurrent depression(s) in the other two areas. Checks should also be performed for the presence of any infraorbital fat herniation or lower eyelid sagging. Caution is required when treating a patient presenting with lax and redundant lower eyelid skin, as loose flaccid skin is not amenable to lifting with small volume injections, while injecting too much volume would invariably lead to visible lumps. Where the patient also presents with flattening of the anterior malar, concurrent volume restoration is advised in the anteromedial cheeks. One pitfall of HA filler, especially when placed in the thin tissues of the tear trough area, is its tendency to absorb water from surrounding tissues and expand. In this respect, patients with high daily fluid intake are more susceptible to developing posttreatment lumpiness due to the swelling of HA. Finally, the presence of any hypertrophy of the medial band of the orbicularis oris m. (located immediately below the tear trough) should be identified, as its contraction during smiling may cause the HA filler placed in the tear trough to clump up and protrude anteriorly (Fig. 1.12).

4.6.3 Injection Technique (Table 4.6)

The use of biphasic HA fillers with small particle size is preferred for injecting the delicate infraorbital area. Monophasic HA fillers are not recommended since they are more prone to absorb water and swell. The use of a thin 30-G × 3-cm cannula is generally preferred for treating the deli-

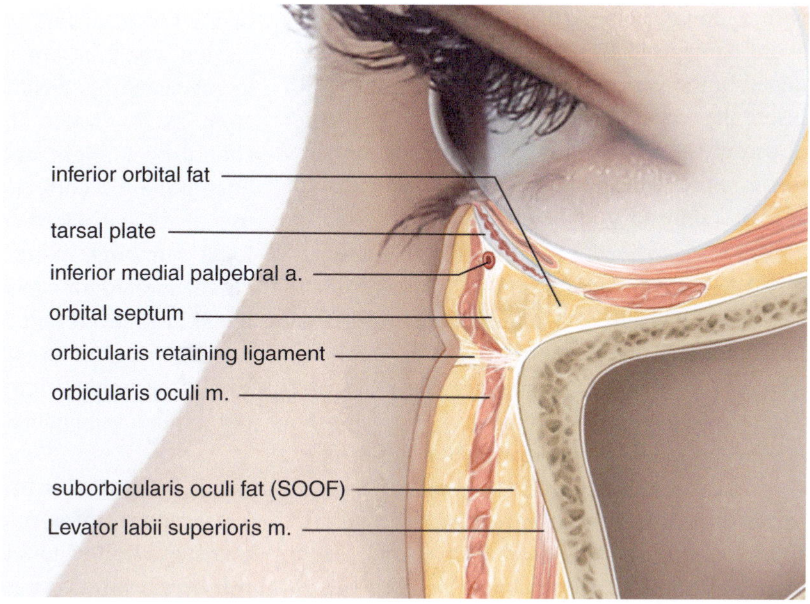

Fig. 4.34 A sagittal section of the infraorbital region

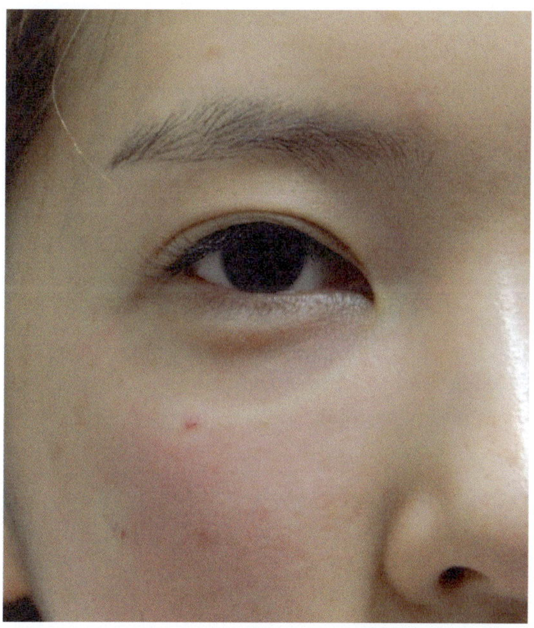

Fig. 4.35 This clinical photo well illustrates the circumference location of the orbital retaining ligament represented in white due to the vasoconstriction induced by diffusion of the epinephrine mixed with lidocaine injected in the cannula entry point

Table 4.6 Summary of infraorbital hollow injection technique

Item	Contents
Needle vs. Cannula	30-G 3-cm cannula for the subdermal layer 27-G or 30-G 3-cm cannula for the deep submuscular layer (preseptal layer)
HA filler	Biphasic filler with fine particles
Amount of HA filler	0.1–0.3 mL per side for the tear trough 0.1–0.5 mL per side for the central inferior orbital hollow 0.3–0.6 mL per side for the palpebromalar groove
Depth of injection	Subdermal layer for superficial correction Submuscular layer for deep injection
Entry point for cannula	0.5–1 cm from the end of the tear trough for the tear trough 1 cm inferolateral to the lateral canthus for the central inferior orbital hollow 1 cm lateral to the lateral canthus for the palpebromalar groove
Target area	Tear trough Central inferior orbital hollow/ palpebromalar groove
Anesthetics	Topical anesthetics
Nondominant hand	Hold the skin in opposite direction to the cannula advancement in order to maintain the skin tension

cate infraorbital area, while the larger 27-G × 3-cm cannula can also be used for performing deep injections. There is a vast network of small vessels underlying the periorbital area, and even a cannula may be capable of damaging any of the weakened vascular walls, causing extensive bruising, particularly when a thin 30-G microcannula is employed. The cannula entry point is created with a 26-G needle. To minimize bruising and avoid damage to the extensive vasculature contained in the periorbital region, it is important to insert the needle slowly with the bevel facing downwards. In the event of any vascular damage, firm compression should be applied to the area for at least 3 mins to stop the bleeding.

4.6.3.1 Tear Trough

The relevant depth of injection is determined by the severity of the tear trough. For mild tear troughs, corrections are made in the subdermal layer superficial to the orbicularis oris m. with a 30-G cannula. For deep tear trough deformities, use of the double-layering technique helps to avoid Tyndalling caused by placing too much HA filler superficially in the subdermal layer. Here, HA filler is placed deep to the orbicularis oris m. into the preseptal fat layer using a 27-G × 3-cm cannula, before detailed refinements are made subdermally using a 30-G × 3-cm cannula (Fig. 4.36). The cannula entry point is made 0.5–1 cm away from the end of the tear trough along a straight line extending from the same (Fig. 4.36). Where the tear trough continues beyond the medial one-third of the infraorbital hollow into the area under the pupil, running horizontally parallel to the orbital rim, a second lateral insertion point is required to address this horizontal portion of the tear trough (Fig. 4.37). Concerning the injection volume, 0.1–0.3 mL of HA in the subdermal level and 0.1–0.3 mL of HA in the preseptal fat layer provide sufficient correction. The thin skin of the tear trough area is apt to reveal any undesired expansion of HA filler from excess water absorption. Thus, the goal should be a slight under-correction rather than attempting full correction in a single session. The use of topical anesthetic cream is sufficient for local numbing. Note, however, that numbing cream applied for a prolonged duration can cause the skin to swell and obscure the appearance of the tear trough to be corrected. As such, the cream should be applied only at the cannula insertion point rather than across the entire treatment area.

4.6.3.2 Central Inferior Orbital Hollow

The central infraorbital hollow refers to the under-eye hollowness located below the pretarsal roll or the inferior tarsus. Here, a 27-G × 3-cm cannula is first inserted into the preseptal fat to substantially fill the depression from the inferior tarsus to the tear trough, before fine-tuning the result with a 30-G cannula maneuvered subdermally. The cannula insertion point is made 1 cm lateral and 1 cm inferior to the lateral canthus (Fig. 4.37). Small volume injection of 0.1–0.5 mL is advised per side, depending on the severity of the depression.

4.6.3.3 Palpebromalar Groove

Using the double-layering approach, a 27-G × 3-cm cannula is introduced first at the supraperiosteal layer deep to the orbicularis oris

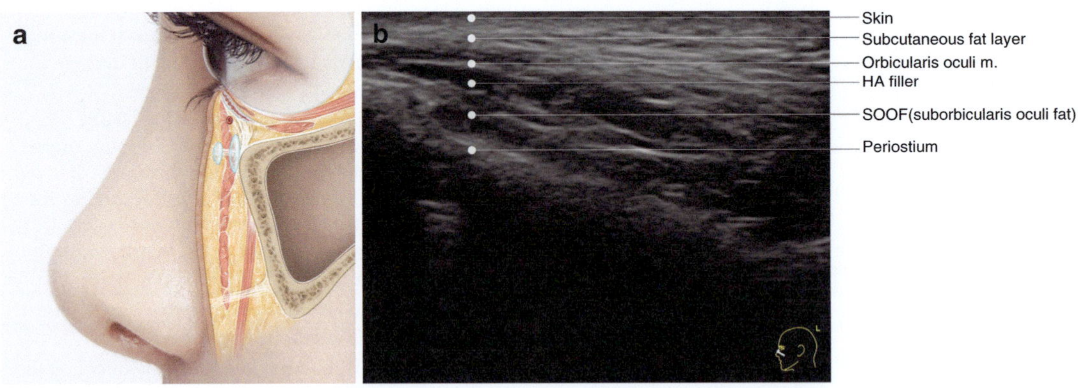

Fig. 4.36 (**a**) Depth of injection for the tear trough, (**b**) sonographic findings of HA filler injected into the tear trough

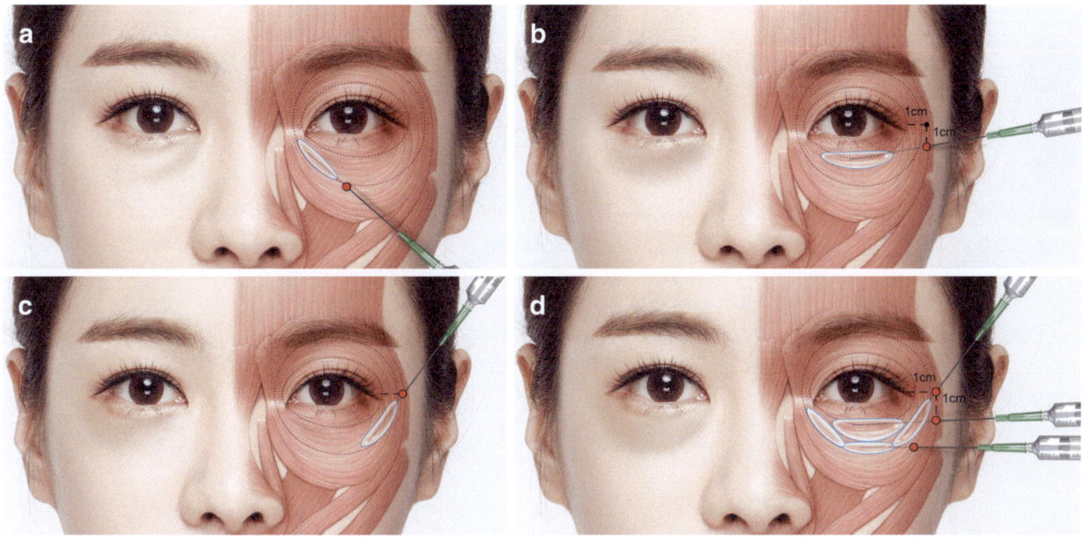

Fig. 4.37 The cannula entry point for (**a**) tear trough (**b**) central infraorbital hollow (**c**) palpebromalar groove, and (**d**) total infraorbital hollow

m. for the primary volumization, before a 30-G cannula is used for making detailed corrections at the subdermal layer (Fig. 4.37). The cannula entry point is made 1 cm lateral to the lateral canthus (Fig. 4.37). The amount of HA filler injected is 0.3–0.7 mL is per side, though a larger volume may be required to fill the deep palpebromalar grooves caused by severe herniation of fat pads with advancing age.

4.6.3.4 Combination Treatment

In patients presenting with a hypertrophic medial band of the orbicularis oculi m. under the eyes, the adjunctive use of BoNT-A in two to three points along the band (1.5–2 U per spot) can further optimize results (Fig. 4.38). Where the patient presents with concurrent depressions in the anterior malar region, make sure to restore also the volume deficit in the anteromedial malar to smoothen the transition at the lid–cheek junction.

4.6.4 Complications

Irregularities: The thin unforgiving skin of the periorbital area makes the region particularly susceptible to contour irregularities. Even a slight overfilling or swelling of the injected HA filler may cause disfiguring lumpiness in the area (Fig. 4.39). The risk is higher with monophasic HA fillers, which are more hydrophilic in nature than biphasic fillers (Fig. 2.23).

Bruising: To prevent damage to the rich vasculature underlying the area while puncturing the cannula entry point insert a 26-G needle slowly with the bevel facing downwards, taking care to avoid visible veins.

Tyndall effect: As is the case with irregularities, the thin skin of the periorbital area also makes this region particularly susceptible to the Tyndall effect. Avoid placing too much HA filler superficially in the subdermal layer.

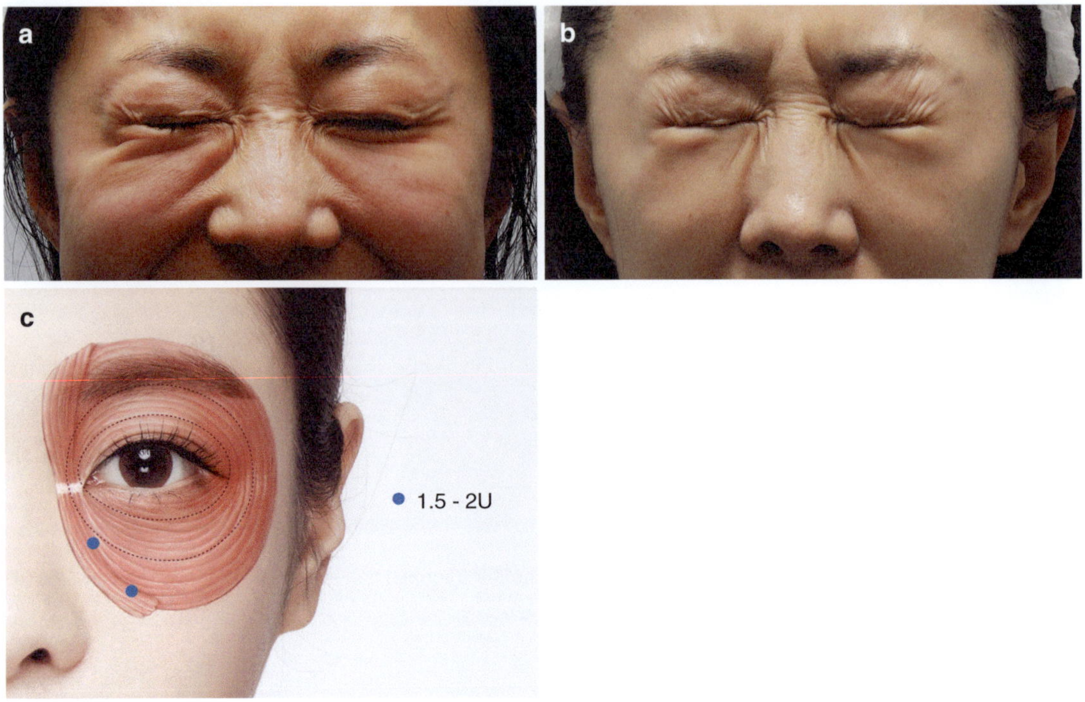

Fig. 4.38 Use of botulinum toxin to treat the hypertrophic medial band of the orbicularis oris m. (**a**) Before, (**b**) after and (**c**). Injection points for the hypertrophic medial band of the orbicularis oris m

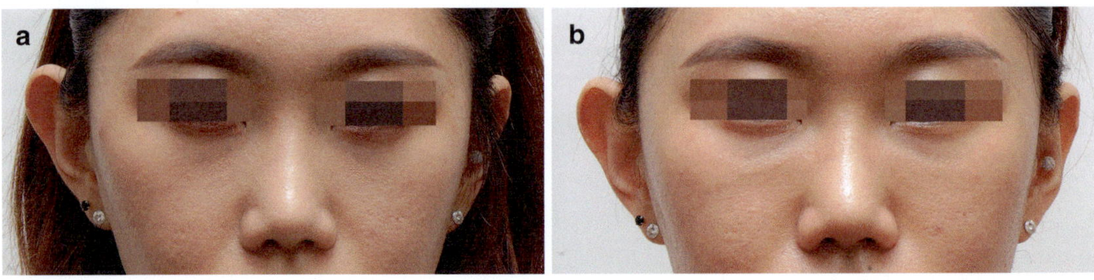

Fig. 4.39 (**a**) Before and (**b**) after tear trough volumization. Note the appearance of lumpiness in the treated area

4.7 Nasojugal Groove

Difficulty Level: A, Effectiveness: A, Complications: B

Summary 1: A23-G × 5-cm cannula is used for deep injections into the SOOF. Both biphasic HA fillers with large particle size and monophasic HA fillers with high viscoelasticity are acceptable for use.

Summary 2: The adjunctive use of BoNT-A can optimize results in patients presenting with a hypertrophic medial band of the orbicularis oculi m. under the eyes. Injection of BoNT-A is advised at two spots (1.5–2 U per spot) along the medial band. In patients manifesting concurrent depression in the tear trough, volume replacement should be performed in the tear trough in conjunction with the nasojugal groove.

> *Summary 3*: In patients concurrently exhibiting sunken cheeks or prominent lateral zygoma, volume should be placed concomitantly in the respective hollows of the cheek to ensure overall facial balance and proportionality.

> *Summary 4*: The combined use of steroid-based fat-dissolving injections can produce more favorable outcomes in patients with a pronounced malar fat pad.

Flattening of the anteromedial malar can exacerbate the appearance of under-eye dark circles and create the perception of facial descent by disrupting the smooth convexity of the face with intervening concavities (Fig. 4.40). Furthermore, the loss of volume in the anteromedial malar region combined with the persistence of fullness in the nasolabial component of the malar fat pad contributes to the formation of a conspicuous groove commencing at the tear trough and running obliquely from superomedial to inferolateral across the medial malar, often intruding into the submalar depressions or cheek hollows below.

This groove is referred to interchangeably as the nasojugal groove, the mid-cheek groove, or the mid-cheek furrow, though "mid-cheek groove" is a broader term that extends to also cover submalar depressions. Nasojugal grooves are also commonly known as Indian bands, as they resemble the painted stripes on the faces of Native American Indians [12]. Tear troughs may sometimes be considered to form part of the nasojugal groove [14] (Fig. 4.41).

Nasojugal grooves can occur due to multiple causative factors, including a congenitally strong fixation of the zygomatic cutaneous retaining ligament (ZCRL), a congenitally weak and underdeveloped maxillary bone, depletion of malar fat volume due to aging or weight loss, hypertrophy of the nasolabial fat with aging, among others. While nasojugal grooves may also be present in young patients with a congenital maxillary deficiency or with an inherently prominent zygomatic cutaneous retaining ligament, in a large majority of cases, the groove becomes more identifiable with advancing age or weight loss, due to the resulting deflation and descent of the malar fat pad. The malar fat pad is separated by the retaining ligament into the lower compartment (nasolabial fat) which progressively slides down and inwards with age toward the nasolabial folds, and the upper compartment (malar fat) which remains suspended in place by the strong ligamentous fixation provided by the zygomatic ligament. Conversely, the hypertrophy of the malar fat pad with aging may cause the fat pad to bulge as two discrete entities, separated by the ZCRL into the malar mound (malar bag) above and the nasolabial fat sitting below. The relative prominence of these structures, in turn, can also accentuate the depth of the nasojugal groove lying in between.

4.7.1 Anatomical Considerations

From the outer to inner, the anteromalar region consists of the following layers: the skin—subcutaneous fat layer/superficial layer of malar fat pad—orbicularis oculi m—SOOF, suborbicularis oculi fat layer/deep layer of malar fat pad—expression muscle layer including the levator labii superioris and zygomaticus minor—infraorbital nerve—periosteum (Fig. 4.42). The malar fat pad is divided by the orbicularis oculi m into the superficial subcutaneous and the deep SOOF layers and separated by the ZCRL into the superior and inferior compartments. The ZCRL runs from superomedial to inferolateral across the medial malar, and it is on the basis of this structure that the malar fat pad is segmented into the malar mound superiorly and the nasolabial fat inferiorly (Fig. 4.43) [14]. Nasolabial fat progressively slides down and inwards with age toward the nasolabial folds and the upper compartment (malar fat) remains suspended in place by due to the strong ligamentous fixation provided by the ZCRL. In 30% of Asians, a detoured branch of the facial artery courses in front of the anteromedial malar region along the medial band of orbicularis oculi m. at the level of SOOF before branching into the angular artery [15].

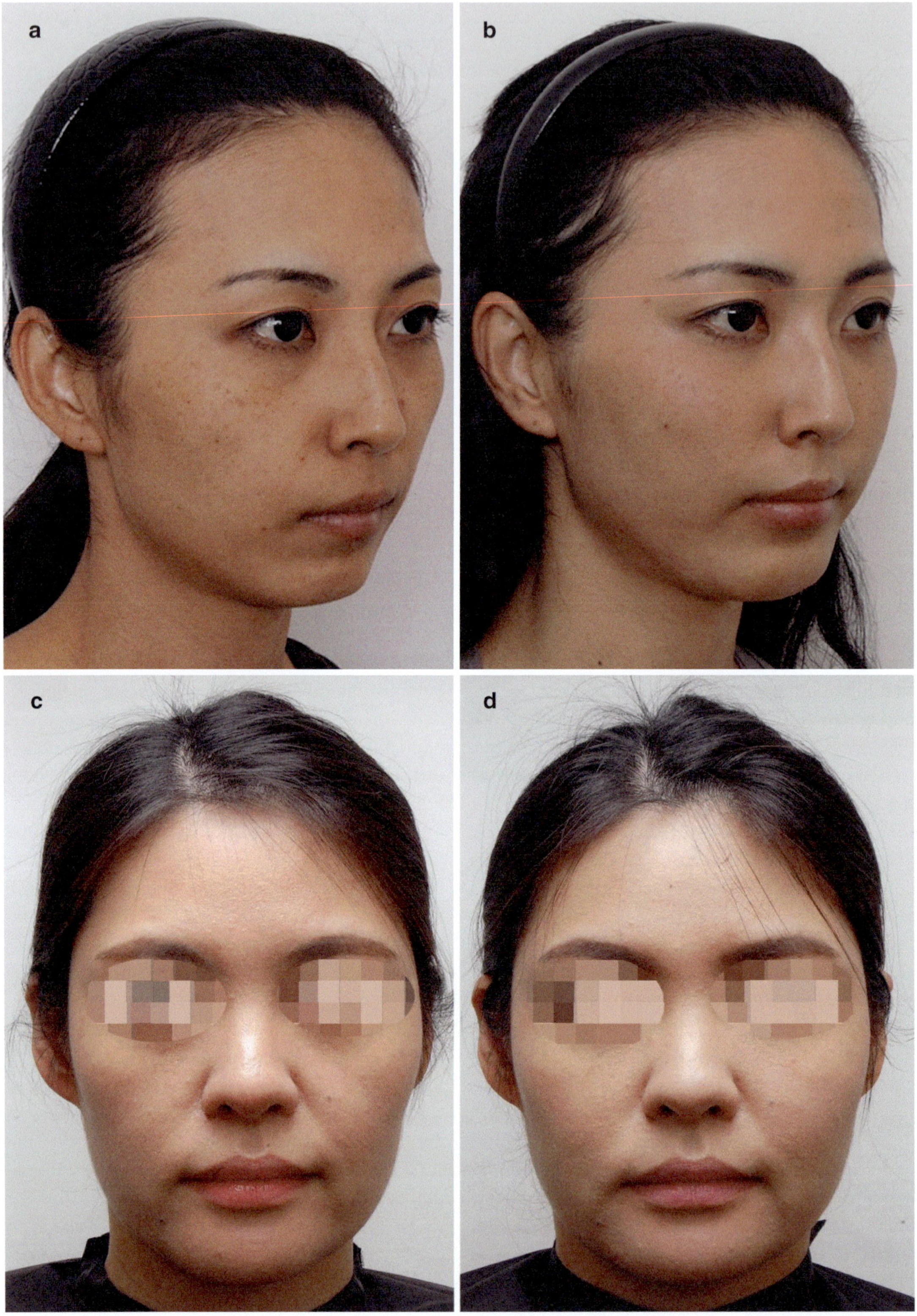

Fig. 4.40 (**a**, **c**) Before and (**b**, **d**) after volumization of the nasojugal groove combined with volumization of the sunken cheeks

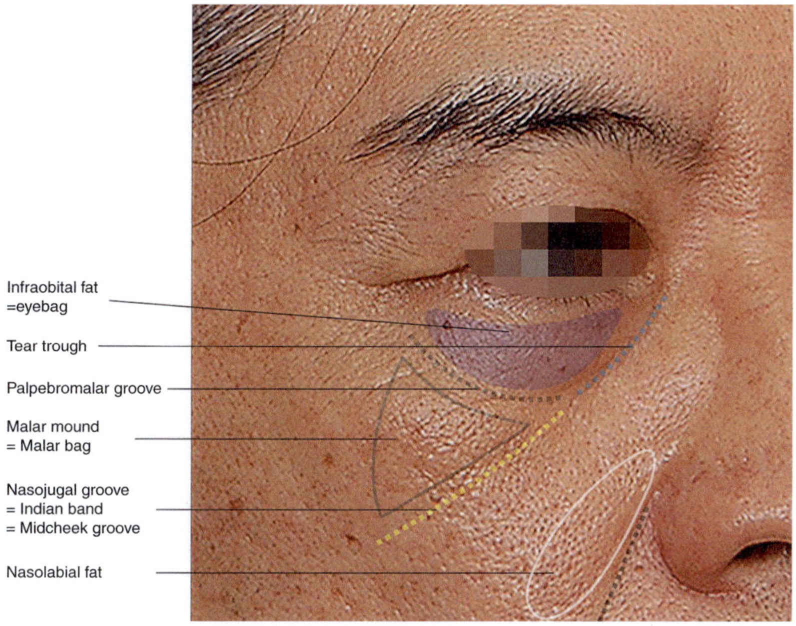

Fig. 4.41 Location of the nasojugal groove and tear trough

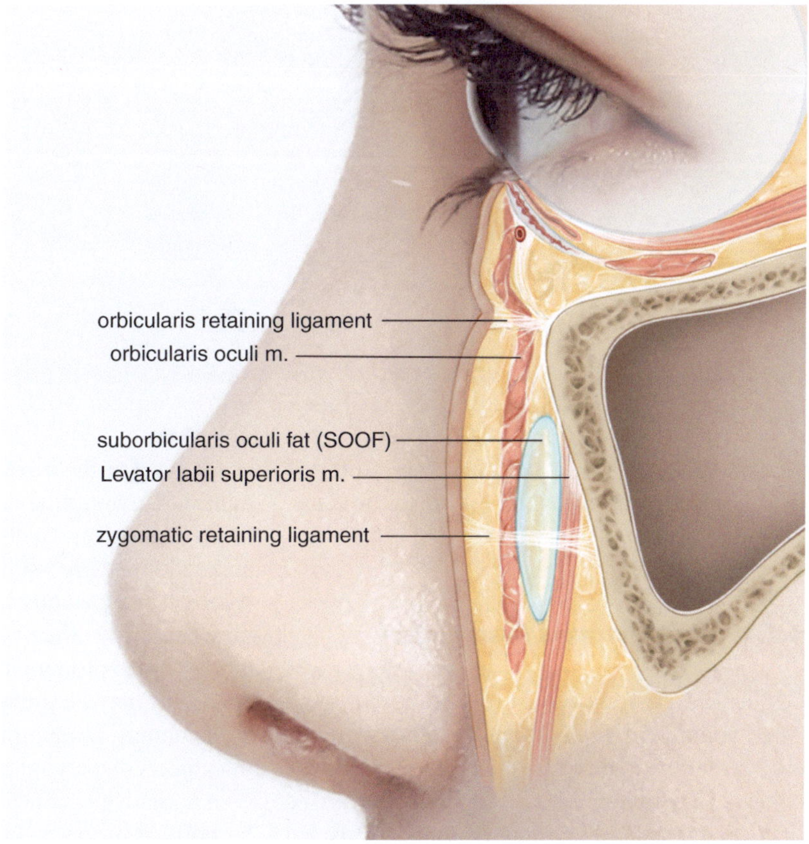

Fig. 4.42 A sagittal section of the anteromalar region

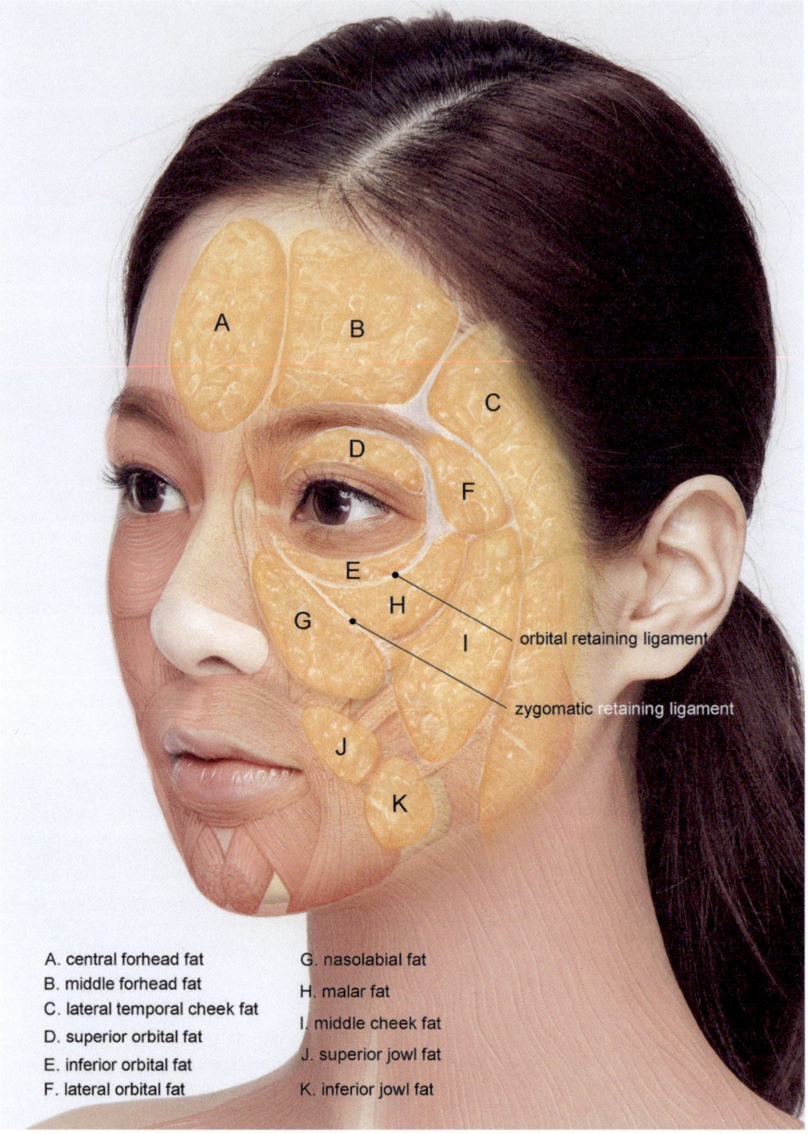

Fig. 4.43 Diagram of the superficial facial fat compartment. The malar fat pad is divided by the zygomatic cutaneous retaining ligament into the superior (malar fat, malar mound) and inferior (nasolabial fat) compartments

Accordingly, the use of a cannula is preferred over a needle for injecting this area in Asian patients.

4.7.2 Pretreatment Assessment

Gender differences should be borne in mind when volumizing the nasojugal groove with fillers in order not to feminize male subjects. In such context, injection of discreet amounts is advised in male subjects, as a slightly rugged chiseled cheek contour is favorably associated with male charisma. On the contrary, more volume in the malar area would be acceptable for female subjects. In subjects with a prominent zygomatic arch, adding extra volume in the malar area, even when placed medially in the anteromedial aspect, may cause the entire zygoma to look wider as a whole. Since prominent zygoma is disfavored by Asians, it may be preferable to inject only minimal amounts, if not omit the treatment altogether, in subjects displaying prominent zygoma.

Alternatively, concurrent filling of the submalar hollows in such subjects can help diminish the appearance of prominent zygoma (Fig. 4.44).

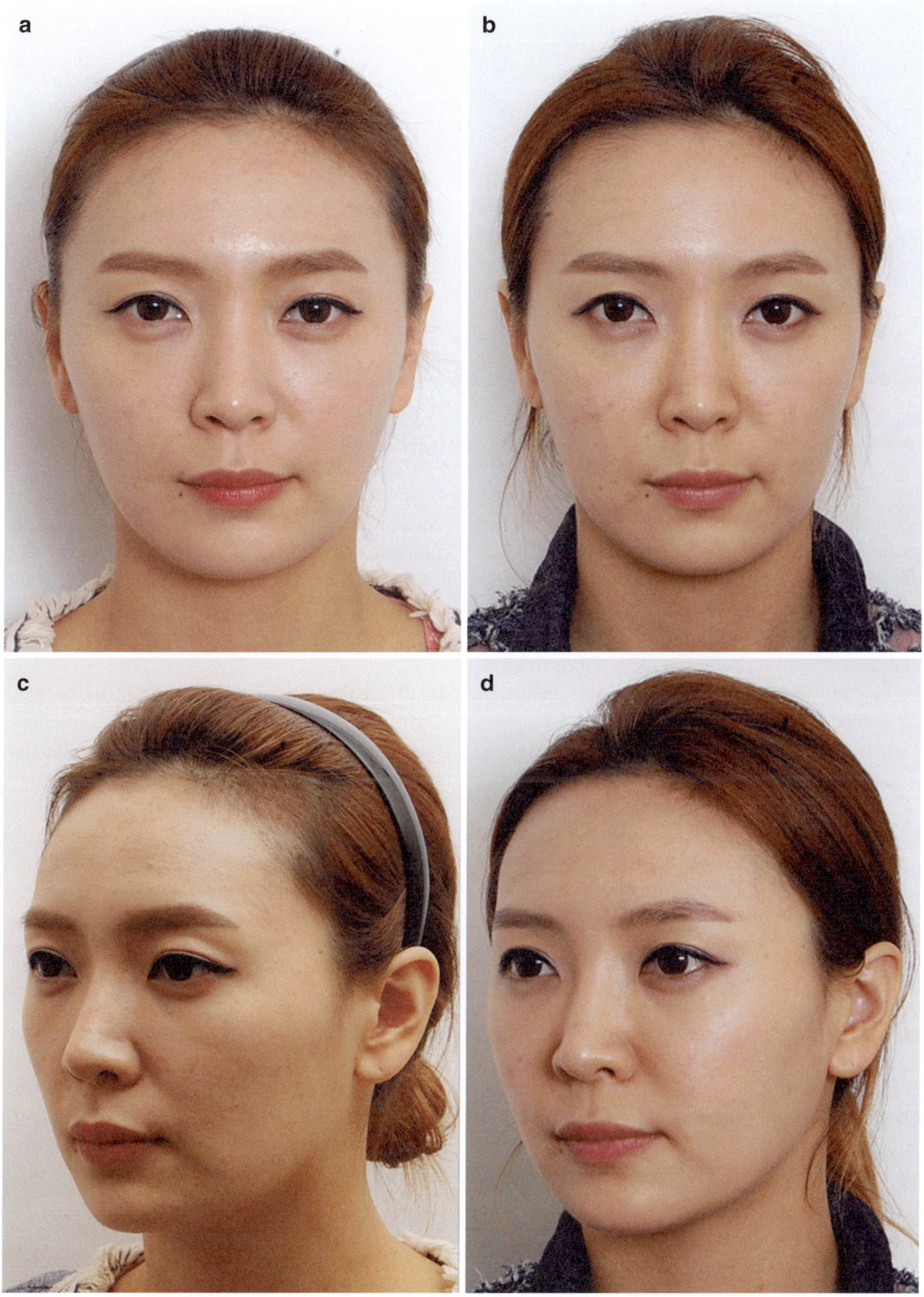

Fig. 4.44 Concurrent flling of the submalar hollows can help diminish the appearance of prominent zygoma caused by the volumization of the nasojugal groove (**a**, **c**) Before and (**b**, **d**) after

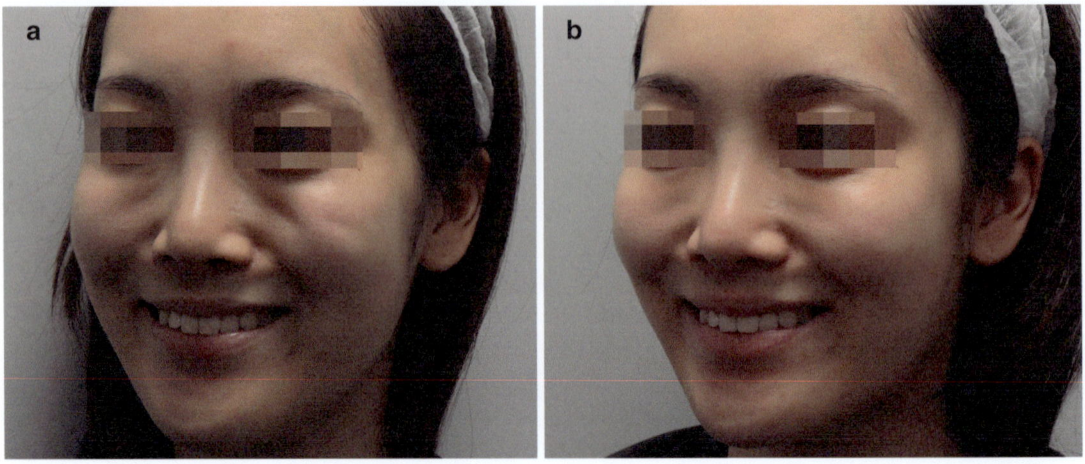

Fig. 4.45 Malar dimples can be improved by the injection of botulinum toxin (1.5U) combined with the injection of botulinum toxin on the medial band of the orbicularis oris m. (**a**) before (**b**) after

Meanwhile, augmenting only the anteromedial malar in patients with concurrent depressions in the tear trough and palpebromalar groove may accentuate the relative prominence of the infraorbital hollows. Accordingly, it is advisable to address the volume deficit in these adjacent areas in tandem to give the face a more balanced appearance.

It is also important to identify the presence, if any, of a hypertrophic medial band of the orbicularis oris m. immediately below the tear trough (Fig. 4.38). The contraction of this band upon smiling may cause the HA filler injected in the anterior malar to bunch together and bulge forward whenever the patient smiles. With repeated contraction, the aggregated HA filler may settle as a conspicuous lump visible even at rest. Adjunctive injection of BoNT-A is advised in such patients to prevent such appearance of lumpiness. In rare cases, the orbicularis oculi may insert into the ZCRL in the mid-cheek, resulting in the formation of dimples on smiling (Fig. 4.45). The injected HA filler, in such case, tends to show a reduced duration of effect.

Where the nasojugal groove has become more conspicuous due to the relative protrusion of the malar fat (malar mound), it is preferable to first reduce the excess volume in the malar fat via subcutaneous steroid injections or facial liposuction before augmenting the volume deficiency in the nasojugal groove (Fig. 4.41).

4.7.3 Injection Technique (Table 4.7)

Both biphasic HA fillers with large particle size and monophasic HA fillers with high viscoelasticity are acceptable for use in the anterior malar area. The used of a 23-G × 5-cm cannula is preferred, while a finer 25-G or 27-G cannula can also be used for layering the HA filler additionally at the superficial subcutaneous level. The depth of injection is the deep SOOF layer deep to the orbicularis oculi (Fig. 4.46). Care should be taken not to inject too deep and hit the levator labii superioris m. lying below the SOOF since it can cause significant pain to the patient. For permanently etched in Indian bands, treatment should also include superficial injection in the superficial subcutaneous fat layer in a double-layering technique.

The cannula entry point is created along the extension of the nasojugal groove, 1 cm away from where groove ends, at the intersection between a vertical line 1 cm lateral from the lat-

Table 4.7 Summary of nasojugal groove augmentation technique

Item	Contents
Needle vs. Cannula	23-G 5-cm cannula for SOOF layer, 25-G or 27-G 5-cm cannula for the superficial subcutaneous fat layer
HA filler	Biphasic HA filer with large particle size or monophasic HA filler with high viscoelasticity
Amount of HA filler	0.5–2 mL per side
Depth of injection	Deep SOOF layer above the muscle layer Superficial subcutaneous layer if necessary
Entry point for cannula	1 cm from the end of the nasojugal groove along the extension of the same
Target area	Mid cheek groove
Anesthetics	Topical anesthetics
Nondominant hand	Hold the skin tightly in the posterior direction to maintain skin tension

eral canthus and a horizontal line running through the nasal base (Fig. 4.47). Insert the cannula deeply into the SOOF layer and inject HA filler using the retrograde linear thread technique along the length of the groove into its deepest central portion for primary volumization. Next, repeating the same process, make parallel retrograde linear injections immediately above and below the first injection to level out the groove shaped in the form of a half-cylinder to yield an even contour. Concerning the injection volume, 0.5–2 mL of HA filler is typically delivered per side depending on the severity of depression, though over 3 mL may be required per side in patients with maxillary deficiency. For anesthesia, the application of topical numbing cream should suffice. The nondominant hand should be used to stretch the skin taut both inferiorly and laterally during the injection to tighten the cheek area to facilitate cannula advancement.

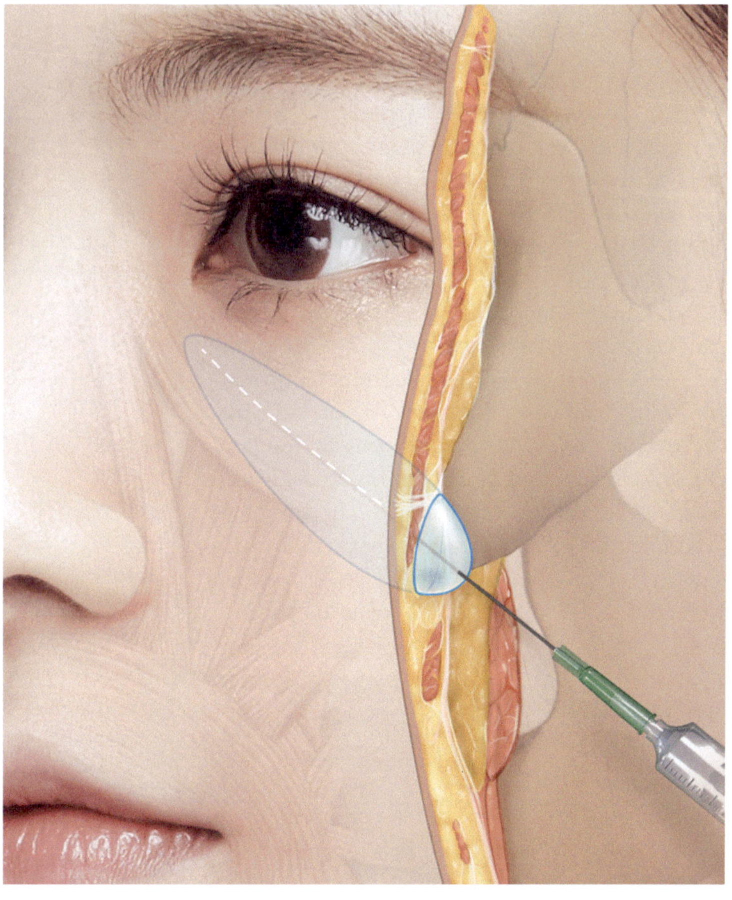

Fig. 4.46 Depth of injection for the nasojugal groove volumization

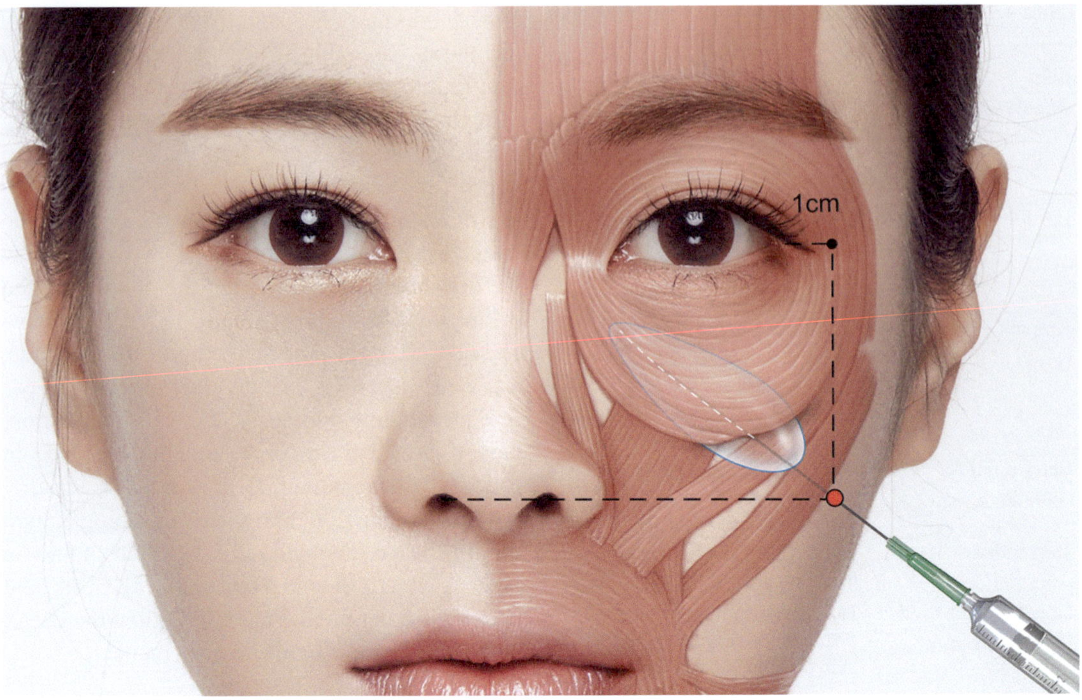

Fig. 4.47 The cannula entry point for the nasojugal groove volumization

4.7.3.1 Combination Treatment

In patients presenting with a hypertrophic medial band of the orbicularis oculi m. under the eyes, the adjunctive use of BoNT-A in two to three points along the band (1.5–2 U per spot) can help to optimize results. Adjunctive injection of BoNT-A at malar dimples is also advised in patients with malar dimples (Fig. 4.45). Where the patient presents with a concurrent tear trough deformity, palpebromalar groove, or submalar depression, volume in these regions should preferably be restored in tandem in order to give the face a more balanced appearance. The combined use of steroid-based fat-reducing injections (dispensed over 2–3 sessions) is advised in patients with substantial fullness in the malar fat pad.

Tip: Corticosteroid Fat-Reducing Injections

A nonsurgical injectable solution promising to melt away unwanted fat can be nothing short of a miracle. A slew of different concoctions has been introduced to this end so far, including injectables that purport to stimulate the neurotransmitters of the sympathetic nervous system to break down localized fat deposits, hypotonic solutions mixed with distilled water which claim to encourage fat dissolution, and hyaluronidase injections for dissolving the hyaluronic acid present in the intercellular substance of the fat tissues. However, the results of these treatments have turned out to be mostly underwhelming. The two nonsurgical treatments tried and tested in their ability to reduce fat are deoxycholic acid and corticosteroid injections, each with its associated drawbacks.

Kybella® (Allergan, USA), containing deoxycholic acid as the active ingredient, represents the first US FDA-approved injectable treatment for addressing the "double chin" or the submental fat present below the chin. However, the results of Kybella® cannot be achieved in a single session, requiring up to 3–6 treatment sessions spaced 1 month apart, each accompanied by significant swelling and tenderness. The appeal of a nonsurgical solution can be outweighed by the substantial downtime involved due to the swelling and pain following each treatment session. In this respect, a facial liposculpture, as a one-time procedure, arguably represent a more efficient option.

Meanwhile, steroid-based fat-reducing injections induce fat reduction by leveraging one of the common side effects of corticosteroids, fat atrophy, for cosmetic purposes. Swelling usually resolves within 2 hrs of injection while bruising can largely be avoided with the use of a cannula. However, given their nature as steroid hormones that are capable of causing systemic side effects including disrupted menstrual cycle, moon face syndrome, and acne, limitations apply in terms of the maximum dose per session, interval between treatments, and the number of consecutive treatments that can be undertaken. Caution must be taken, as these steroids may cause atrophy not only in the subcutaneous fat but also in the dermis when used in high concentrations or doses, leading to dermal thinning and atrophic indentations on the skin surface (Fig. 4.48).

Note that in areas of excess facial fat, when the HA filler is injected to fill the hollows in an adjacent area, the injected volume may serve to exaggerate the existing fullness as it pushes against the surrounding tissues. By way of example, HA filler placed in the buccal hollows or the nasolabial folds may exacerbate the appearance of sagging jowls, while the volume added in the nasojugal grooves may aggravate the bulge of the malar mounds or the malar fat pad sitting above the nasolabial fold.

In such cases, the combined use of steroid-based fat-reducing injections can help achieve a smoother and more natural appearance. Steroid based fat-reducing injections can be safely administered based on the following guidelines. The use of a cannula can help to avoid bruising. Deep injection into the subcutaneous layer helps to prevent dermal atrophy. In the case of dexamethasone injections, 1–2 mL is injected per spot at a concentration of 1.25 mg/mL to a maximum of 8 mL per session. Dexamethasone can be dispensed in up to three consecutive sessions spaced 1 week apart, though, given its short half-life of 3 h, the interval may be shortened to 3 days.

In comparison, triamcinolone has a longer half-life; 1–2 mL is injected per spot at a concentration of 5 mg/mL to a maximum of 8 mL per session. It can be dispensed in up to three consecutive sessions spaced 2 weeks apart. While triamcinolone is more efficacious than dexamethasone, it is more prone to the risks of dermal atrophy and systemic complications. For this reason, dexamethasone is the preferred choice of steroid injections for inducing fat reduction.

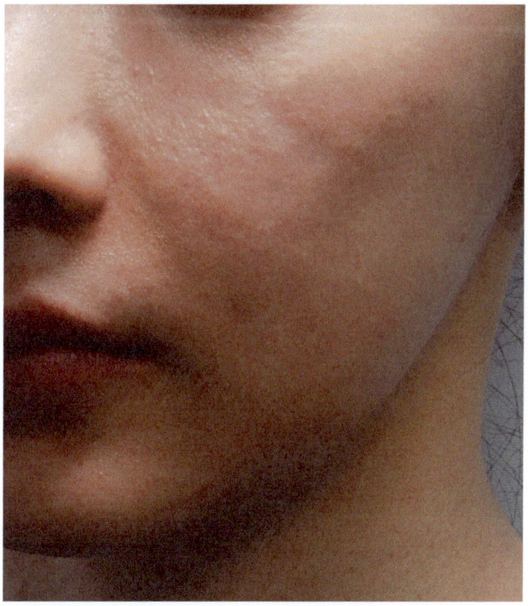

Fig. 4.48 Dermal atrophy caused by fat reducing injection

4.7.4 Complications

Irregularity: Volume restored in the medial malar needs to be proportionate to the rest of the face. Augmenting the mid cheeks alone without considering the transitions to the adjacent areas or the hollowness in the tear trough above can results in unnaturally abrupt transitions in the facial contour. Meanwhile, repeated contraction of a hypertrophic medial band of the orbicularis oris m. may lead to the subsequent migration and bunching of the HA filler. Further, discrepancy in the HA filler duration in different facial regions may create an obvious "step" in the lid–cheek junction 6–12 months following treatment as the volume deeply placed in the anterior malar area dissipates more quickly while the superficially implanted volume in the tear trough remains intact (see Sect. 5.2).

Episode: Sure, We Hire Based on Looks
Patients occasionally ask if I happen to hire my staff based on their looks, as a well-meant joke to compliment my immaculately presented staff. Each time, I respond with a ready comeback "Of course. In fact, that's our sole criteria" to which both the patient and the staff burst out laughing. Needless to say, comments like this, in this day and age, can border on workplace sexual harassment, but I am pleased to report that so far, no such complaints have been raised by any of my staff. Notably, one critical element of a sexual harassment claim is the subjective feeling of the aggrieved employee, that is, how the individual felt after what was said or done. Accordingly, a casual offhand joke can constitute harassment if the victim took offense from it. Conversely, to the extent that the comment was not considered as an insult by the employee, then there is no case for a harassment claim. Needless to say, my responses have so far been taken by my staff as nothing more than a witty compliment.

As aptly noted in the book *Whale Done!*, everybody appreciates a good compliment, and that includes doctors too. After performing filler treatments, I make it a rule to pass a mirror to the patient to obtain their immediate assessment and feedback. While invariably, the results are instantaneous and changes visible, the response from patients are varied and diverse. Some would stick both thumbs up in delight and exclaim "No wonder you are the Master of Fillers!" Others stare intently into the mirror scrutinizing their faces for any odd asymmetry or imperfection. Granted, Koreans are not best known for their expressiveness and can be rather tight with compliments. The majority of my patients are therefore either nonresponsive if not fall into the latter category of tough critics. So in the occasional event I get a patient who happens to be generous with compliments, that can really make my day.

Upon obtaining my medical license I had originally set out to become a professor at a university hospital where, hopefully, I could engage in both research and patient consultation. Things did not exactly work out according to plan and in the end I ended up starting my private practice. My biggest qualm regarding that decision was whether I could draw the same sense of purpose and fulfillment as a physician when most of my daily practice would revolve around performing aesthetic procedures for clients rather than getting down to the serious business of treating diseases for patients. This coming from a dermatologist may come across as a frivolous concern compared with the work of general surgeons or cardiologists whose entire practice is built around dealing with matters of life and death. To my relief, however, such concerns became a moot point within a few years of opening my own clinic. Soon enough I was receiving positive feedback from clients genuinely pleased with their rejuvenated and refined appearances, which I found to be just as gratifying and rewarding as those received from patients treated for their illness.

"Getting the procedure was the best decision I've made this year."

"It's as if somebody's turned the clock back by 10 years"

"Magical!"

"Absolutely addictive"

Truth be told, I have a sweet spot for short yet captivating plaudits like these. Sometimes I would go the extra mile simply for the joy of eliciting more such response by adding extra doses or addressing facial areas that extend beyond the original treatment plan at no extra charge. Apparently, positive feedback from patients is what motivates me to go to these lengths to achieve the best possible result.

In Whale Done!: The Power of Positive Relationships MIT professor and top business consultant Ken Blenchard describes how animal trainers pay positive attention to killer whales rather than punishing their unwanted negative behavior to encourage these massive unwieldy creatures, weighing more than three tons, to leap several meters above water as per the trainer's instructions. This approach is also is backed up by the famous study by Robert Rosenthal, Professor of Psychology at the Harvard, where students at an elementary school were given a disguised IQ test, of which 20% (selected at random) were represented to the teachers as having a particularly higher IQ. Interestingly, students who were described as having higher IQs actually showed significant gains in both their IQ score and exam results in subsequent tests taken 8 months later. Dubbed the Rosenthal effect, this establishes how positive expectation and attention on the part of the teacher can positively affect the performance of the student by encouraging the students to live up to teacher expectations.

Humans, like all other animals, are social learners. We learn to perform behaviors in such a way to gain reward and to avoid sanctions. In retrospect, I realize my entire life too has been shaped by my endeavors to win the approval and praise of my parents as a child, my teachers as a student, my professors as a medical resident, and my patients for the past 20 years as their aesthetic physician. Positive feedback is in my mind is the most powerful driver for boosting higher performance. So the next time you feel inclined to applaud someone on their strengths, don't be shy. After all, there's nothing like a good compliment to bring out the best in all of us (September 2019).

4.8 Malar Eminence

Difficulty Level: A, Effectiveness: A, Complications: B

Summary 1: A 23-G × 5-cm cannula is used for injection in the supraperiosteal layer deep to the SOOF. Both biphasic HA fillers with large particle size and monophasic HA fillers with high viscoelasticity are acceptable for use.

Summary 2: Volume is enhanced in the zygomatic arch lying lateral to a line connecting the lateral canthus and the oral commissure.

Summary 3: Augmentation of the zygomatic arch is not suited for northern facial type Asians with an inherently pronounced zygoma, as accentuating the zygomatic prominence serves to broaden their wide faces.

Enhancement of the malar eminence can complement a thin dolichocephalic Caucasian face by creating definition and adding balance to the horizontally narrow facial appearance [16].

And also a slight convexity of the lateral zygoma is a feature highly coveted by Caucasian females, as it forms an integral element of the "Ogee (Ω) curve" or the "triangle of beauty" upheld as the aesthetic ideal in this population [17] (Fig. 4.13).

4.8.1 Anatomical Considerations

From the outer to inner, the relevant tissue layers of the lateral cheek can be divided as follows: the skin—subcutaneous fat layer or the superficial layer of the malar fat pad—orbicularis oculi m.—SOOF or the deep layer of the malar fat pad—mimetic muscles including the zygomaticus minor and major—periosteum (Fig. 4.49).

4.8.2 Pretreatment Assessment

Malar eminence augmentation is a prime example where ethnic differences must be considered when performing filler injection (see Sect. 1.3). Accentuating the zygomatic arch works best for a Caucasian female subject presenting with a long, narrow dolichocephalic face, as it brings the midface closer to achieving the aesthetic ideal of the Ogee curve. By contrast, the procedure is not recommended for a northern facial type Asian dem-

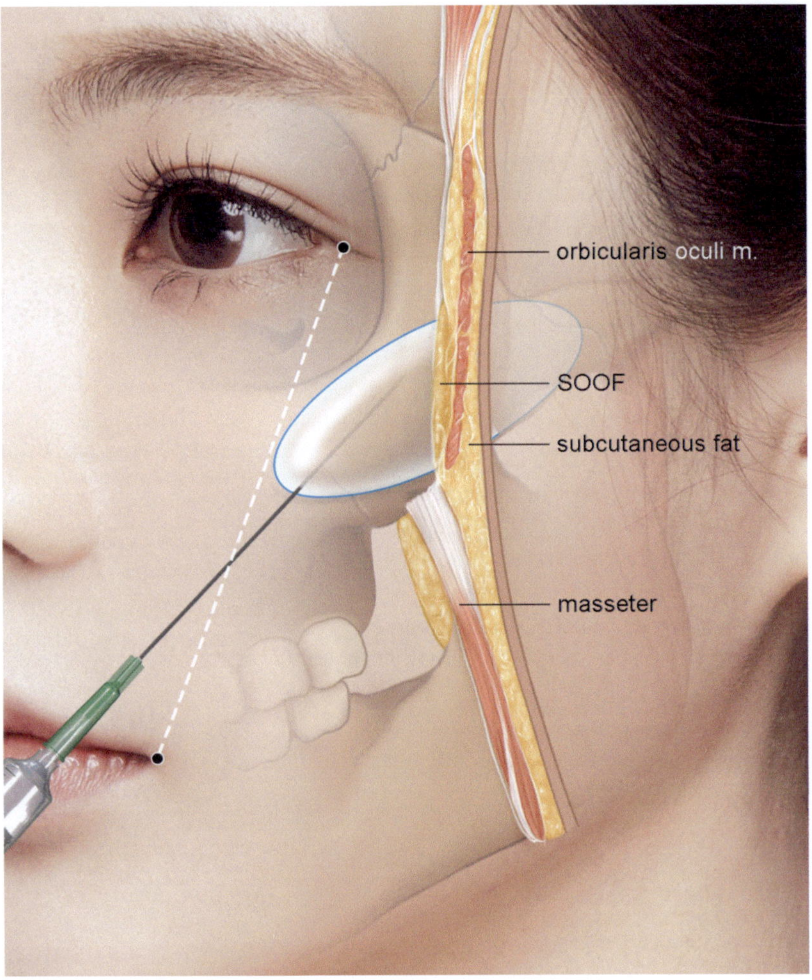

Fig. 4.49 Depth of injection for the malar eminence

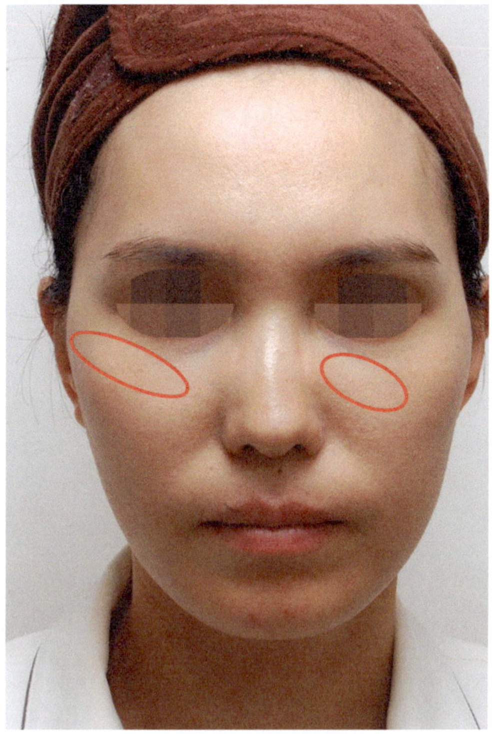

Fig. 4.50 Differences in malar augmentation between West and East. Accentuating the zygomatic arch is not recommended for a Northern Facial Type Asian demonstrating a brachycephalic face, as highlighting the zygomatic prominence would only serve to make their broad faces appear bigger and wider

onstrating a brachycephalic face, as highlighting the zygomatic prominence would only serve to make their broad zygoma appear bigger and wider [18] (Fig. 4.50). That being said, a slight elevation of the malar eminence may be of benefit to a southern facial type Asian patient manifesting a small narrow face (Fig.1.16). It is therefore prudent to consult with each patient regarding their individual aesthetic preferences before proceeding with the augmentation of the malar eminence.

Episode: A must-do in Korea

It has long been the case that two of the top things to do when a Korean female residing in the U.S. visits Korea are getting a medical check-up and undergoing an aesthetic procedure. Health screening programs in Korea are efficient, of good quality, and affordably priced. A comprehensive medical screening program inclusive of both upper GI endoscopy *and* colonoscopy typically costs around $1500, the equivalent of what it costs to get a GI endoscopy alone in the United States. In this respect, getting a medical package in Korea makes better economic sense for overseas Koreans even considering the cost of the round trip airfare.

Aesthetic procedures represent another must-do in Korea as treatments performed by Western physicians tend to miss the subtle nuances of the aesthetic ideal pursued by Koreans. Even in the most skilled and capable hands, Asian patients tend to find aesthetic outcomes produced by their Western-trained doctors less than satisfactory due to the differences in beauty standards to which they aspire. This typically occurs in the context of Asian double-eyelid surgeries or augmentation rhinoplasty performed overseas. The purpose of the double-eyelid surgery is to create a pretarsal crease (i.e., "double eyelid") in an upper eyelid that is naturally without a pretarsal crease. However, double-eyelid surgeries performed by Western-trained plastic surgeons tend to create lid creases too tall for the narrow Asian eyes. Meanwhile, rhinoplasty undertaken in Caucasians is known to be geared primarily toward reduction rhinoplasty indicated for decreasing a humped or an overly large nose in contrast to augmentation rhinoplasty highly requested by Asian patients to elevate their flat noses.

The same can be said of BoNT-A treatments. Whereas smaller doses of BoNT-A are more appropriate for Asians given the relatively reduced activity and mass of their facial mimetic muscles, the use of high BoNT-A dosages typically described for Caucasians tends to result in an unnatural frozen appearance in Asian patients. Also, while the preferred shape of eyebrows for a Korean woman is horizontally straight and flat, failure to appreciate such aesthetic preferences on the part of the Western practitioner will lead to highly arched brows that are disfavored by Koreans as it gives their faces a harsh and severe appearance. Whereas a Caucasian physician may favor effacing the under-eye pretarsal fullness in Asians with BoNT-A believing it to cause the relatively small palpebral aperture in Asians to appear even smaller upon smiling, a Korean aesthetic patient would instead elect to have their pretarsal roll augmented with HA fillers, as the presence of this roll imparts a soft, friendly, and smiley impression. In a nutshell, mapping the BoNT-A treatment strategies and dosages described for Caucasians directly onto an Asian patient can create a face that appears aggressive and unnatural, devoid of any feelings or expressions.

The same applies to filler treatments. Taking the popular treatment of cheek augmentation as an example, when cheek filler is indicated for a Caucasian patient, volume is typically added laterally in the malar eminence and zygomatic arch to accentuate the triangle of beauty or the Ogee (Ω) curve upheld as the aesthetic ideal in this population. However, a prominent lateral zygoma set against sunken cheeks is a feature largely disfavored by an average Korean female whose perception of facial beauty consists of an oval babyish face with full plump cheeks. Where the physician and patient are not on the same page in terms of their facial aesthetic standards and preferences, the well-meaning Western physician may believe he provided satisfactory augmentation of the patient's lateral cheeks, while the Korean patient is left displeased with the wider zygoma she ended up with. Obviously, this is what causes the overseas Korean resident to seek out HA filler treatments in Korea where she can find a practitioner whose aesthetic style resonates with her better. Fortunately, it is a welcome development that a growing proportion of Western physicians practicing in the United States and elsewhere are becoming increasingly appreciative of the ethnic variations in aesthetic standards and are differentiating their HA filler and BoNT-A treatments to ethnic patients accordingly.

4.8.3 Injection Technique

Both biphasic HA fillers with large particle size and monophasic HA fillers with high viscoelasticity are acceptable for use (Table 4.8). The use of a 23-G × 5-cm cannula is generally preferred for treating the lateral cheeks. The relevant plane of injection is the supraperisoteal layer at the deepest level of the SOOF below the orbicularis oculi (Fig. 4.49). The cannula entry point is made at the intersection between a vertical line dropped from the lateral canthus and a horizontal line running through the nasal base (Fig. 4.51). Insert the cannula deep into the SOOF of the zygomatic arch and place the filler along the zygomatic arch from the midpoint of the arch to the point sitting lateral to the line connecting the lateral canthus and the oral commissure. Augment the zygomatic arch to the desired height by depositing HA via retrograde linear threading for primary volumization. Next, using the same approach, place smaller amounts of HA immediately above and below the first injection to smoothen the curvature of the malar eminence. The injection volume should range between 0.5 and 2 mL, depending on the deficiency of lateral cheek volume. The nondominant hand should be used to stretch the cheek inferomedially during the procedure to maintain tension on the skin overlying the lateral zygoma. Concerning anesthesia, application of topical numbing cream should suffice. Where the patient presents with concurrent depression in the anteromedial malar or a palpebromalar groove, volume should be added concurrently in these adjacent regions for a more favorable aesthetic balance.

Table 4.8 Summary of injection technique for lateral cheek augmentation

Item	Contents
Needle vs. Cannula	23-G 5-cm cannula for SOOF layer
HA filler	Biphasic HA filer with large particle size or monophasic HA filler with high viscoelasticity
Amount of HA filler	0.5–2 mL per side
Depth of injection	Deep SOOF layer above the periosteum
Entry point for cannula	The point where a vertical line from lateral canthus meets the horizontal line from the nasal base
Target area	Zygomatic arch from the midpoint of the arch to the point sitting lateral to the line connecting mouth corner and the lateral canthus
Anesthetics	Topical anesthetics
Nondominant hand	Hold the skin inferiorly in order to maintain the skin tension

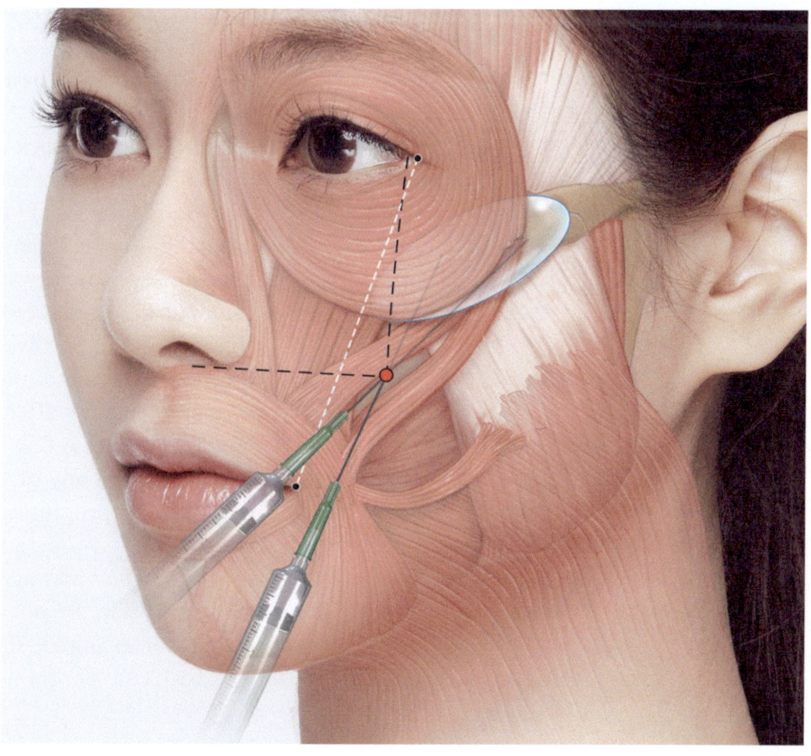

Fig. 4.51 Cannula entry point for malar eminence augmentation

4.8.4 Complications

Irregularities: Augmenting the lateral cheeks without regard to the concurrent anteromedial malar depression, submalar depression or a palpebromalar groove may lead to unfavorable contour irregularities. Note that the procedure may exacerbate the appearance of a wide zygoma in those with a prominent zygomatic arch.

4.9 Nose

Difficulty Level: B, Effectiveness: A, Complications: C

Summary 1: Injection is performed primarily with a 23-G 5-cm cannula. The cannula entry point is created at the infratip lobule. Needles may be used only for performing deep supraperiosteal placement of HA filler in the radix. Regarding the choice of HA filler, use only biphasic HA fillers with large particles.

Summary 2: The ideal nasal length corresponds to three quarters (3/4) the length of the lower facial third while the nasal dorsal width at the radix should approximate the height of the palpebral fissure or 60% of the width of the nasal tip. The ideal aesthetic range for the NLA is between 90° and 110° and is generally wider in females than in men.

Summary 3: Dorsum augmentation is indicated for correcting a flat, short nose, a nasal hump, saddle nose, or any other irregularities in the nasal dorsum. Nasolabial angle correction is ideal for treating a low-set, plunged nose, as it gives anterior projection and cephalic rotation to a droopy, under projected nasal tip.

Summary 4: Preferably, patients should be monitored in the office for approximately 30 min postinjection for any ischemic skin changes such as greyish or violaceous skin discoloration. Where any vascular occlusion is suspected, subcutaneous injection of hyaluronidase in sufficient volume (> 3000 U) and high concentration (750 U/mL) is required along the entire nasal dorsum (from nasal tip to radix) where the ischemic signs are present.

The nose represents the central feature of the face with an aesthetically profound effect on the overall balance of other facial components including the eyes and the mouth. Accordingly, reshaping a flat and poorly defined nose can add definition and sophistication to the overall face. It is not surprising then that surgical rhinoplasty for enhancing the nose has long been practiced as a popular procedure in Asians whose nose is generally flatter and less pronounced than that of Caucasians. It is for this same reason that filler rhinoplasty, which allows convenient reshaping of the nose without the downtime involved in surgery, has become one of the most popular injectable filler procedures among Asians [19]. While the need for repeat treatments due to the dissipation of the injected HA filler over time may appear as a drawback against traditional operative rhinoplasty, this becomes a moot point when considering the good longevity of HA filler in the nasal region which may last for up to 5–10 years. Instead, the countervailing advantages of filler rhinoplasty are numerous and compelling. Most significantly, it involves minimum social downtime since there is almost no bruising or swelling even immediately after the procedure. Moreover, in terms of its safety profile, filler rhinoplasty does not entail any of the risks arising from surgery such as progression of nasal deviation over time due to postoperative scar contracture or an overly pinched and narrow nasal tip. That being said, HA fillers are not suited for reduction rhinoplasty, for example, sharpening a bulbous nose, reducing the size of a large nose, eliminating a nasal hump, or narrowing a wide nasal dorsum, etc., since such outcomes can ultimately be accomplished only by surgical procedures [19]. This chapter aims to provide an overview of the techniques, useful tips, and precautions involved in performing nose augmentation with HA filler.

4.9.1 Anthropometry of the Nose

While there is no uniform standard for an ideal nose that works for every face, an aesthetic nose may generally be characterized as featuring a high dorsum and projected tip, though subtle differences exist between the sexes, ethnic groups, and changing aesthetic trends. An ideal nose is also one that is well proportioned for the individual's face, as facial beauty is a function of the balanced and harmonious relationship among various facial components. In this regard, the metrics for defining ideal facial ratios are by no means absolute and notions such as the "golden ratio" does not universally hold true in every case. Nonetheless, having a general sense of facial balance and proportionality can be instrumental in the planning and treatment of filler rhinoplasty in individual patients, as will be detailed as follows.

The nose is divided into several anatomical subunits including the dorsum, sidewall, nasal tip, ala nasi, and columellar (Fig. 4.52). In addition, there are certain topographic landmarks of the nose used for cosmetic and reconstructive procedures as shown in the illustration. Although the term "nasion" is sometimes used mistakenly to refer to the deepest point of the nasal root, technically speaking, the nasion represents the midpoint of the nasofrontal suture line. Instead, when referring to the most posterior point of the

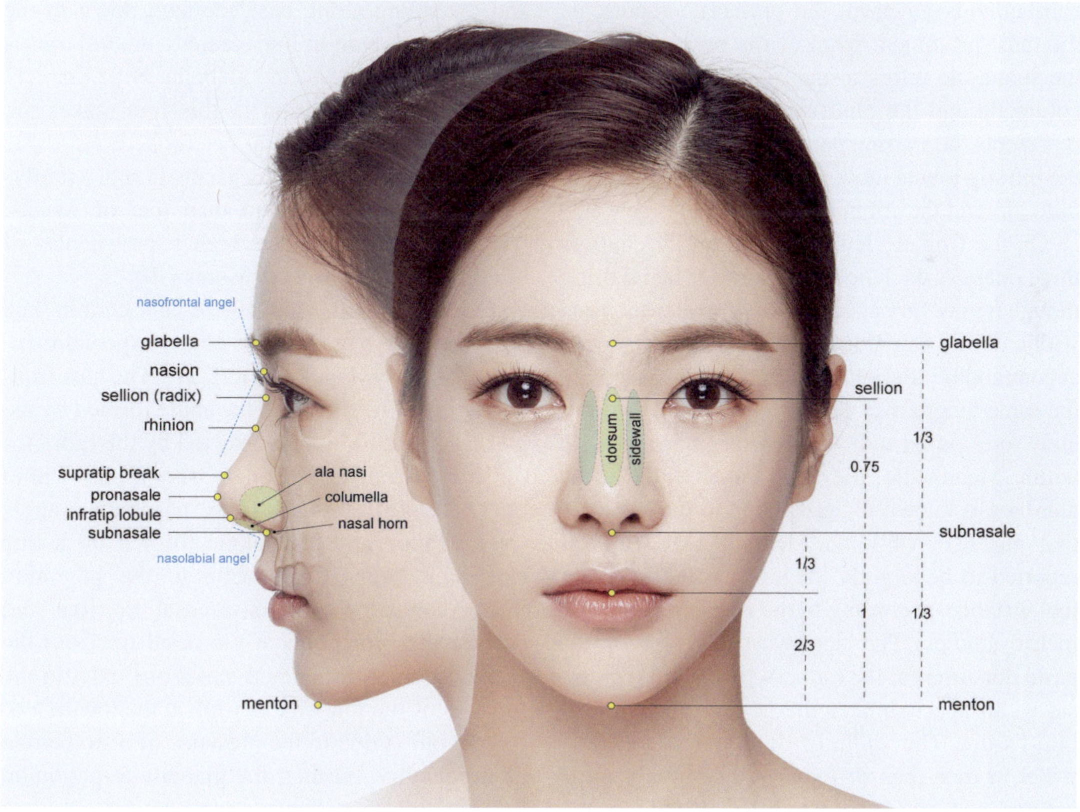

Fig. 4.52 Topographical facial landmarks and ideal facial proportions

Table 4.9 Anthropometric factors for filler rhinoplasty

Indication	Anthropometric Factor	Definition
Nasal dorsum augmentation	Nasofrontal angle	angle between the nasal dorsum line and the glabella line
	Modified nasofacial angle	angle between the nasal dorsum line and the line perpendicular to the Frankfurt horizontal line (PFHL)
	Radix height increment (RHI%)	Radix height (RH) is the distance between the radix and the line parallel to the PFHL drawn at the anterior margin of the lower eyelid. RHI (%) represents the rate of increase (%) in the RH measured before and after treatment.
Tip rotation	Nasolabial angle	angle between the line tangent to the columella and the subnasale-to-labial limb line
Hump correction	Rhinion angle	angle between the nasal dorsum line and the rhinion-to-nasal tip line

Reproduced from Ref. [20]

nasal bone or the nasofrontal angle, the proper term should be the "sellion" [19]. However, since the sellion represents a bony landmark, the more relevant term for describing the "soft tissue sellion" or the deepest point of the nasal root corresponding to the surface anatomy would be the "radix." Meanwhile, the rhinion marks the osseocartilaginous junction, the pronasale represents the most prominent point of the nasal tip, while the subnasale refers to the junction between the columella and the philtrum. The supratip break represents the starting point of the nasal tip, while the infratip lobule marks the junction between the nasal tip and the columella.

On the frontal view, the ideal nasal length is three quarters the length of the lower facial third, though it may vary according to the relevant nasal width. While individuals with a wide nose can accommodate a slightly increased nasal length, the same length may appear to be disproportionately long on an individual with a narrow nasal width. Meanwhile, the ideal nasal width at the alar base is known to correspond to the intercanthal distance, while the actual nasal width is reported to be slightly longer than the intercanthal distance, according to the relevant anthropometric studies. The narrowest segment of the nasal dorsum is at the radix, where the nasal dorsal width approximates the height of the palpebral fissure. The width of the radix is generally wider in men than in females, but should in no case exceed 60% of the nasal width at the alar base even in males. Precaution must be taken, in this regard, against placing too much volume in the radix/upper nasal dorsum with the intent of elevating the nasal height, as the excess volume would end up spreading sideways broadening the nasal dorsum as a consequence. Meanwhile, a gentle curvilinear arch emanating from the medial brow toward the lateral border of the radix and extending along nasal dorsum down to the nasal tip in a straight line creates a natural transition from the nose to the glabella. Note that any irregularity or deviation in this line makes the nose appear asymmetrical or crooked. As a side note, the nasal tip in Caucasians is more thinly-skinned and well defined than that of Asians, which accounts for the higher prevalence of bilobed nasal tips in Caucasians [19].

On the lateral view, there are certain key anthropometric factors that deserve special mention (Table 4.9; Fig. 4.53) [20, 21]. The nasofrontal angle (NFrtA) reflects the angle formed by the glabella-to-radix line intersected by the radix-to-tip line. Ideally, this angle should be within the 115°–130° range. The nasofacial angle (NFcA) represents the angle formed by a line extending from the glabella to the pogonion intersected by the radix-to-nasal tip line and defines the projection of the nasal tip from the face. However, individual variations exist in the fullness of the glabella as well as the location of the pogonion due to the presence of retrognathia or prognathia. Further, the glabella-to-pogonion line is subject to change where the patient were to undergo any forehead glabella and/or chin

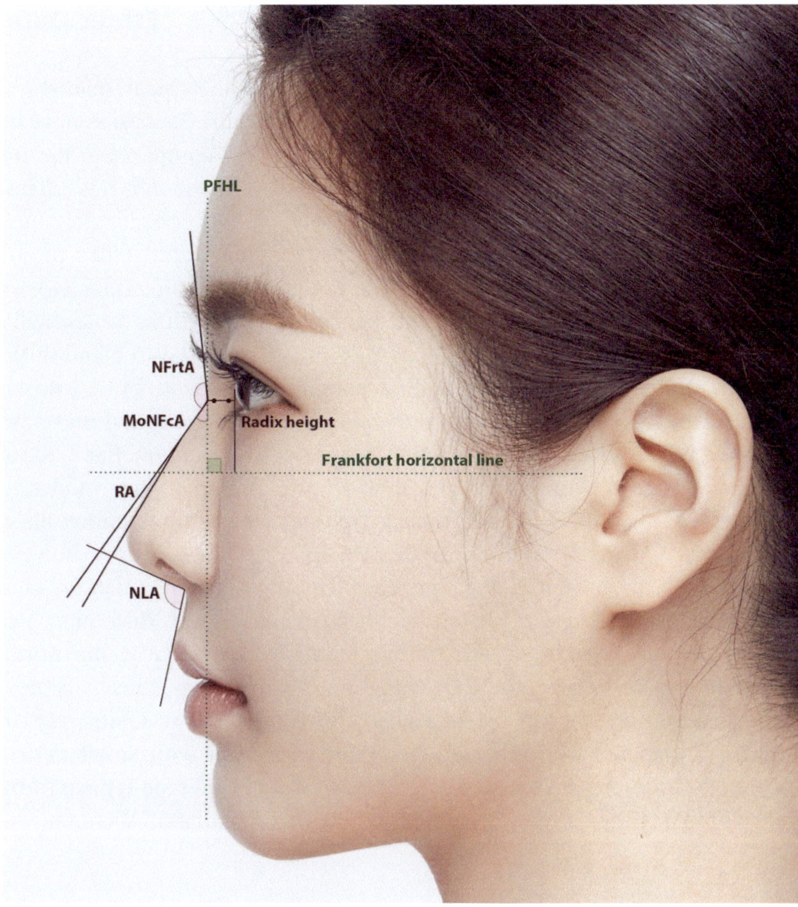

Fig. 4.53 Anthropometric factors related to the nose. *MoNFcA* modified nasofacial angel, *NFrtA* nasofrontal angle, *RA* rhinion angle, *NLA* nasolabial angle

augmentation. That being the case, the line perpendicular to the Frankfort horizontal line (PFHL) is more suitable as the reference rather than the glabella-to-pogonion line for defining nasal tip projection. The resulting angle formed by the intersection between the radix-to-tip line and the PFHL is referred to as the *modified NFcA* (MoNFcA) [20]. The aesthetic ideal for MoNFcA is 35°–40°. Meanwhile, the nasolabial angle (NLA), useful for assessing the effectiveness of nasal tip rotation, represents the angle formed by the line tangent to the columella intersected by the subnasale-to-labial limb line [19]. Opening the nasolabial angle beyond 90° can create a more refined and sophisticated nasal contour on the profile view. The ideal aesthetic range for the NLA is between 90° and 110°, though it may differ by ethnicity and sex, with the female NLA being wider than that of males. The ideal NLA of males is reported to be less than 90°.

To date, the efficacy of nasal radix/dorsum augmentation via surgery or filler rhinoplasty could only be inferred indirectly by reference to the changes in the nasofrontal or nasofacial angles. A direct comparison of the nasal dorsal height pre- and posttreatment was hard to make due to the lack of prior literature providing objective anthropometric assessments. It was against this backdrop that the author developed an indicator for objectively establishing the incremental increase in nasal dorsal height posttreatment via anthropometric measurement, termed as the Radix Height Increment (RHI) [20]. The RHI represents the rate of increase

(%) in the distance between the radix and the line parallel to the PFHL drawn at the anterior margin of the lower eyelid measured before and after treatment. In addition, the author also developed the concept of the rhinion angle (RA), defined as the angle between the radix-to-rhinion line intersected by the rhinion-to-nasal tip line to ensure an objective anthropometric assessment of nasal hump correction. The RA is 0 in those with no nasal humps and becomes higher with increased severity.

In the anthropometric study of 242 patients who received HA filler rhinoplasty at the author's clinic, the NFrtA was found to have increased on average by 5.7° from 138.7° ± 6.1° to 144.4° ± 4.9°, the MoNFcA to have decreased on average by 1.9° from 30.2° ± 4.6° to 28.3° ± 4.1°, while the NLA showed a 9.4° increase from 87.4° ± 10° to 96.8° ± 10° [20] (Table 4.10). In patients who received nasal dorsum augmentation at the author's clinic, the RHI was found to have increased on average by 78.3% postinjection. In 25 patients who received HA filler for hump correction, the RA showed a decrease of 8° from 11° to 3° [20].

4.9.2 Ethnic Differences

The typical features of a leptorrhine (tall and thin) Caucasian nose have been described above. By comparison, the platyrrhine (broad and flat) African nose is characterized by a low radix, short concave dorsum, widened alae base, a bulbous and under projected tip, flared alae with round nostrils, and extremely thick skin. The mesorrhine (intermediate) Asian nose is characterized as a blend of the two; it is typically characterized by a low broad dorsum, short nasal bone, a round under projected and under-rotated tip, columellar recession, somewhat rounded nostrils, and moderately thick skin [19]. The nasal tip is unilobular rather than sharp and well defined. Note, however, that even within the Asian population, stark distinctions are found among different facial morphotypes [18]. Specifically, the northern facial type common among those from Mongolia, Korea, and Northern China, etc. manifest a high nasal dorsum with small narrow nasal ala; the southern facial type typical of those from The Philippines, Thailand, Vietnam, and other Southeast Asian

Table 4.10 Comparison of anthropometric factors pre- and postfiller rhinoplasty

Subgroup	Anthropometric factors (°)	Preinjection	Postinjection	Difference
Nasal dorsum augmentation	NFrtA	138.0 ± 6.2	144.7 ± 4.5	6.7 ± 4.3**
	MoNFcA	30.8 ± 4.9	28.3 ± 4.1	−2.5 ± 2.8**
	RHI	100%	186%	86%
Tip rotation	NLA	80.0 ± 12.3	91.3 ± 9.3	11.3 ± 5.1**
Whole nose augmentation	NFrtA	139 ± 6.1	144.2 ± 5.1	5.2 ± 3.7**
	MoNFcA	29.7 ± 4.3	28.1 ± 4.0	−1.6 ± 2.8**
	NLA	87.6 ± 9.6	96.9 ± 10	9.3 ± 4.5**
	RHI	100%	176.2%	76.2%
Hump Correction	RA[c]	10.9 ± 2.7	3.3 ± 2.9	−7.6 ± 2.6**
Total	NFrtA[a]	138.7 ± 6.1	144.4 ± 4.9	5.7 ± 4.1**
	MoNFcA[a]	30.2 ± 4.6	28.3 ± 4.1	−1.9 ± 2.9**
	NLA[b]	87.4 ± 10	96.8 ± 10	9.4 ± 4.5**
	RHI[a]	100%	178.3%	78.3%

[a]Measured only among the nasal dorsum augmentation group and whole nose augmentation group (234 among 242)
[b]Measured only in the tip rotation group and the whole nose augmentation group (130 among 242)
[c]Measured only in the hump correction group. (25 among 242)
NFrtA nasofrontal angle, *MoNFcA* modified nasofacial angle, *RHI* radix height increment, *NLA* nasolabial angle, *RA* rhinion angle
**$p < 0.01$
Reproduced from Ref. [20]

countries exhibit a flat nasal dorsum with wide, round nasal ala, while the intermediate facial type representative of those from Hong Kong, Taiwan, Southern China represent a combination of the other two. As such, applying a strict ethnic classification becomes increasingly less meaningful, as differences arise even within the same ethnic population, distinct ethnic features become more muted due to increased interracial marriages, and standards of beauty become increasingly universal. That notwithstanding, a general appreciation of such ethnic differences can lend some precious insight when providing filler rhinoplasty to ethnic patients.

4.9.3 Anatomical Considerations

The soft tissue of the nose consists of the following five layers from the outer to the deep: skin—subdermal fatty layer—fibromuscular layer including the procerus m. and nasalis m.—deep fatty layers—and periosteum/perichondrium layers [21]. The upper nasal dorsum is covered by the smooth, pliable, and mobile soft tissue envelope which allows sufficient space for HA filler placement both above and below the fibromuscular layer, that is, at the subdermal fat and the muscular/deep fatty layers. In contrast, the tight connection between the dermis and the fibromuscular layer at the nasal tip restricts the placement of HA filler in the subdermal fatty layer and requires most of the volume to be deposited instead in the deep fatty layer (Fig. 4.54). The use of a needle is best avoided during filler rhinoplasty, as the vascular supply in the nasal area runs extensively throughout the fibromuscular layer as well as the fatty layers lying both superficial and deep to it. That said, needles may be used for injecting HA filler deep into the supra-

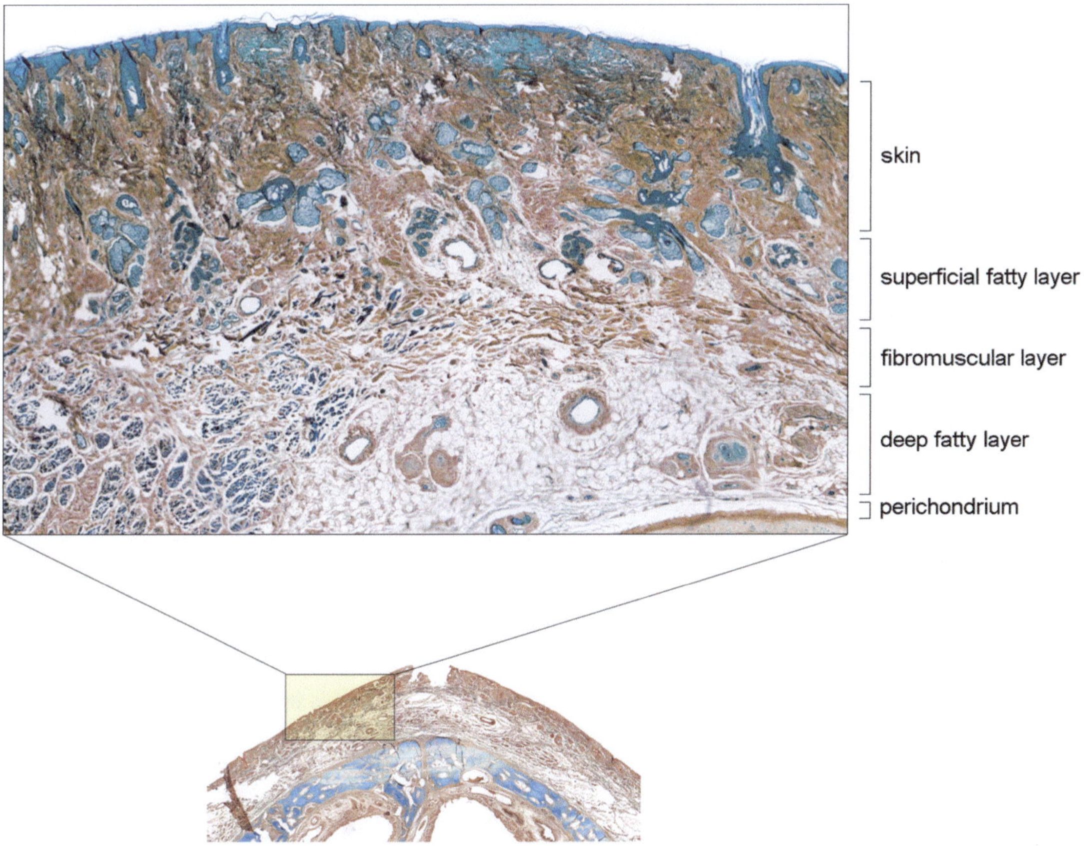

Fig. 4.54 Cross section of nose (courtesy of Pf. Kim Hee-Jin)

periosteal layer of the radix (located at the upper nasal dorsum) where the vasculature runs superficially between the fibromuscular and the subdermal fatty layer.

The blood supply to the external nose is provided largely by the ophthalmic artery, a branch of the internal carotid system, and the facial artery, a branch of the external carotid system.

The upper nasal dorsum is principally supplied by the dorsal nasal artery, a branch of the ophthalmic artery and the angular artery branching out from facial artery (Fig. 4.17). The blood supply to the lower nasal dorsum including the nasal tip originates primarily from the lateral nasal artery, while the columellar is supplied by the columellar branch of the superior labial artery and the inferior alar branch of the facial artery (Fig. 4.17) [21]. These arteries form broad-based anastomosis among themselves at the nasal dorsum. Therefore, any inadvertent intravascular injection of HA filler at the nasal tip is capable of causing skin necrosis across the entire nasal dorsum or, worse still, traveling through the dorsal nasal artery into the ophthalmic artery, leading to blindness as consequence.

4.9.4 Pretreatment Assessment

Perform an objective assessment of the nasal shape and size, before consulting with the patient on what they subjectively consider to be an aesthetic and balanced nose. First, evaluate the nose from the frontal view on the basis of the nasal dorsal length and height, nasal dorsal width, width of the nasal bone, width and size of the ala nasi, size and shape of the nasal tip, extent of columella show, nostril shape, and extent of nos-

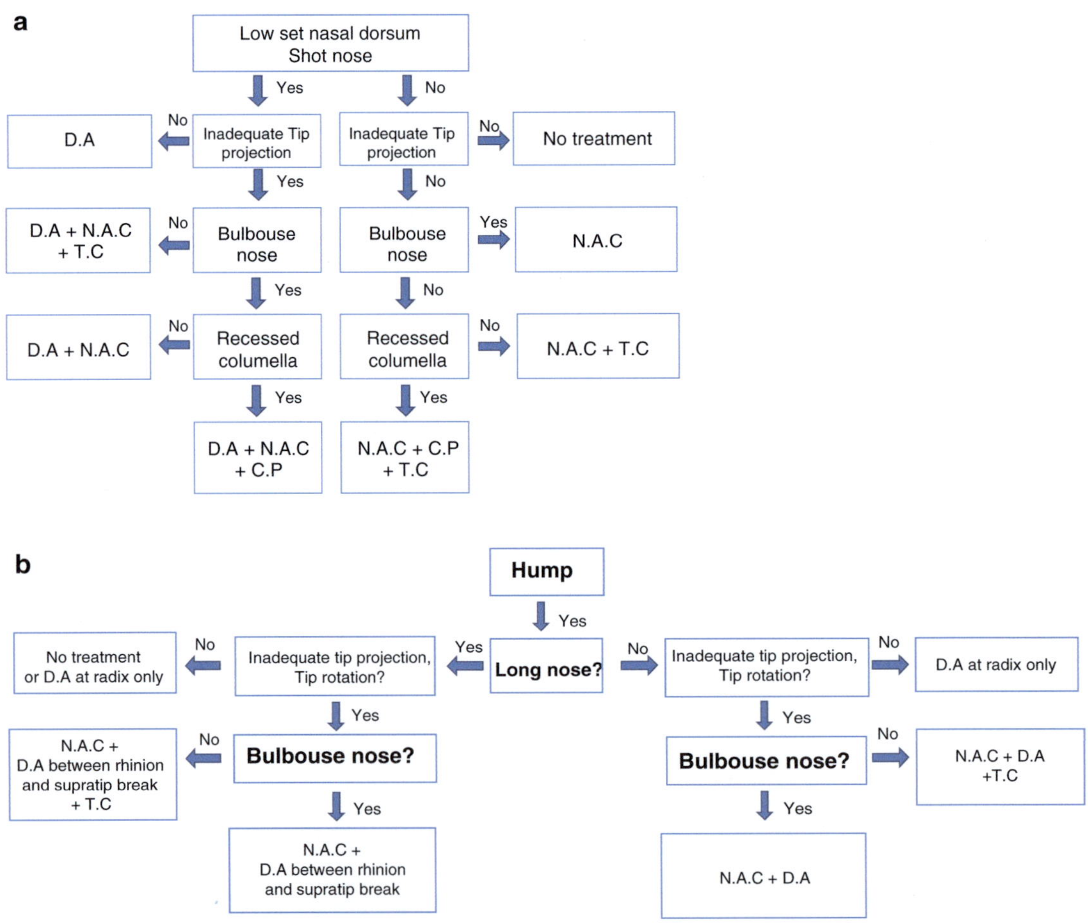

Fig. 4.55 Flow chart of pretreatment assessment for nose filler. (**a**) General assessment, (**b**) hump assessment (**N.A.C.* nasolabial angle correction, **T.C.* tip correction, **D.A.* dorsum augmentation, **C.P.* columella plasty)

tril show. Consideration must also be given to the adequacy of the nasal length relative to the length of the face, forehead, and the lower facial third. Consider also whether the nasal length is in adequate proportion to the nasal width; and also whether the width of the nasal dorsum is in adequate balance with the width of the ala base. The nasal tip should be also appraised for the presence of any bifid, bulbous, or plunging tip or inadequate tip projection.

Next, from the profile view, establish the presence or absence of dorsal humps or depressions lying between the rhinion and the nasal tip. Also, assess the nose for the adequacy of nasal dorsal height, nasal tip rotation, tip projection, columella length and columella show. The activity of the depressor septi nasi m. during speaking or smiling is also more visible from the lateral view.

Gender-specific differences as well as the ethnicity of the patient must also be reflected in the treatment plan. For an Asian patient, it should be further determined whether the patient belongs to the northern, southern or intermediate facial morphotype. Respecting different ethnic aesthetic preferences can be relevant, for example, when shaping the nasal tip with HA filler. While Asians tend to feature a nasal tip relatively larger and more rounded than that of Caucasians, and thus favor augmenting a bifid or overly sharp nose tip to bring it into better conformity with the prevailing aesthetic norm, a Caucasian patient may prefer instead to retain his/her bifid nasal tip. Meanwhile, skin in Asians tends to be generally thicker, thus allowing for an easier injection than in Caucasians. On the other hand, when treating an Asian patient, keen attention should be paid to the patients' past medical history, in particular, for any reference to a previous nose surgery, a procedure popular among Asians. Filler rhinoplasty should be avoided in areas where a nasal implant is placed; great caution is required even where the implant had been subsequently removed as it heightens the risk of vascular complications.

It is also imperative to confirm with the patient beforehand what they deem as the ideal nasal dorsal height. In most cases, however, patients tend to lack a clear idea of the desired dorsal height as they typically undergo the procedure for the very first time. For ease of communication, therefore, the author customarily presents the patient with the following three options; (a) maximal enhancement of the nasal dorsum as long as results appear natural in the eyes of a stranger, (b) subtle enhancement of the nasal dorsum perceptible only to the patient herself, or (c) somewhere in between. The patient's subjective preferences are also important in defining the ideal nasal width. Note that an aesthetic male nose can be wider than that of a female. Meanwhile, when performing a nasolabial angle correction with HA, it is advisable to identify and disclose to the patient prior to treatment any nostril show they may present, and inquire whether the patient would be comfortable with a slightly greater increase in nostril show following the procedure. Also, patients who have a wide nasal dorsum largely attributable to the width of the underlying nasal bone should be forewarned that nasal dorsum augmentation with HA filler may serve to further expand their nasal width.

4.9.4.1 Pretreatment Assessment Flowchart (Fig. 4.55)

As the first step, determine whether the patient has a low-set nasal dorsum or a short nose. Next, evaluate the nose for the adequacy of nasal tip rotation and projection. Patients presenting a low nasal dorsum with a short nasal length require nasal dorsum augmentation, while patients with an underprojected or underrotated nasal tip are candidates for columella and nasolabial angle correction. Nasal tip correction (i.e., augmentation of the nasal tip) may or maynot be indicated depending on the bulbousity of the nasal tip. The decision whether to create the arch-shaped transition between the glabella and the dorsum can be deferred until during the treatment of nasal dorsum. When treating a humped nose, consideration must first be given to the length of the nose relative to the overall facial length. Where the nasal length is disproportionately long for the face, nasal hump correction should be confined to the lower portion of the nose (i.e., between the rhinion and the nasal tip) combined with nasolabial angle correction. Corresponding augmentation in the upper dorsum (i.e., the radix) is best avoided in such patients, as it can make the nose appear even longer.

4.9.5 Injection Technique (Table 4.11)

Filler rhinoplasty can be broadly divided into five subcategories based on the injection site, namely nasal dorsum augmentation, glabella correction, nasal tip correction, columella correction, and nasolabial angle correction (Fig. 4.56). Dorsum augmentation is indicated for patients with a flat or short nose, a nasal hump, saddle nose or any other irregularities in the nasal dorsum, and is performed by injecting HA filler from the radix to the supratip break along the nasal dorsum. Glabella correction is often undertaken in conjunction with nasal dorsum augmentation to create a confluent arch-shaped transition extending from the medial brow of the glabella region to the nasal dorsum. Nasal tip correction is suitable for patients with bifid or otherwise blunt nasal tip, in which small volumes of HA filler are directly injected to augment the weak nasal tip, and incidentally allow mild cephalic rotation and slight projection. For columella correction, HA filler is injected in the columella to project the recessed columella; the procedure is often performed in conjuction with nasolabial angle correction. Nasolabial angle correction is performed by injecting HA filler deep into the anterior nasal spine of the subnasale. This helps to increase the nasolabial angle to more than 90°, causing not only nasal tip projection but also cephalic rotation of the nasal tip. As previously mentioned, nasolabial angle correction is routinely performed in tandem with columella correction, the combined effect of which is equivalent to a columellar strut insertion in surgical rhinoplasty. The procedure is ideal for patients with a plunged or pulling nose, as it projects the low and droopy nasal tip away from the face as well as rotating the tip upwards in a superior direction. Injection of HA in the anterior nasal spine also helps to narrow the nasal base on the frontal view while visually shortening a long nasal dorsum by tilting the nasal tip upwards. Further, an obtuse nasolabial angle wider than 90° combined with a slight protrusion of the columella contributes to a more sophisticated nasal contour on the profile view.

Table 4.11 Summary of Injection Technique for nose augmentation

Item	Contents
Needle vs. Cannula	23-G 5-cm cannula
HA filler	Biphasic HA filer with large particle size
Amount of HA filler	0.5–2 mL
Depth of injection	Deep subcutaneous layer above the periosteum.
Entry point for cannula	Infratip lobule
Target area	nasal dorsum augmentation, glabella correction, nasal tip correction, columella correction, and nasolabial angle correction
Anesthetics	Epi-lidocaine local anesthetics at entry point
Nondominant hand	Pinch the dorsum of nose to prevent lateral migration of HA filler during dorsum augmentation

Use only biphasic HA fillers with large particle size for injecting the nose. Note that HA filler has a propensity to attract water from surrounding tissues and the overlygin skin of the nasal dorsum is thin. To prevent lateral expansion of the nasal dorsum due to the undesired swelling of the HA filler, the use of biphasic HA filler, which is less hydrophilic in nature, is preferred over monophasic type HA filler. Also, in situations where the use of a needle is inevitable, biphasic HA fillers better lend themselves to preinjection blood aspiration tests. Meanwhile, in order to avoid inadvertent intravascular injection of HA filler, the use of the cannula is recommended instead of a needle. The practitioner may use a combination of different cannula sizes from among the 23-G 5-cm, 25-G 5-cm, and 27-G 3-cm as appropriate, depending on the relevant injection site and indication.

The cannula entry point is created at the infratip lobule located below the pronasale. The desired depth of injection is the deep fatty layer or supraperiosteal layer. Where necessary, additional injection in the subdermal superficial fatty layer may be performed subsequent to the primary augmentation in the supraperiosteal layer. In case where the use of a needle is inevitable, a 27-G or 30-G needle may be used for the injection. In such case, aspiration should be performed prior to each injection to ensure that the needle is

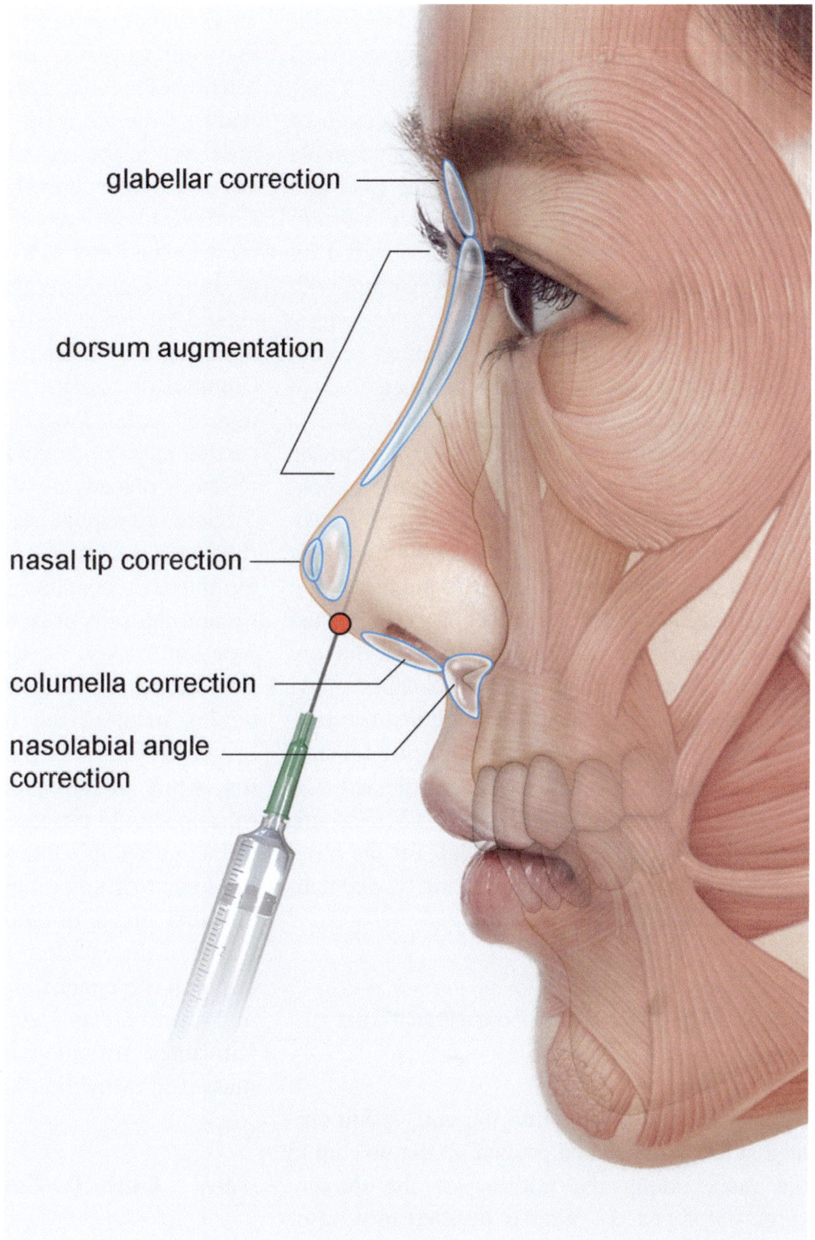

Fig. 4.56 Filler rhinoplasty can be broadly divided into five subcategories based on the injection site, namely nasal dorsum augmentation, glabella correction, nasal tip correction, columella correction, and nasolabial angle correction

not accidentally placed in the vessel. Note, however, that a negative aspiration does not necessarily guarantee 100% safety, as finer needles with smaller inner diameter may not adequately draw reflux blood even when it has entered a blood vessel [22]. According to one study, needles sized 27G or thinner were shown to be not amenable to aspiration [22].

As a general preventative strategy against intravascular injection, therefore, it is best to avoid the use of a needle altogether in the region between the nasal tip and the rhinion, as the vasculature in this area traverses even in the deep subcutaneous fat layer and muscular layers. Not coincidentally, in the five incidences involving intravascular injections encountered in the author's practice, a 30-G needle was used at the nasal tip. By comparison, the radix is a relatively safer area to inject as the blood supply runs mostly superficial to the musculature and thus intravascular injections can be avoided by injecting deep to the muscle at the supraperiosteal layer (Fig. 4.54).

With respect to anesthesia, prior injection of dental lidocaine with epinephrine in the cannula entry point is advised to help reduce pain and bleeding during the procedure. Wait for 3–5 min for the onset of dermal blanching triggered by epinephrine to create the needle entry point with a 21-G needle. When injecting HA filler using a 30-G needle, an anesthetic numbing cream applied 20–30 min in advance can help reduce discomfort during the procedure.

The adequate volume of HA filler to be injected varies widely depending on the indication and extent of correction required by each patient. In the anthropometric study involving 242 patients who underwent nose augmentation with HA filler at the author's clinic, the injected volume range was 1 ± 0.4 mL for nasal dorsum augmentation, 0.9 ± 0.3 mL for nasolabial angle correction, and 1.6 ± 0.5 mL for whole nose augmentation [20]. Broken down by specific subsites of injection, the range of volume injected was 0.3 ± 0.2 mL for the glabella area, 0.8 ± 0.4 mL for the nasal dorsum, 0.4 ± 0.2 mL for the nasal tip, and 0.7 ± 0.3 mL for the columella and subnasale, respectively.

4.9.6 Nasal Dorsum Augmentation (Fig. 4.57)

The cannula is inserted into the entry point created at the nasal tip and pushed all the way up to the radix, along the midline of the dorsum (Fig. 4.58). The HA filler is injected in a retrograde manner from the radix to the supratip breakpoint to build a "column" of injected HA filler to elevate the nasal dorsum to the desired height (Fig. 4.59). Subsequent HA filler injections are made on either side of the column to the desired width using the same technique, so that the transition to the nasal side wall is natural. Any unwanted contour irregularities between the heightened nasal dorsum (i.e., the injected HA filler column(s)) and the nasal side wall can be smoothened out with detailed corrections using a 30-G cannula from the nasal sidewalls. Note that the width of the nasal dorsum should be the narrowest at the radix, approximating 60–70% of the width of the nasal tip in an ideally proportioned nose. While the radix in an Asian face typically sits on the inter canthal line connecting the medial canthus of both eyes, injection of HA filler should relocate the radix 3–5 mm superior to its original position. Consequently, the repositioned radix should sit on a horizontal line connecting the highest points of the left and right eye lash-line or supratarsal crease. While HA filler may be injected as far down as the nasal tip in case concurrent nasal tip augmentation is required; otherwise it is placed only down to the supratip break.

Generally speaking, HA filler injection in the rhinion is best avoided if not limited to the minimum extent, considering the slight anterior protrusion naturally present at the osseocartilaginous junction as well as its very thin skin envelope. For the purpose of enhancing the nasal dorsal height, most of the volume should be placed instead at the radix located superior to the rhinion, while injection of the area inferior to the rhinion should proceed no further than the point immediately above the nasal tip, limited only to the extent of smoothening the transition to the elevated upper dorsum. The thumb and index finger of the nondominant hand should be used to pinch the upper nasal dorsum at the intercanthal line to prevent lateral migration of HA filler. Unwanted irregularities in contour should be massaged away via postinjection molding.

4.9.7 Glabella Correction

To ensure a smooth transition from the reshaped upper nasal dorsum to the orbital rim, arches naturally extending from the medial eyebrows toward the radix of the augmented nasal dorsum are created by injecting HA fillers into the glabella-to-radix region using a 27-G cannula (Fig. 4.60). Incidentally, heightening of the upper nasal dorsum may cause an obvious "step" at the junction where the elevated radix meets the relatively low-lying central glabella. Accordingly, the depression in the center of the glabella should be

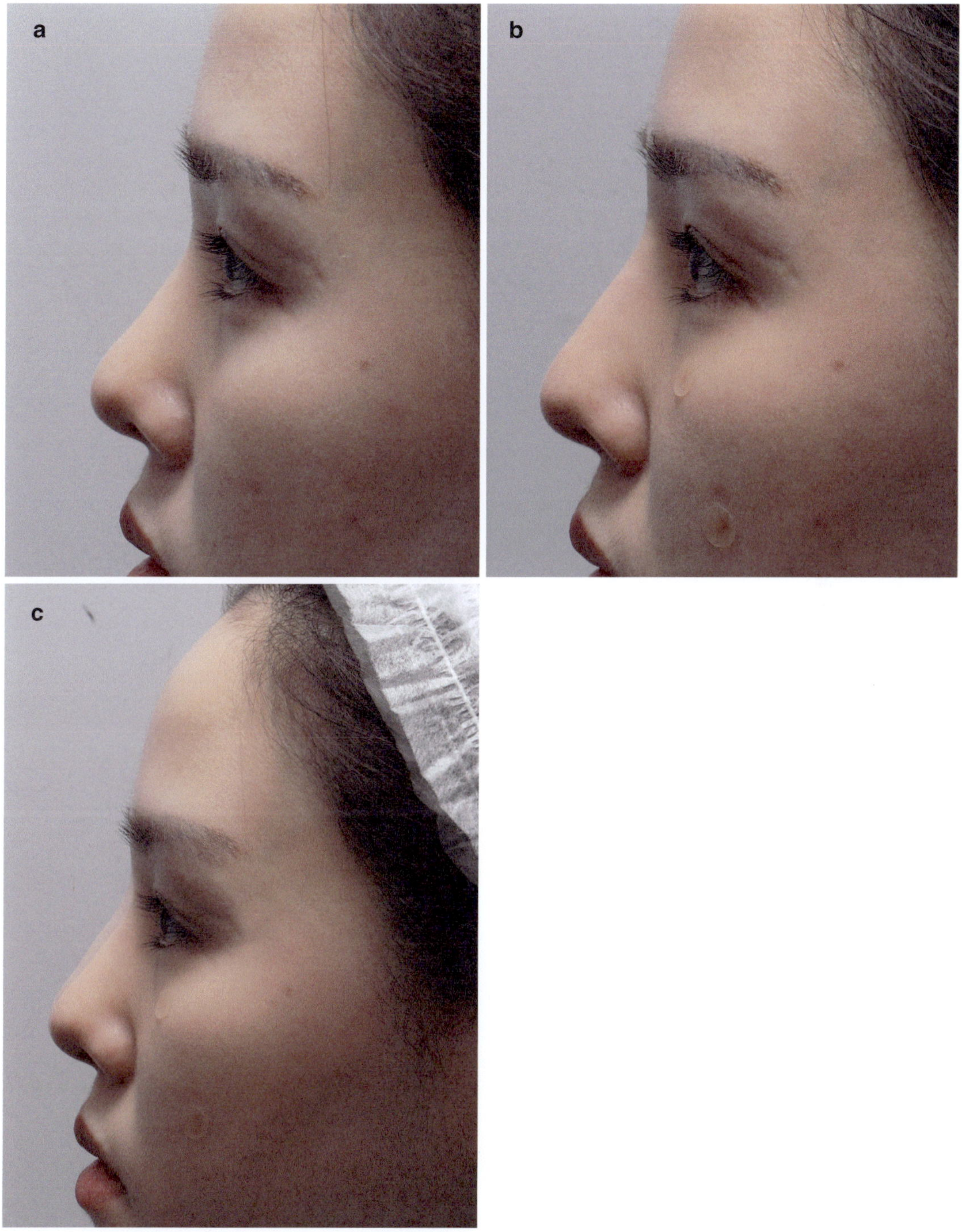

Fig. 4.57 (**a**) Before and (**b**) after nasal dorsum augmentation (**c**) Superimposed image of nasal dorsum before and after augmentation clearly domonstrates the heightened dorsum of nose

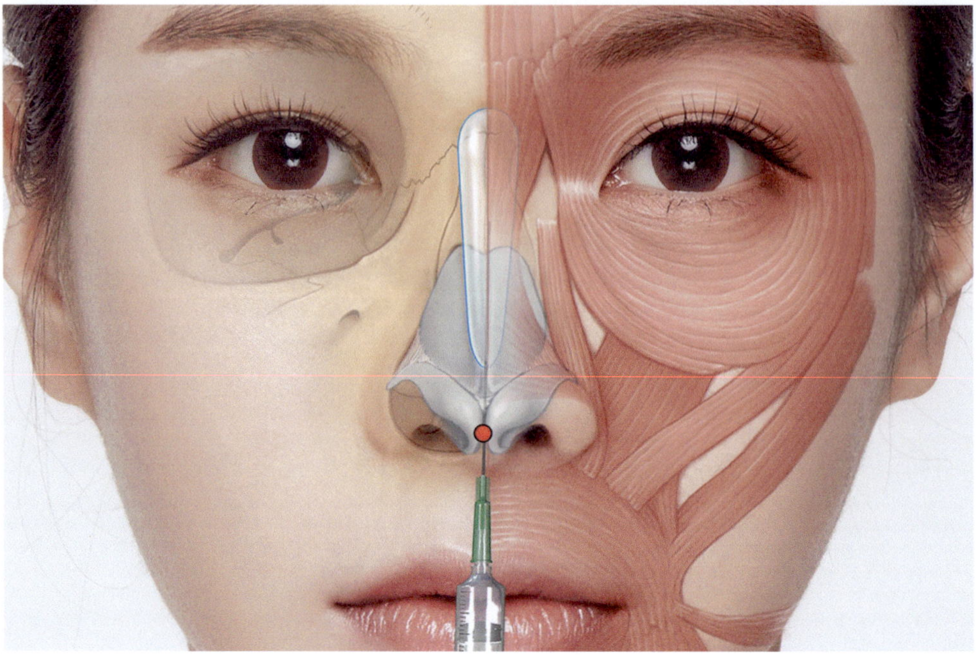

Fig. 4.58 The cannula entry point for nasal dorsum augmentation

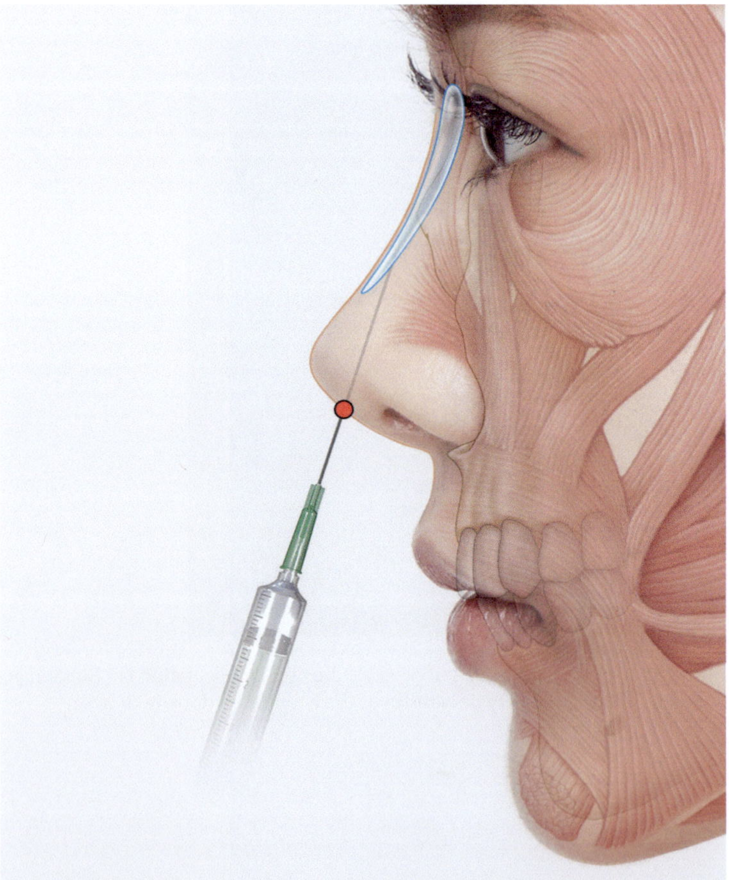

Fig. 4.59 Depth of injection for nasal dorsum augmentation

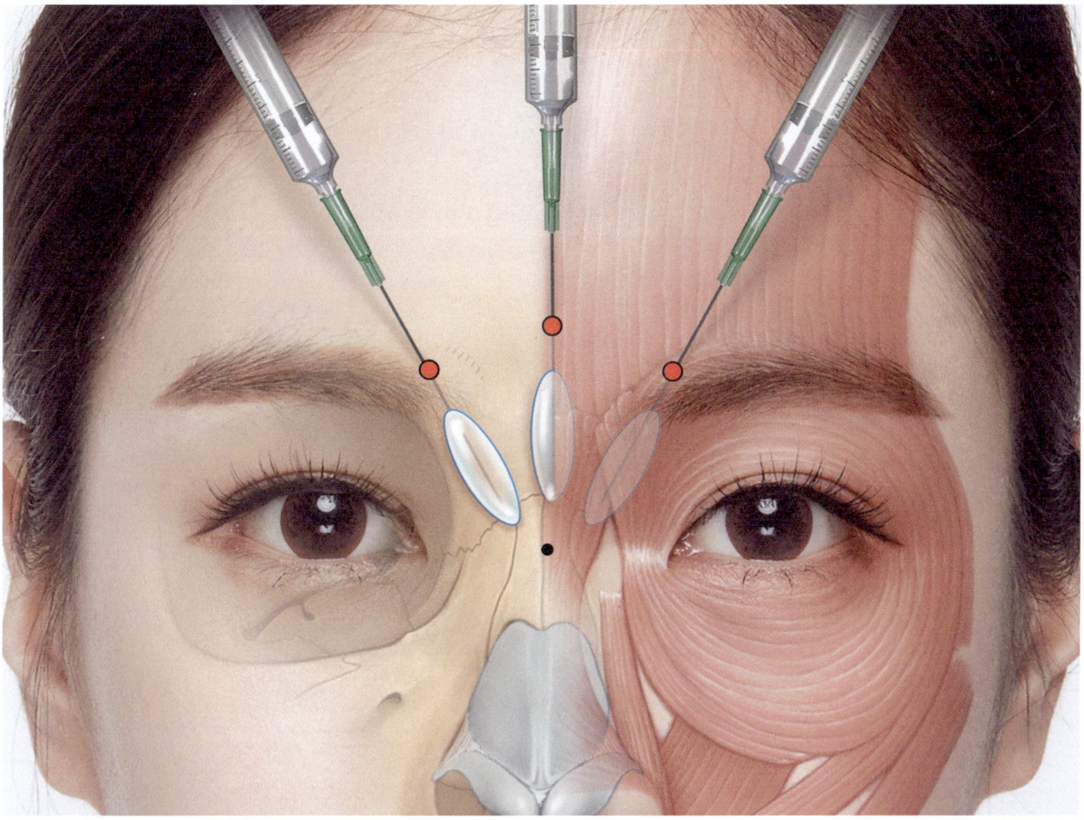

Fig. 4.60 The cannula entry point for glabella correction

filled in so as to remove such irregularity and to ensure an appropriate nasofrontal angle when viewed from the side. Note, however, that overfilling the arch connecting the glabella to the radix can widen the nasal dorsum, giving rise to the appearance of the "Avatar nose" or a "lion nose." Hence, care must be taken to ensure that the thickness of radix does not exceed 60% of the total width of the nose measured at the nasal base.

The same approach may be employed on a patient with a previous augmentation rhinoplasty to address any demarcations or "step" present between the inserted silicone implant and the glabella.

4.9.8 Nasal Tip Correction

A weak and overly pointy nasal tip can be corrected by placing HA filler into the interdomal area. It must be pointed out, however, that the size of the augmented tip should not be bigger than that of the ala nasi, since an excessively prominent nasal tip would be just as undesirable from an aesthetic perspective. HA filler injection into the interdomal area can also be beneficial for patients with a bifid nasal tip, as it smoothens the visible indentations in the nasal tip. Conversely, nasal tip augmentation is not advised for patients with a large round nasal tip, since they would end up instead with a prominently bulbous nose.

In principle, filler rhinoplasty is not indicated for sharpening a bulbous nasal tip. That said, HA filler placed in discrete amounts (0.1–0.2 mL) subdermally at the pronasale with a 27-G cannula or intradermally using the 30-G needle can add subtle projection to the pronasale, effecting a slightly sharper, better defined nasal tip (Fig. 4.61). This also has the effect of improving nasal tip projection and rotation from the lateral view. Of course, it bears reminding that where

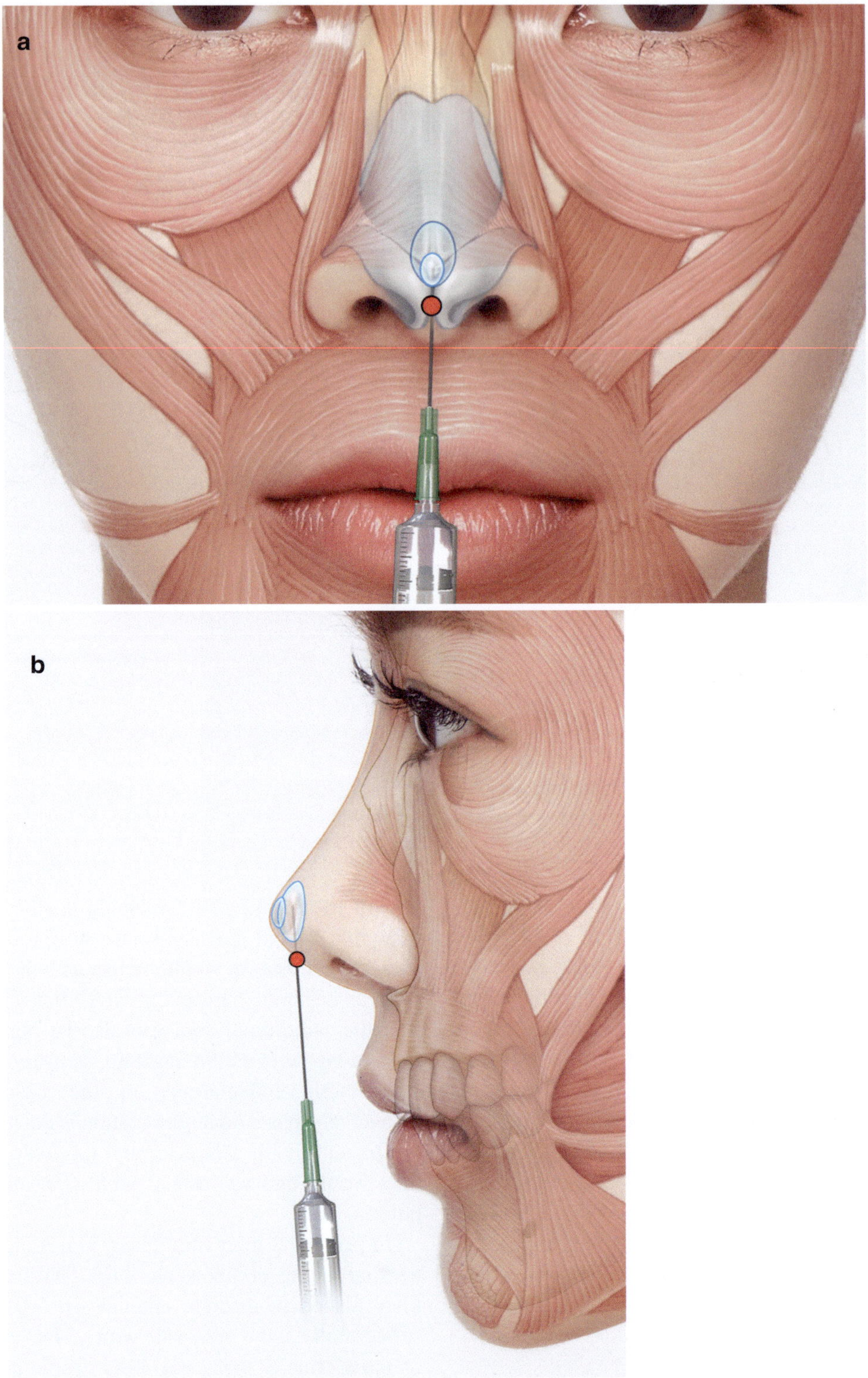

Fig. 4.61 (**a**) The cannula entry point for nasal tip correction. (**b**) Depth of injection for nasal tip correction

nasal tip rotation is the primary goal, concurrent corrections should preferentially be made to the columella and the nasolabial angle rather directly to the nasal tip itself.

4.9.9 Columella Correction

Too little columella show when observed in the lateral view is undesirable; instead, a slight protrusion of the columella creates a much more refined and sophisticated appearance. To this end, subcutaneous injection of HA filler in volume ranging from 0.2 to 0.5 mL into the columella helps to project the retracted columella (Fig. 4.62).

4.9.10 Nasolabial Angle Correction

The nasolabial angle is known to range between 95° and 120° in Caucasians, while the corresponding angle in Asians often falls below 90°. Injecting 0.3–1 mL of HA filler in the subcutaneous layer of the subnasale (i.e., on the nasal spine side) (Fig. 4.63) opens the nasolabial angle to beyond 90°, creating cephalic rotation of the nasal tip (Fig. 4.64). Enhancing the nasolabial angle not only refines the nasal contour on the profile view by everting the nasal tip and improving tip projection, but also has the effect of visually shortening a long nasal dorsum on frontal view. As the procedure is regularly performed in conjunction with columella correc-

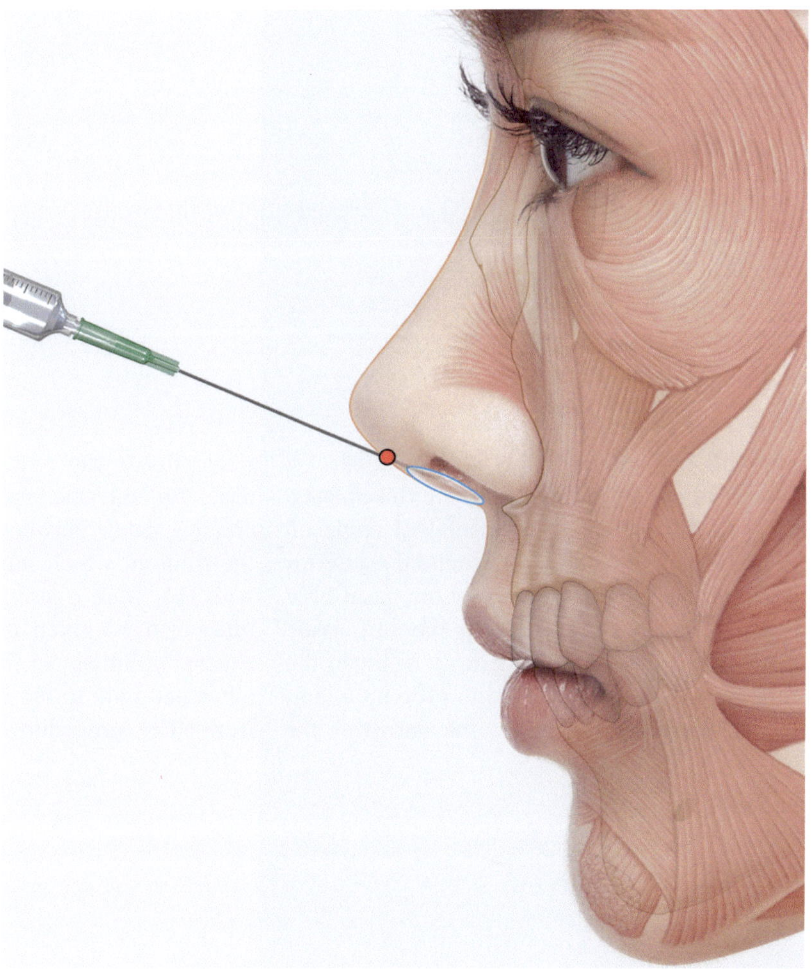

Fig. 4.62 Depth of injection for columella plasty

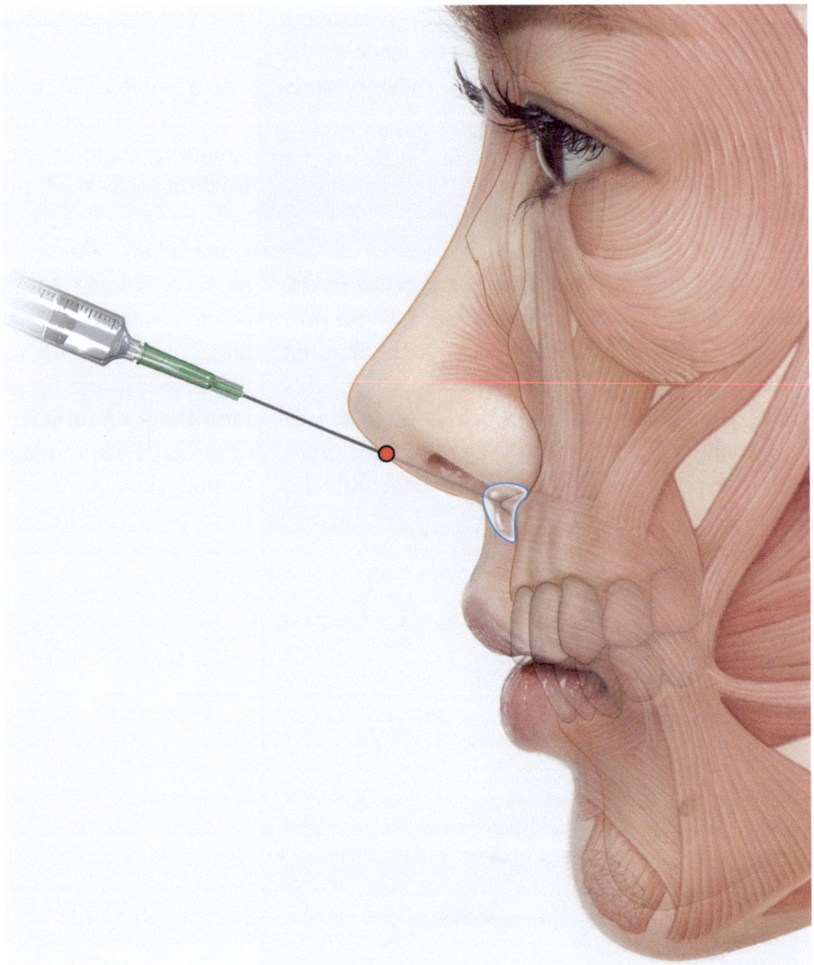

Fig. 4.63 Depth of injection for nasolabial angle augmentation

tion with HA, the net effect is equivalent to a columellar strut graft in surgical rhinoplasty. Apart from increasing the nasolabial angle on profile view, injection of HA around the anterior nasal spine also helps to narrow the nasal base on the frontal view, by tenting the soft tissue layers of the nasal base superiorly in much the same way tent poles are used to prop up a tent; that is, the taller the poles, the narrower the space inside the tent. Incidentally, lifting the nasal tip via nasolabial angle correction may create a saddle between the rotated nasal tip and the rhinion, which must be filled concurrently with HA filler to straighten the nasal profile. It must also be noted that HA filler injected in excess volumes in the subnasale may add unwanted bulk to the upper portion of the philtrum. The procedure is also advised against

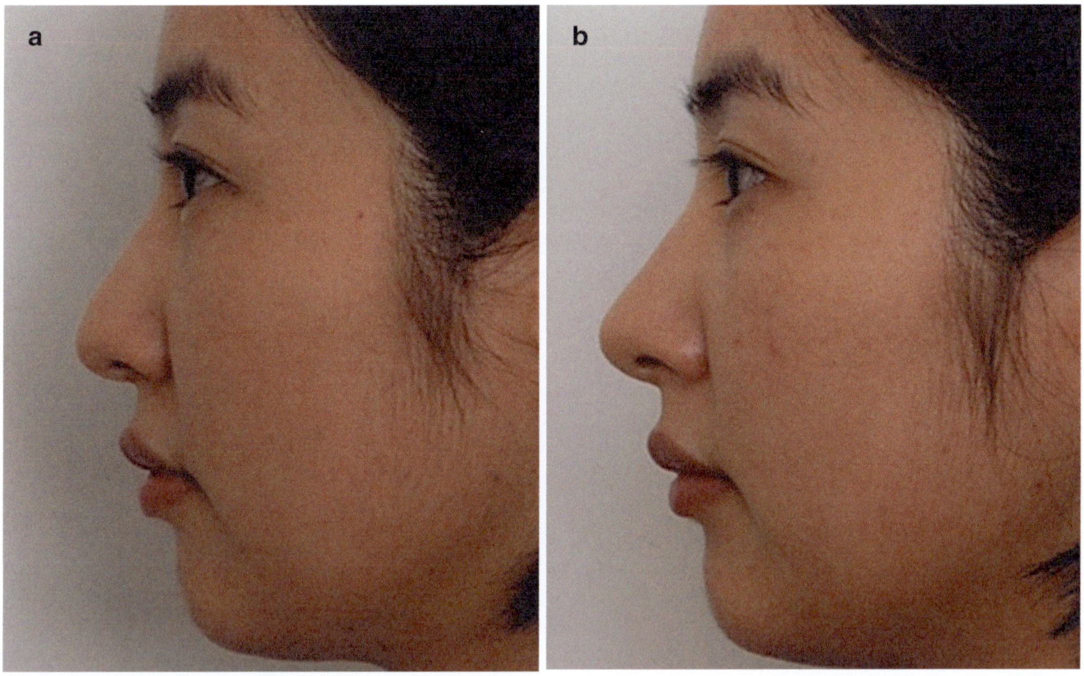

Fig. 4.64 (**a**) Before and (**b**) after nasolabial angle augmentation

patients with upturned nostrils or over rotated nose, as it can cause excessive nostril show. The thumb and index finger of the nondominant hand should be used to pinch the nasal tip to prevent any superior migration of HA filler from causing unwanted bulbosity at the nasal tip.

4.9.11 Injection Techniques for Special Indications

4.9.11.1 Humped Nose (Fig. 4.65)

A mild nasal hump is easily corrected by injecting HA filler only in the upper nasal dorsum near the radix (i.e., the area just above the hump). However, in the case of a severe hump, concurrent HA filler injection into the nasolabial junction and the columella is required. This is because correcting the radix only without the corresponding elevation of the nasal tip can cause the nasofrontal angle to detract beyond the natural range of 140°, and visually elongate the nasal dorsum. For partial correction of the upper nasal dorsum only (i.e., around the radix), a 30-G needle may be used instead of a cannula. Deep injections in the supraperiosteal layer must be performed when injecting with a needle.

4.9.11.2 Wide Nasal Base (Fig. 4.66)

Concurrent use of HA filler in the columella and the nasolabial angle can help to narrow the nasal

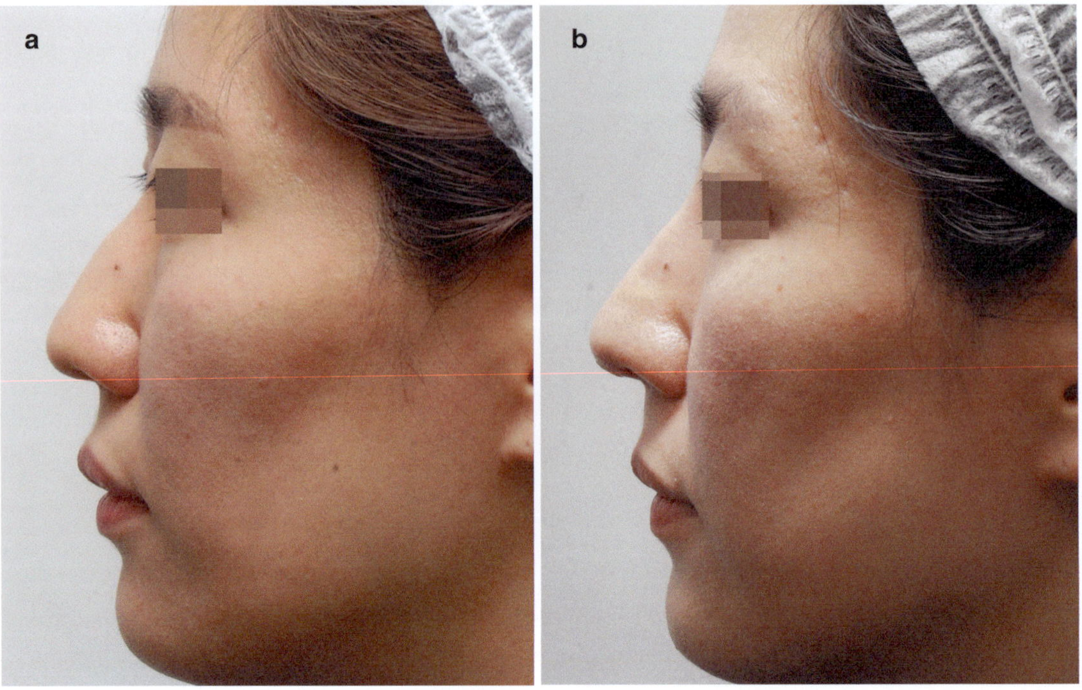

Fig. 4.65 (a) Before and (b) after correction of humped nose. (Dorsum augmentation combined with nasolabial angle augmentation)

base by increasing the projection and upward rotation of the nasal tip. Further, elongating the nose via nasal dorsum augmentation can also give the visual illusion of a slimmer nose. In this regard, it may be worthwhile to maximize the length of the radix during nasal dorsum augmentation so that the ratio between the length of the nose and the width exceeds the range of 1:1.4–1.5.

4.9.11.3 Bulbous Nose

As a general rule, filler rhinoplasty is not indicated for sharpening a bulbous nose prevalent among Asians. However, injecting very small amounts of HA filler intradermally in the pronasale using a 30-G needle may be attempted to effect subtle definition and sharpness to the nasal tip. Also, a visual illusion of a narrower nose can be effected by increasing the length of the nose with nasal dorsum augmentation.

4.9.11.4 Pulling Nose (Arrow nose) (Fig. 4.67)

Priority should be placed on enhancing the nasolabial angle and the columella. Augmentation of the nasal dorsum may or may not be performed depending on the individual case. Notably, nasal dorsum augmentation is not recommended for patients with a long dorsum.

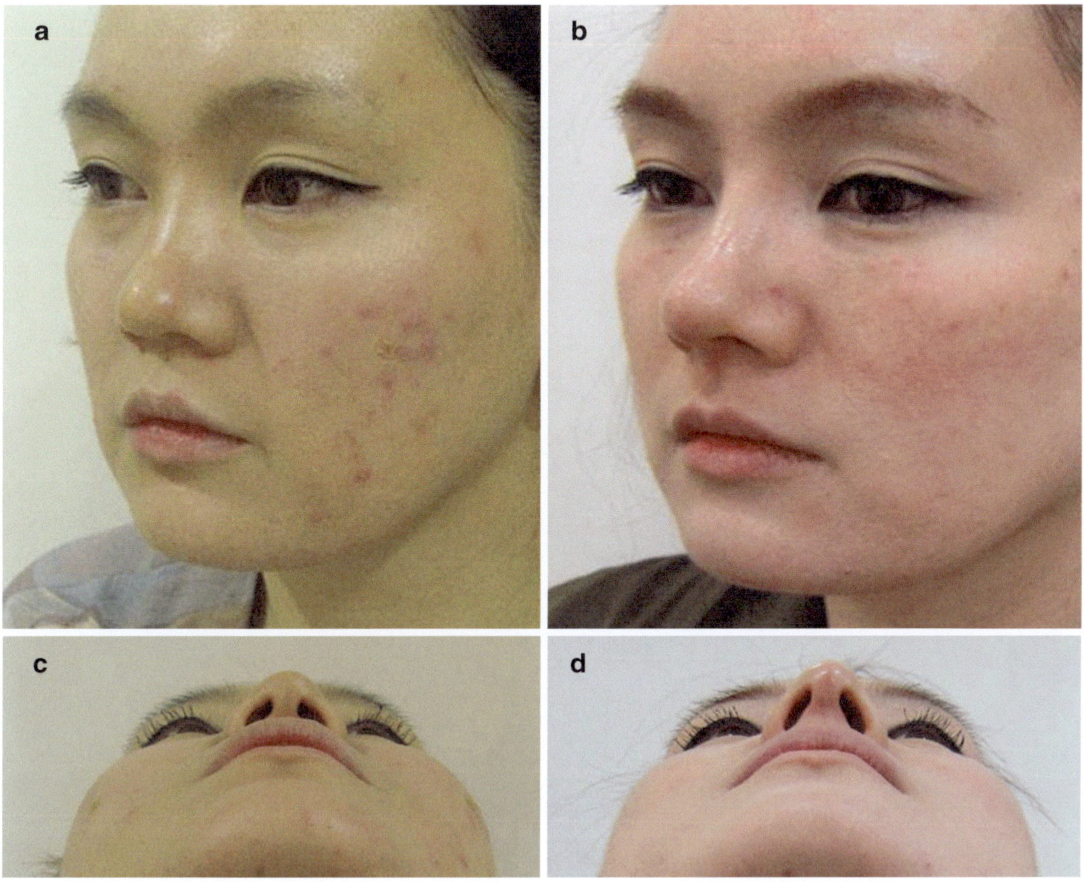

Fig. 4.66 (**a**, **c**) Before and (**b**, **d**) after correction of Wide Nasal Base. (Dorsum augmentation combined with nasolabial angle augmentation)

4.9.11.5 Deviated Nose

Curved Nose

The nasal profile can be straightened by filling the concavity present in the mid portion of the nose and filling the contralateral depressions at the radix and the nasal tip. Precaution should be taken against creating an overly thick radix or dorsum (Fig. 4.68).

Slanted Nose (Deviated Septum)

HA filler should be injected into the contralateral side of the deviated septum at the supratip break point behind the nasal tip and ipsilateral side at the radix (Fig. 4.69).

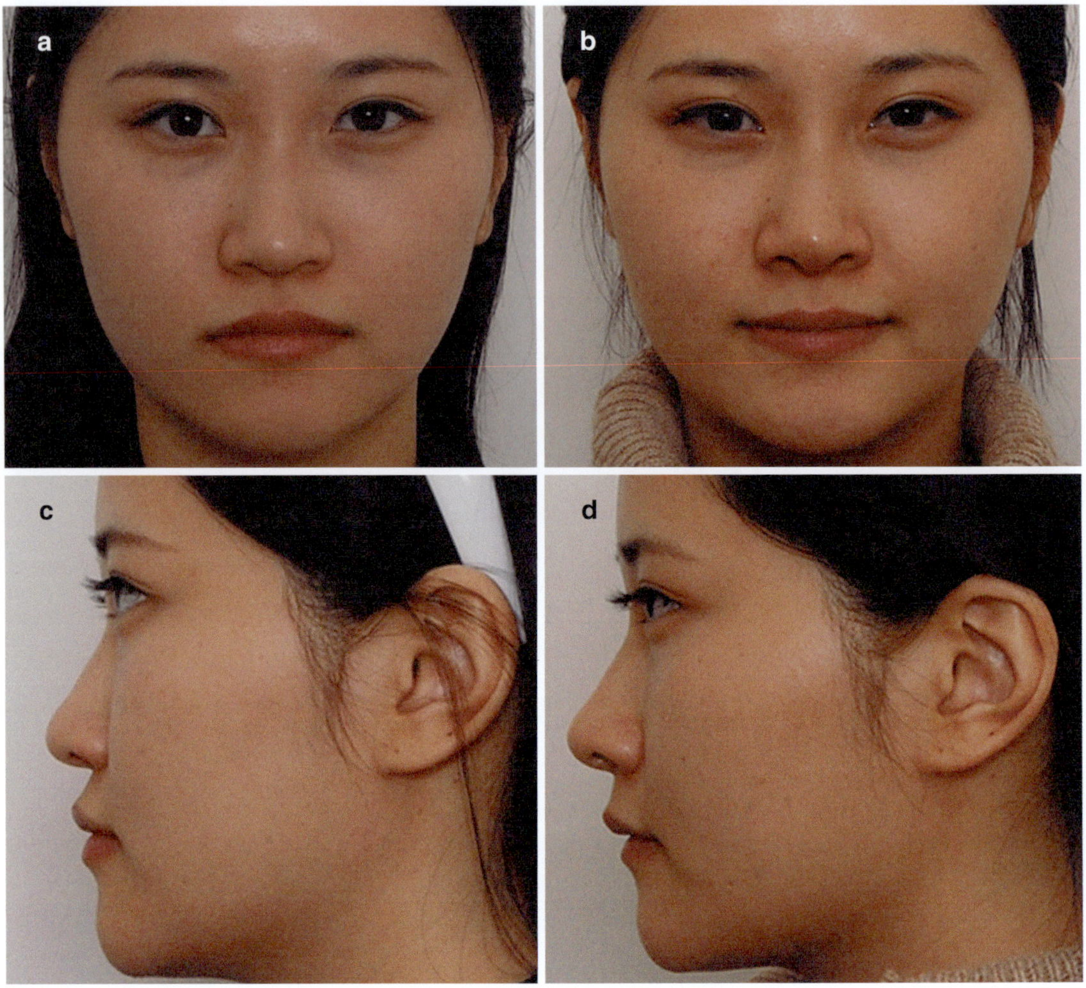

Fig. 4.67 (**a**, **c**) Before and (**b**, **d**) after correction of pulling nose (arrow nose)

4.9.12 Combination Treatment

Additional HA filler injection into the glabella may be necessary in patients with deep glabellar grooves. Patients demonstrating pronounced activity of the depressor septi nasi m. may require adjunct injection of BoNT-A (4 U) in the subnasale to prevent the downward pull and drooping of the nasal tip during speaking or smiling [23].

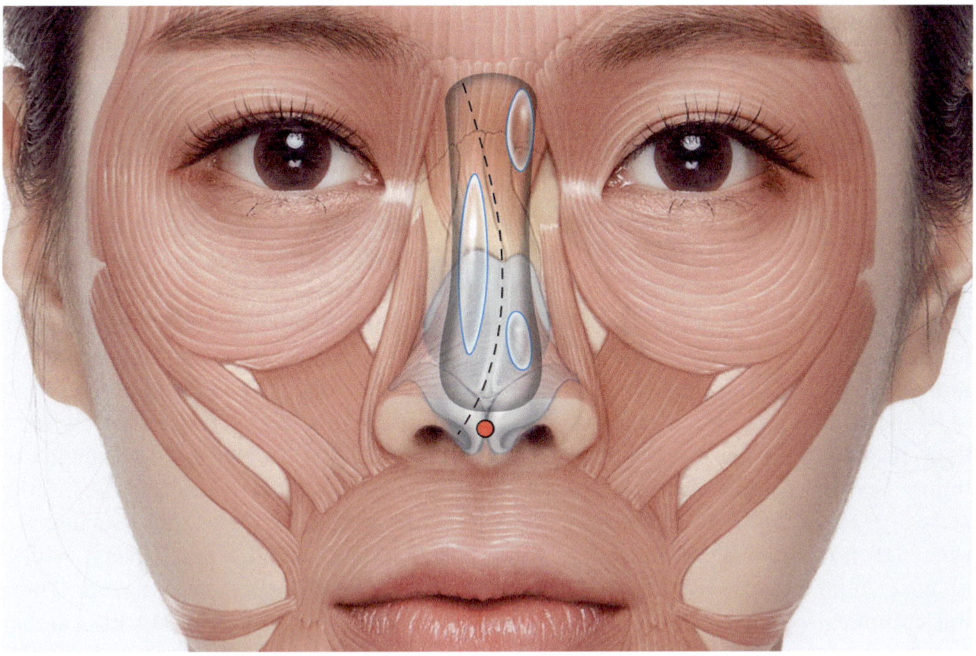

Fig. 4.68 Injection technique for the correction of curved nose

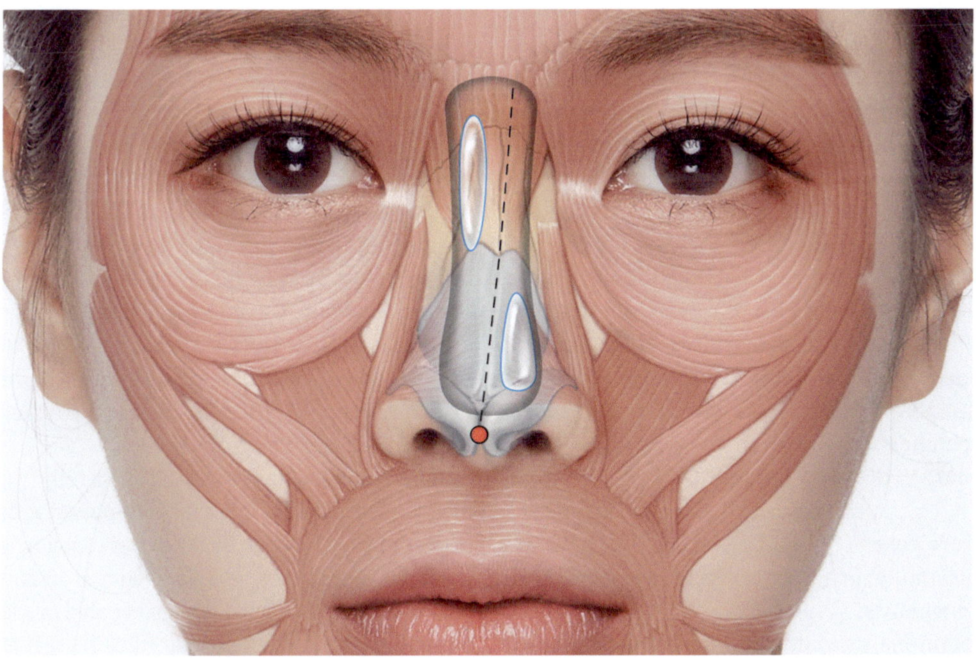

Fig. 4.69 Injection technique for the correction of slanted nose

4.9.13 Complications

There may be mild transient complications following HA filler injection in the nose including temporary swelling and erythema, bruising, headache, as well as rare incidences of infection. On occasion, erythema may persist for several months in peripheral regions such as the nasal tip. This is presumed to arise from the capillary dilatation triggered as a secondary reaction to compensate for the impaired blood circulation from the vascular compression caused by the HA filler injection into the dense and tight tissue of the nasal tip. Symptoms continuing beyond several weeks should be reversed by injection of hyaluronidase. However, the most serious adverse event following nose augmentation with HA filler is vascular complication. The causes of vascular compromise are largely two-fold, that is, vascular compression from the pressure exerted by injected filler material and the intravascular embolization from inadvertent intravascular injection of fillers. Extreme care must be taken to avoid intravascular injection of HA filler which, though rare, may bring about skin necrosis and even blindness in the most disastrous case. Ischemic color changes such as immediate postinjection blanching or violaceous or grayish skin discoloration (Fig. 4.70) occurring 20–30 min after HA filler injection should be considered as a sign of vascular embolization, for which timely and adequate treatment must be administered (Fig. 4.70). If left unaddressed, multiple reticular erythematous patches may develop the next day across the nasal dorsum, glabella and forehead (Fig. 4.71), accompanied by multiple pustules in severe cases (Fig. 4.72). In the extreme, the pustules may progress to skin necrosis with crust formation (Fig. 4.73a).

Practitioners should also be vigilant of the risk of blindness following HA filler injection in the nasal region. According to the literature review by Beleznay et al., the nose was the second most common site for filler induced blindness representing 25.5% of all cases after the glabella (38.8%).

Notably, HA filler injected under strong pressure into the dorsal nasal artery may migrate in reverse direction to the proximal ophthalmic artery and occlude the distal branches of the ophthalmic artery such as the retinal artery and the posterior ciliary artery, leading to blindness (see Sect. 5.1.4). While the blood supply to the upper nasal dorsum is mainly provided by the dorsal nasal artery and the angular artery, the lower part of the nose receives blood supply primarily from the lateral nasal artery, whereas the nasal tip is supplied by the the columellar branch of the superior labial artery and the inferior alar branch of the facial artery. The dorsal nasal artery communicates extensively with these arterial branches at the nasal dorsum. Therefore, any inadvertent injection of HA filler at the nasal tip or even at the columella may travel retrograde through the dorsal nasal artery into the ophthalmic artery via the broad-based anastomosis at the nasal dorsum and contribute to blindness as well.

Vascular complications are more likely to occur in patients whose vascular circulation has already been compromised due to a previous nose surgery, or whose blood vessels are adhered to the scar tissue in the operated area. Note that vessels trapped inside scar tissue adhesions become easy targets for needle penetration during filler rhinoplasty, and are substantially more vulnerable to the risk of intravascular filler injection. Hence, particular care must be taken when treating a patient with history of a nose surgery even if the nasal implant had been subsequently removed.

The cannula technique is generally recommended when injecting the nose to minimize the risk of vascular occlusion. That said, precaution is still required even when injecting with a cannula as small-diameter cannulas remain capable of piercing through a vessel. As a general rule, the use of cannulas sized 25 or larger, gentle movement, and slow injection speed help reduce the risk of intravascular filler injection. In case the use of a needle is inevitable, needles should be used only for delivering HA

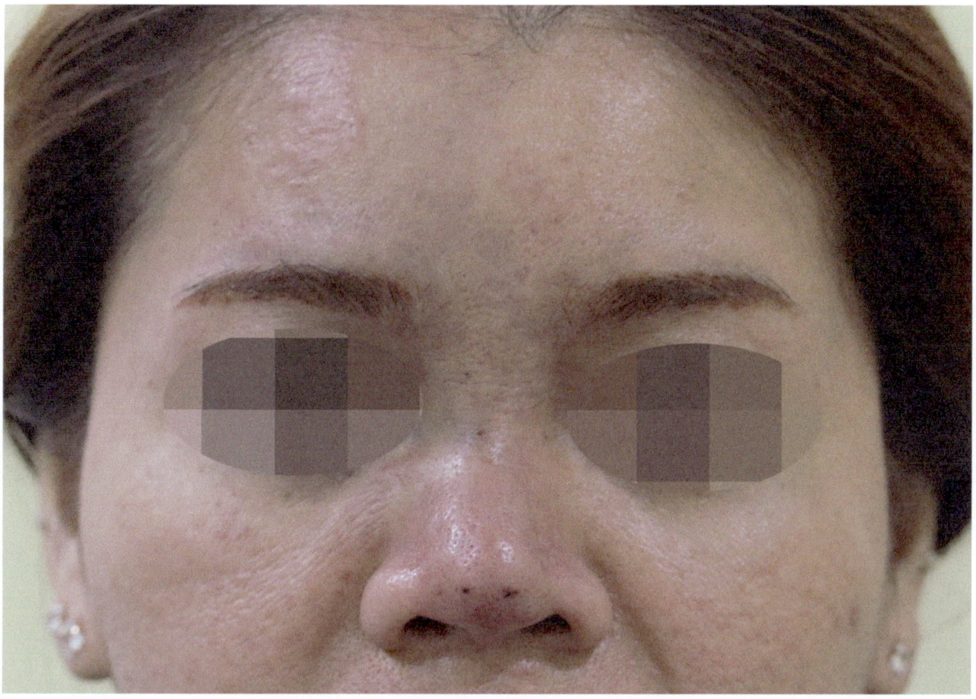

Fig. 4.70 Ischemic color changes such as immediate postinjection blanching or violaceous or greyish skin discoloration occurring 20–30 min after nose filler injection should be considered as a sign of vascular embolization. (Photo: courtesy of Dr. Kim Sang-Yon)

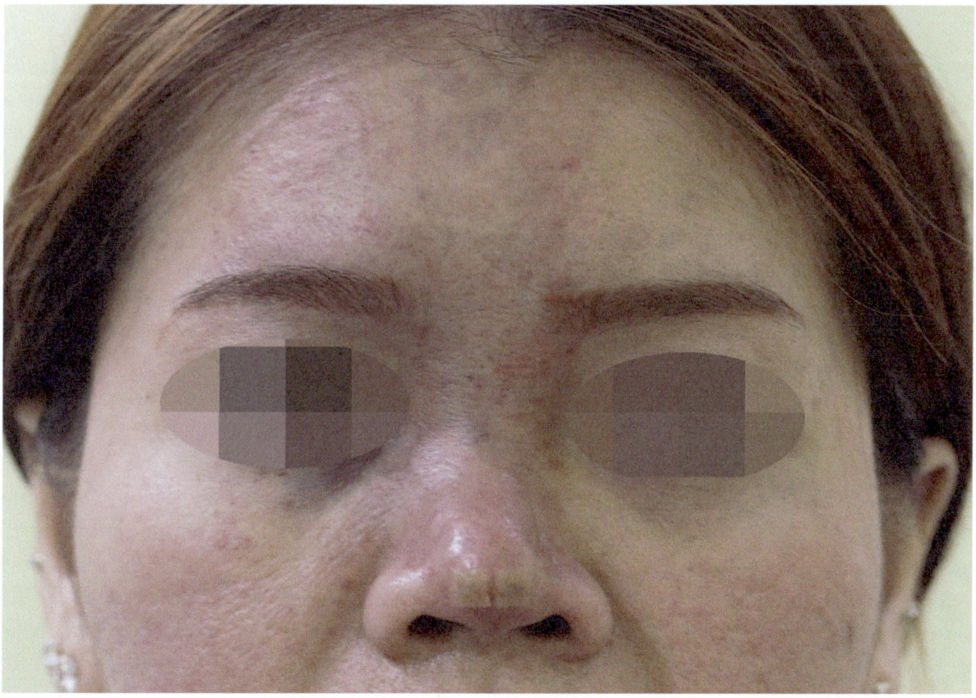

Fig. 4.71 Multiple reticular erythematous patches may develop across the nasal dorsum, glabella and forehead the next day after nose filler injection. (Photo: courtesy of Dr. Kim Sang-Yon)

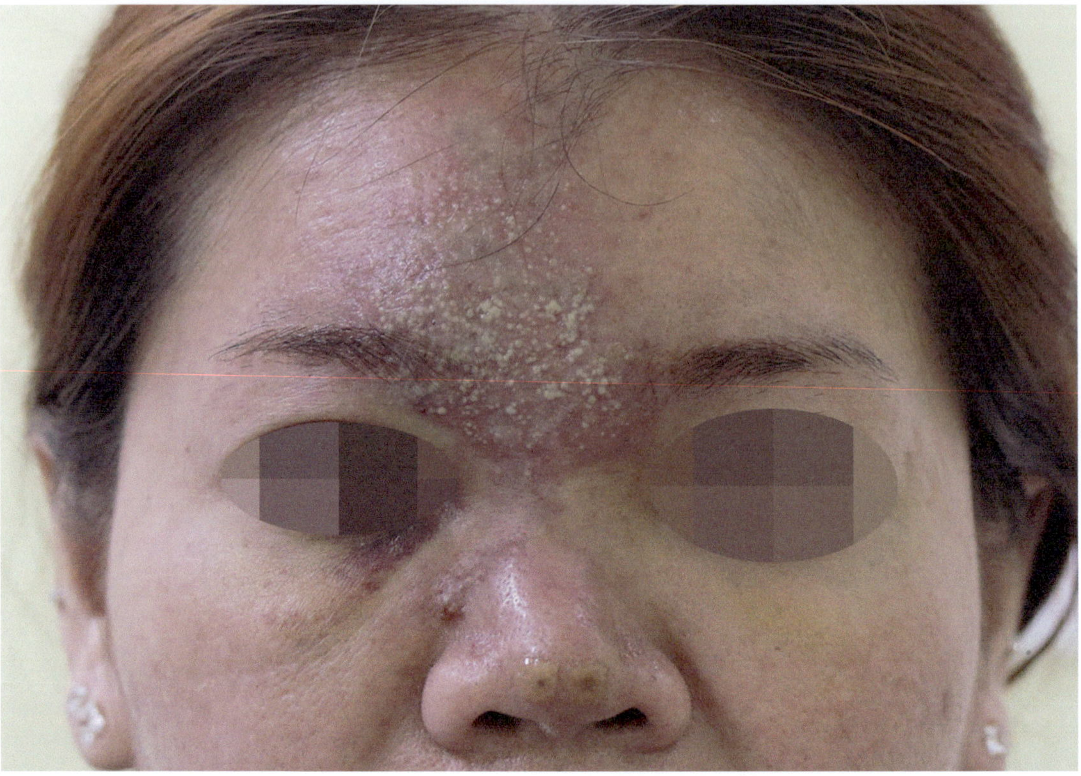

Fig. 4.72 Multiple pustules may develop in severe cases. (Photo: courtesy of Dr. Kim Sang-Yon)

supraperiosteally in the radix where the vasculature runs superficially close to the skin surface. Aspiration should be performed prior to each injection in such case to ensure that the needle was not accidentally placed in a blood vessel. Note however, that the results of blood aspiration tests are not fail proof, as the test may produce false negatives, especially where the injection was performed using gel-type HA fillers or small diameter needles. In the five cases of vascular occlusions from filler rhinoplasty encountered by the author, HA fillers were injected at the nasal tip with a needle instead of a cannula. Not coincidentally, gel-type HA fillers (newly released at the time) had been injected in five cases. In three cases out of five, the event went unnoticed during the treatment, and it was not until the next day that mottled erythematic patches began appearing on the patient's face, which took approximately 1 month to fully disappear. Fortunately, all three patients recovered without experiencing any severe sequelae such as pustule formation or skin necrosis.

Since then, the author has made it a rule to use only cannulas and particulate-type biphasic HA filler in the nose. It is also the policy of the clinic to have the patient remaining in the office for 30 min after injection of nose filler to ensure prompt detection of any ischemic skin changes, and to advise the patient to revert back to the clinic immediately upon noticing any violaceous changes in the skin 1–2 hrs of their departure.

While it may prove elusive to pinpoint the exact location of the arterial occlusion in which to inject hyaluronidase, hyaluronidase is known to diffuse *across* the arterial wall to reach the hyaluronic acid held in the blood vessel when infiltrated in large volumes [23]. Hence, subcutaneous injection of hyaluronidase at high volumes (>3000 U) and high concentration (750 U/mL) is advised along the entire nasal dorsum (from nasal tip to radix) where ischemic symptoms such as blanching, greyish decolorization, or mottled erythema are present.

Where vascular events are suspected, the effective window of treatment using hyaluronidase is within 24 hrs of HA filler injection. Administration of sublingual nitroglycerin tablets twice at 30 min' intervals (i.e., two tablets given 30 min apart), together with oral aspirin and sildenafil (or tadaifil) is necessary to facilitate peripheral blood circulation. In case the patient presents to the clinic *after* the golden hour of treatment (i.e., the first 24 h) has passed, with severe symptoms including multiple pustules, skin necrosis, and scab formation, concurrent injection of PRP (platelet rich plasma), stem cell extracts, or placenta extract once daily during the first week and twice weekly thereafter is also helpful (Fig. 4.73b). For reference, the relevant prevention and management strategies against filler induced vascular complications are summarized in Table 5.1 (see Sect. 5.1.3).

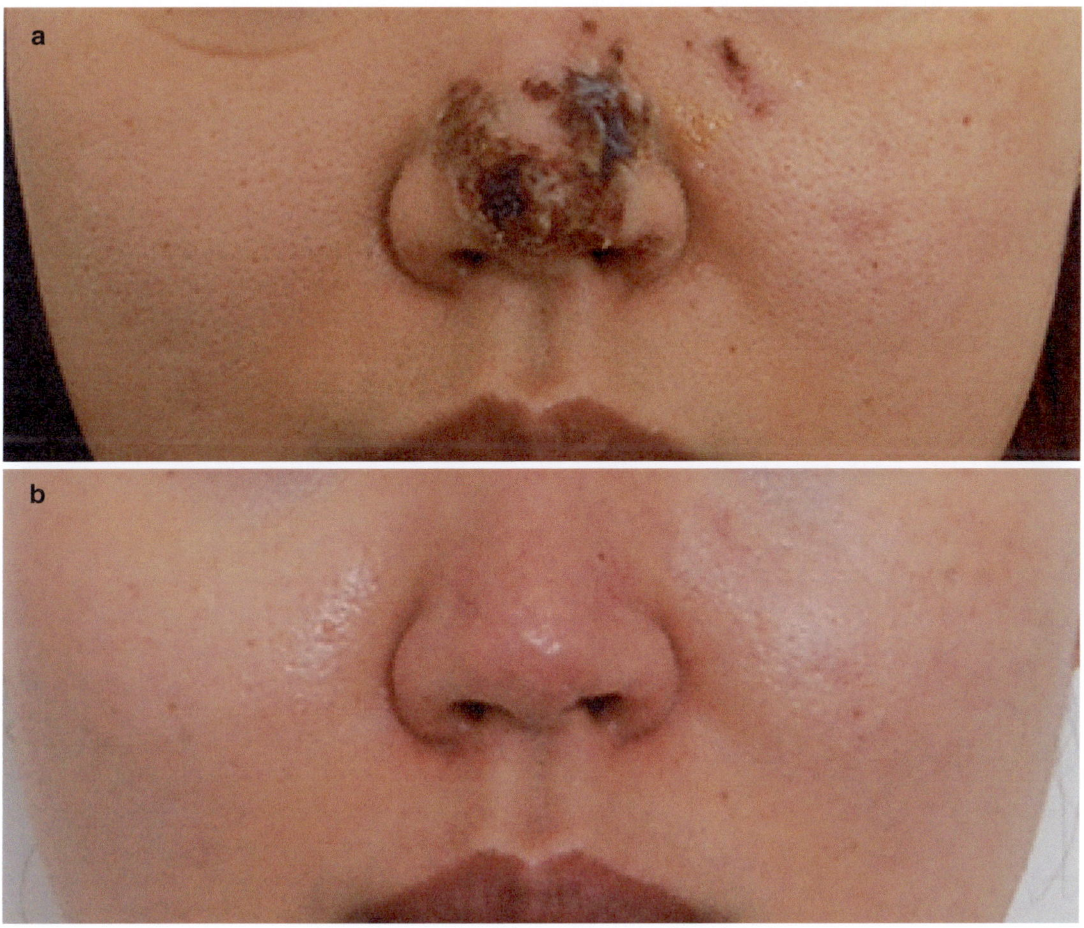

Fig. 4.73 (**a**) The pustules may progress to skin necrosis with crust formation in the extreme case. (**b**) Improvements after 6 months following PRP and placenta extracts injections combined with fractional laser treatment and laser toning with NdYAG laser

4.10 Sunken Cheek Augmentation

Difficulty Level: A, Effectiveness: A, Complications: B

> *Summary 1*: The use of a cannula is advised for cheek augmentation. The target injection plane is the superficial subcutaneous fat layer underlying the skin surface as opposed to the deep buccal fat pad.

> *Summary 2*: When creating the cannula entry point for anterior cheek augmentation, the needle should be introduced slowly with a downward-facing bevel to prevent hematoma formation from injury to the facial artery which runs superficially beneath the skin surface.

> *Summary 3*: Different aspects of the cheek can be addressed according to different aesthetic goals. To diminish the prominence of the lateral zygoma on the frontal view and achieve an oval face, volume should be directed at the posterior cheek, that is, the area inferior to the zygomatic arch. To offset the pronounced zygoma from the oblique view or to improve the saggy jowls, volume should be placed in the lateral aspect of the anterior cheek also referred to as the submalar hollow. Where improvements in the nasolabial folds are desired, the medial aspect of the anterior cheek should be restored.

> *Summary 4*: In patients in their mid-40s and above presenting with pronounced buccal fat pads or preexisting jowls, judicious placement of HA filler in conservative amounts is advised.

Deflation of cheek volume is primarily the result of facial aging or weight loss, though it can also be caused due to congenital volume deficit. Depression of the cheeks creates the appearance of sagginess and age, as the relative prominence of the zygomatic arch, the nasolabial folds, and the saggy jowls serve to disrupt the smooth continuity in facial contour seen in a youthful face.

Restoring volume deficiency in the cheeks not only brings the overall face closer to the ideal oval shape by obscuring the cheek bones but also gives the face a more tightened and uplifted look (Fig. 4.74).

4.10.1 Anatomical Considerations

The cheek is divided by the masseteric ligament anterior to the masseter m. into two separate segments, namely the anterior cheek, a.k.a. the buccal area or submalar area, and the posterior cheek, a.k.a. the lateral cheek, or the subzygomatic region (Fig. 4.75) [24]. Accordingly, the depressions of the anterior cheek (the buccal hollows) and the posterior cheek (the subzygomatic hollows) should also require separate consideration. While the volume depletion in anterior cheek is usually accompanied by a corresponding loss of volume in the posterior cheek, patients who received BoNT-A treatment for masseter reduction 1–3 months before may present with a more significant degree of hollowing in the posterior cheek.

The anterior cheek consists of the following soft tissue layers arranged in the order of the outermost to the deepest as follows: the skin—subcutaneous fat—facial expression muscles and SMAS—buccal fat pad—buccinator m—oral mucosa [24]. The fat compartments of the cheek are made up of the subcutaneous fat lying beneath the skin surface and the buccal fat pad located deep to the facial expression muscles/SMAS. The buccal fat pad is readily distinguishable from the subcutaneous fat not only based on the relevant tissue planes, but also because it is wrapped in a distinct envelope of thin fascia. The buccal fat pad is supported inferiorly by the risorius muscle, and it is the loosening and ptosis of the risorius

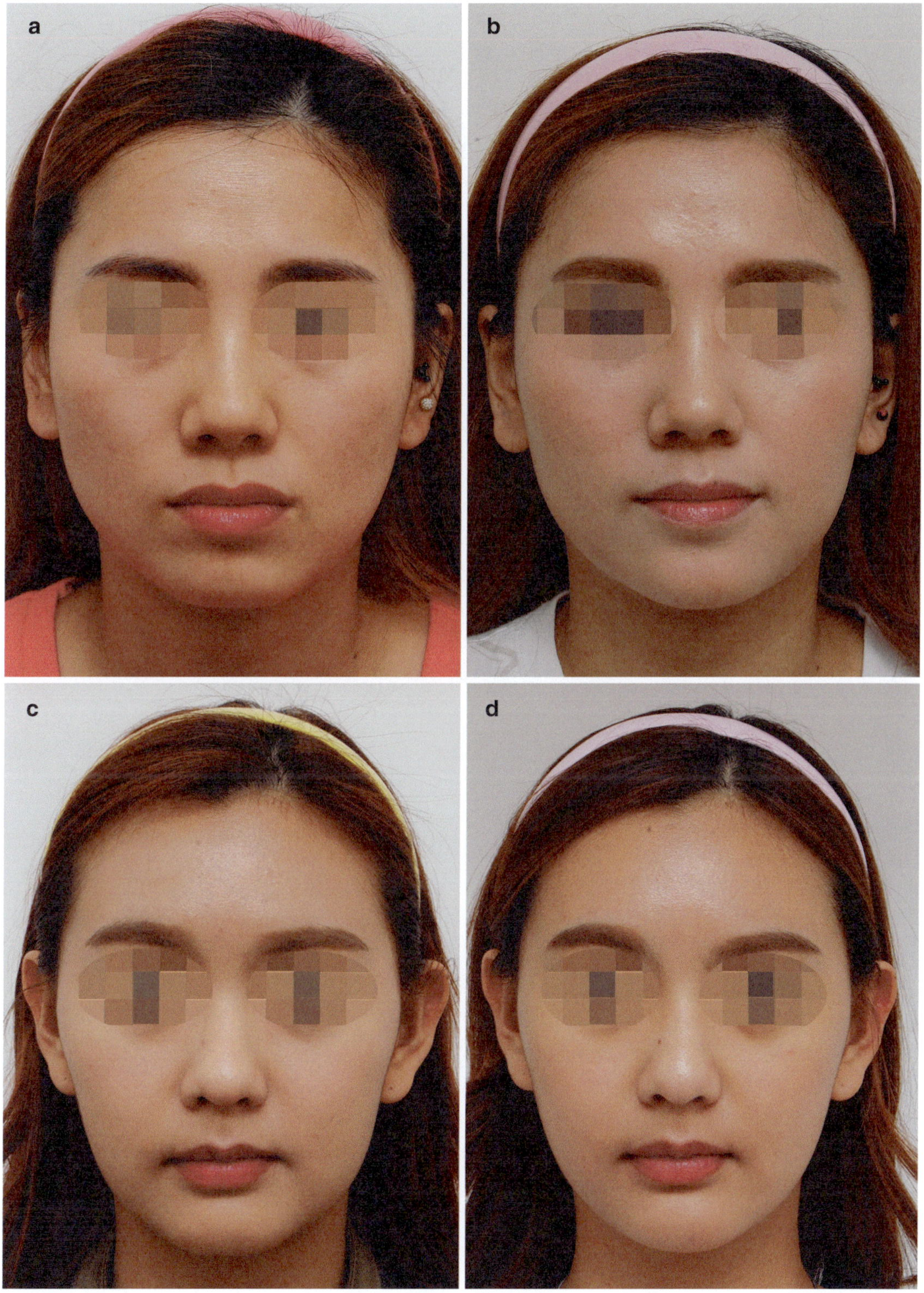

Fig. 4.74 (**a**) Before and (**b**) after sunken cheek augmentation. (**c**) Before and (**d**) after posterior cheek augmentation

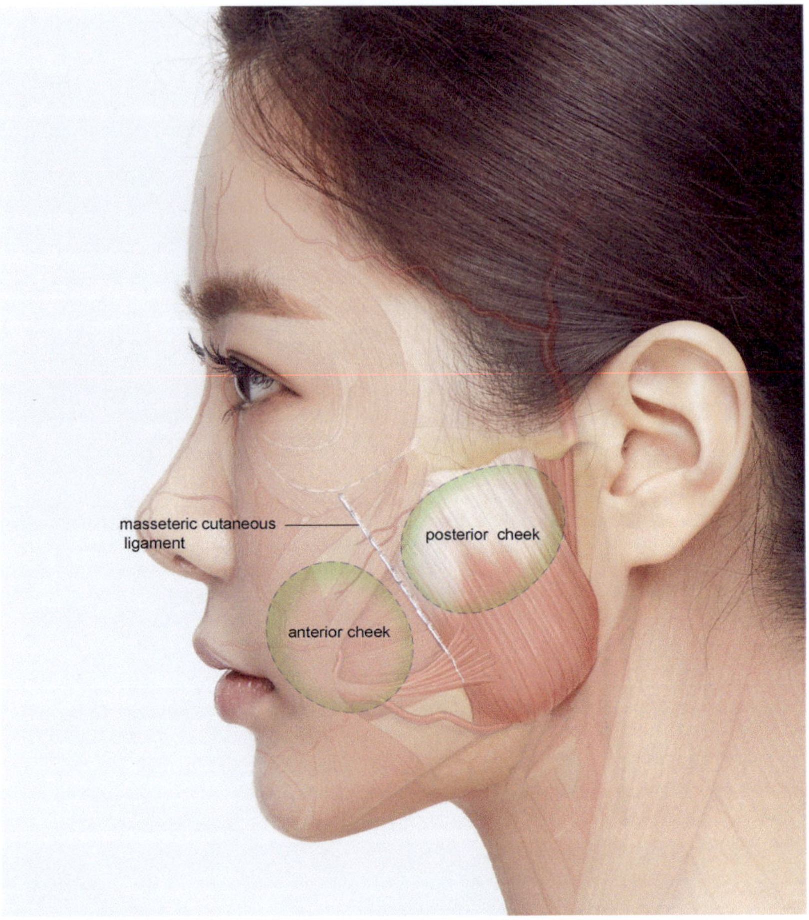

Fig. 4.75 The cheek is divided by the masseteric ligament anterior to the masseter m. into two separate segments, namely, the anterior cheek, a.k.a. submalar area or the buccal area, and the posterior cheek, a.k.a. the lateral cheek, or the subzygomatic region

due to aging which results in the descent of the buccal fat pad, exacerbating the appearance of jowls. While both the subcutaneous fat and the buccal fat pad are affected by the loss of volume in the cheek, volume restoration is to be undertaken primarily at the subcutaneous fat compartment, as direct injection of volume into the buccal fat pad may cause the material to weigh down the face, accentuating the saggy appearance in patients with prominent jowls.

Caution should be exercised while puncturing the cannula entry points for anterior cheek augmentation since the facial artery runs superficially in proximity to the potential entry point, the damage to which can cause extensive bruising [24] (Fig. 4.76). In posterior cheek augmentation, care should be taken not to injure the transverse facial artery branching from the superficial temporal artery emerging 1 cm inferior to the zygomatic arch toward the anterior cheek [25].

4.10.2 Pretreatment Assessment

As a preliminary matter, it is important to establish the location and severity of the volume deficiency in the anterior and/or posterior cheek. Consideration must also be given to the patient's subjective aesthetic concerns, as it determines both the target site(s) to be addressed and injection volume. Confirm with the patient whether the aim is to ovalize the face on the frontal view by diminishing the prominence of the lateral zygoma, or to deemphasize the zygoma from the 45° angle, or to improve the appearance of nasolabial folds or saggy jowls by restoring the perioral region (Fig. 4.75); notably, sunken cheek volumization is not often practiced in Caucasians since a moderate undulation in facial contour from the convexity of the lateral zygoma to the concavity of the subzygomatic region ("Ogee curve") is a trait considered aesthetically desir-

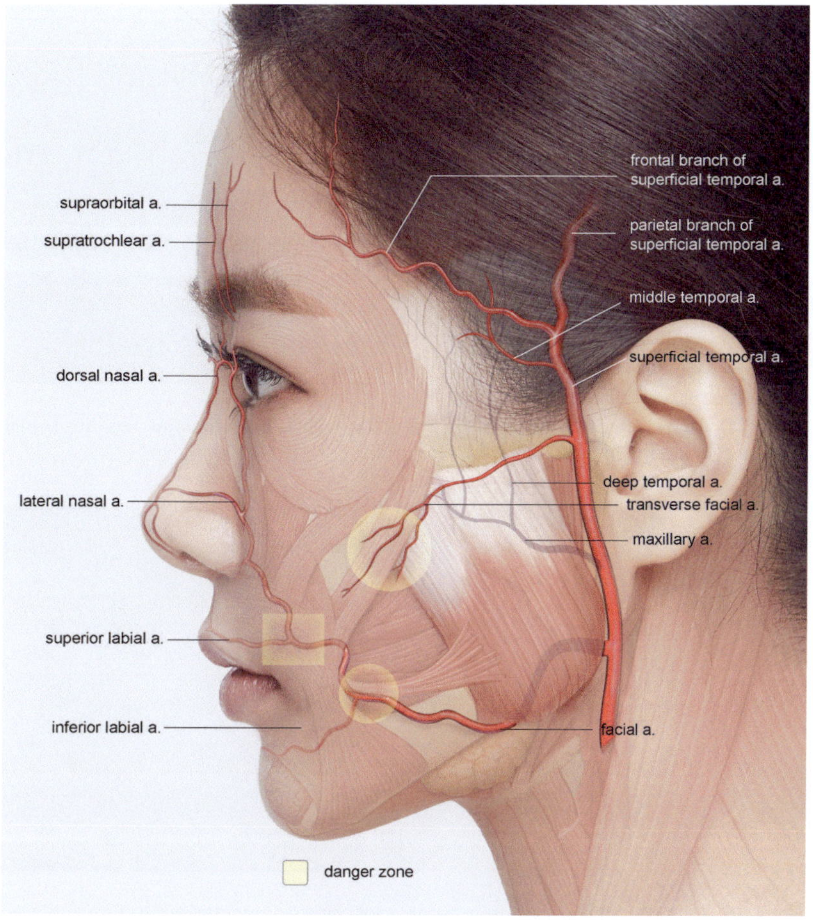

Fig. 4.76 Danger zones for bruising by needle insertion

able by Caucasians (Fig. 4.13) [17]. Therefore, when performing this indication in a Caucasian patient, injection of discreet amounts is advised just enough to improve the severity of submalar depression or irregular lateral facial contour. Likewise, when treating a male cheek, the goal should be simply to mitigate the severely gaunt, hollowed-out appearance of the patient instead of achieving full correction since a mildly rugged, angulated facial contour is considered manly and desirable in men.

4.10.3 Injection Technique (Table 4.12)

In sunken cheek augmentation, different compartments of the cheek are injected depending on the patient's aesthetic need. Posterior cheek

Table 4.12 Summary of cheek filler injection technique

Item	Contents
Needle vs. Cannula	23-G 5 cm Cannula
HA filler	Monophasic HA filler
Amount of HA filler	2–5 mL per side for ant. Cheek 1–2 mL per side for post. Cheek
Depth of injection	Subcutaneous level
Entry point for cannula	Ant. cheek: 3 cm lateral and 1 cm inferior to the mouth corner Post. cheek: point where vertical line drawn 2 cm lateral to the lateral canthus meets the imaginary line connecting the mouth corner and the tragus
Target area	Ant. cheek for the nasolabial fold and the submalar depression Post. cheek for the subzygomatic depression
Anesthetics	Topical anesthetics

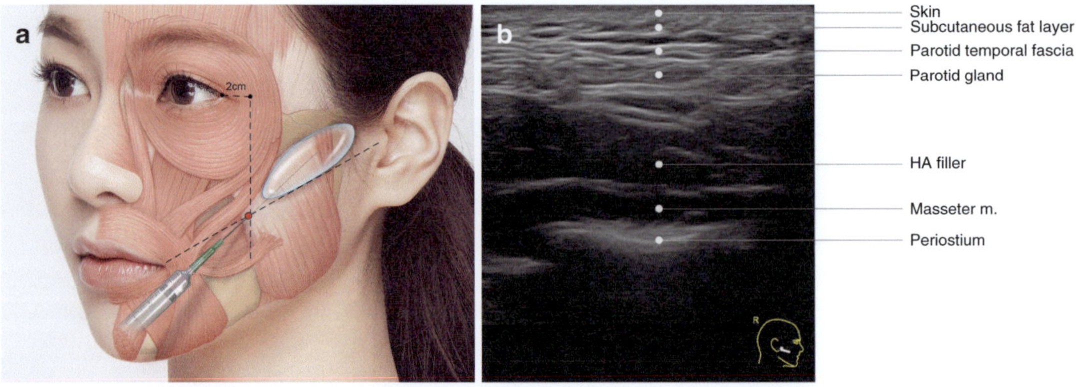

Fig. 4.77 (**a**) The cannula entry point for posterior cheek augmentation. (**b**) Proper placement of HA filler in the posterior cheek confirmed by sonography evaluation

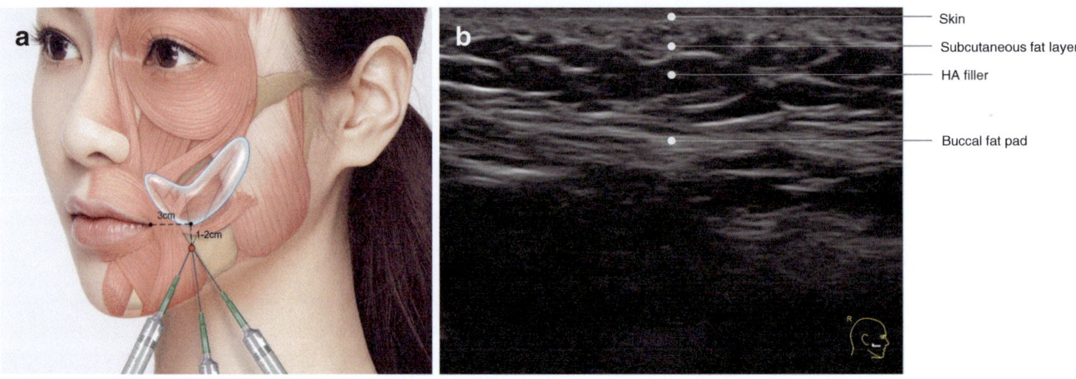

Fig. 4.78 (**a**) The cannula entry point for anterior cheek augmentation. (**b**) Proper placement of HA filler in the anterior cheek confirmed by sonography evaluation

augmentation is indicated for creating an oval face on the frontal view by diminishing the visibility of the lateral zygoma (Fig. 4.77). To offset the pronounced zygoma from the oblique view or to improve the saggy jowls, volume should be placed in the lateral aspect of the anterior cheek also referred to as the submalar depression (Fig. 4.78). Finally, to improve the appearance of nasolabial folds, volume should be restored in the medial aspect of the anterior cheek (Fig. 4.78).

Injection is performed with a 23-G cannula. The relevant plane of injection is in the subcutaneous adipose layer. When augmenting the anterior cheek, the ideal entry point is located 3 cm lateral and 1 cm inferior to the oral commissure. For posterior cheek volumization, the cannula entry point is at the intersection between the vertical line drawn 2 cm lateral to the lateral canthus and an imaginary line connecting the oral commissure and the tragus [25]. When treating the anterior cheek, the relevant sequence of injection is to first fill the lateral aspect (i.e., the submalar depression) of the anterior cheek before proceeding to address the medial part (i.e., nasolabial fold. For the posterior cheek, start by addressing the deepest point of the subzygomatic hollow, with subsequent gradation in volume inferiorly to achieve a smooth taper toward the jawline. Note, however, that the thick ligamentous tissue lying behind the masseteric ligaments may, similarly to scar tissues, hinder the smooth and even distribution of HA filler. Aggressive filling is to be avoided, as it can cause unwanted bulging of the region inferior to the ligamentous tissue. While the subcision technique can be employed to create space for HA filler placement, bruising is to be expected.

The standard amount of HA filler injected for anterior cheek volumization is 1 mL medially in the nasolabial fold and 1 mL laterally in the submalar depression totaling a minimum of 2 mL per side subject to individual variations. For more severe depressions, the injection volume can be increased to as much as 3–5 mL per side. For posterior cheek depressions, 1–2 mL is required depending on the severity of the condition. The use of topical anesthetic cream is sufficient for numbing the treatment.

4.10.4 Complications

Irregularity: The posterior cheek lies posterior to the masseteric ligament, and as such, patients with naturally large ligamentous tissue may have a slight bulge 1–2 cm under the zygomatic arch at baseline, which they may not have noticed previously (Fig. 4.79). This must be brought to the patient's attention before treatment and documented in the pretreatment photos. Otherwise, the patient may attribute the bump to HA filler placement.

Bruising: The facial artery is at risk during the puncture of the cannula entry point for anterior cheek augmentation, while the transverse facial artery is in danger when making the relevant access point for filling the posterior cheek. When creating the cannula entry point for anterior cheek augmentation, the needle should slowly enter the skin with the bevel facing down to avoid injuring the facial artery running superficially below the skin surface. In the case trauma to the facial artery is suspected, press the area hard for at least 3 min to prevent a hematoma.

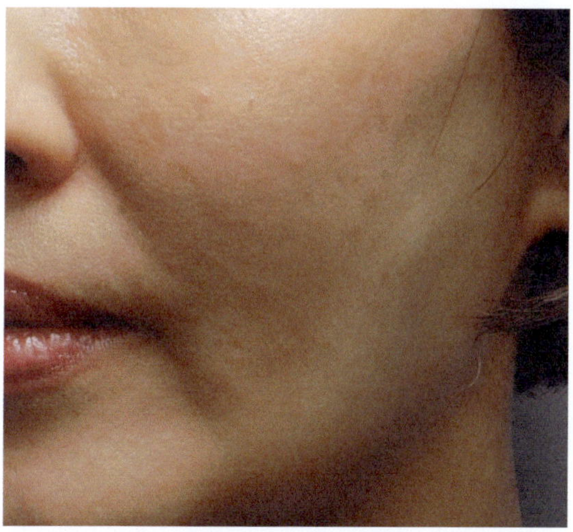

Fig. 4.79 Irregularity due to masseteric ligament

Sagging Jowls: In patients in their mid-40s and above with preexisting saggy jowls or bulging buccal fat, cheek augmentation can result in the exacerbation of jowl descent. While this is caused mostly by placement of HA filler directly into the deep buccal fat pad, in patients with severe jowls, sagging can occur even from subcutaneous HA filler placement. Accordingly, care must be taken to place cheek filler only in the subcutaneous fatty layer and in minimum amounts in patients with preexisting jowls. Concominant steriod fat reducing injection for the sagging jowl and butulinum toxin injection for the masseteric reduction should be performed.

Bogus Face (Fig. 1.13): Occasionally, patients seeking cheek augmentation may present with cheek dimples formed by the action of bifid zygomaticus major m. Repeated contraction of the zygomaticus major m. each time the patient smiles can progressively push the implanted HA filler away from its original location. This, in turn, may cause the cheeks to stick out laterally when the patient smiles, like the cartoon character Mr. Bogus with characteristically bulging cheeks (Fig. 1.13). In such patients, most of the volume should be placed medial to the dimples with only minimum amounts applied in the lateral aspects.

Vascular Adverse Effect: Patients previously treated with fat graft, Sculptra, or collagen stimulators in the cheek are often left with scar tissue adhesions in the subcutaneous fat, with blood vessels trapped inside. Vessels trapped by scarring lie vulnerable to the risk of rupture, or intravascular embolization even when a blunt cannula is used for the injection. The 40-year-old female patient in the photo developed mottled erythema in the posterior cheek the day following posteriors cheek augmentation; even though the damage to transverse facial artery was highly suspected, 48 hrs had already passed since the onset of symptoms, and symptoms were mild enough not to justify taking further interventions apart from medication for improving blood circulation. Fortunately, full recovery was achieved within a week without reversing the HA (Fig. 4.80).

Pain: Patients with enlarged masseteric ligaments may develop bruising and pain persisting for more than 2 weeks due to the rupture of the ligament caused by the cannula movement.

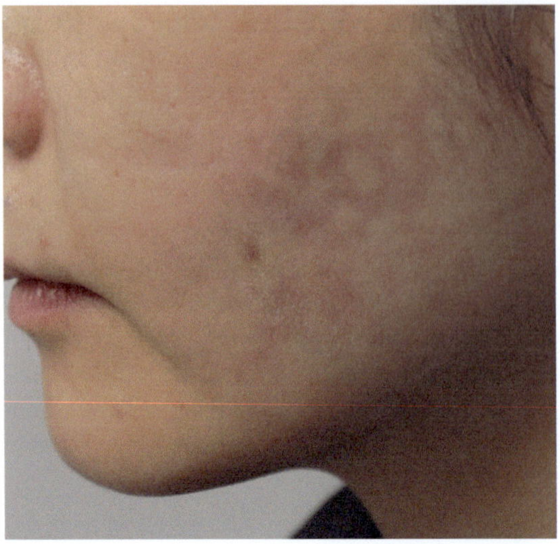

Fig. 4.80 The 40-year-old female patient developed mottled erythema in the posterior cheek the day following posterior cheek augmentation due to the damage to transverse facial artery

4.11 Nasolabial Folds

Difficulty Level: A, Effectiveness: B, Complications: B

Summary 1: Inject using a thick 23-G 5-cm cannula to minimize trauma to the facial artery running along the nasolabial fold. Both biphasic HA fillers with large particle size and monophasic HA fillers with high viscoelasticity are acceptable for use.

Summary 2: Nasolabial folds constitute one of the three-dimensional arcs that make up the human face. Correspondingly, correction of the alar groove located lateral to the nasal ala is best avoided if not provided sparingly only in severe cases. Most of the volume correction should instead be directed at the lower two-thirds of the nasolabial fold.

Summary 3: Both the dynamic and the static components of the nasolabial fold should be considered. The appropriate injection method should be tailored according to the nature (i.e., static vs. dynamic) of the nasolabial fold.

Summary 4: Concurrent volume restoration is recommended if any marionette lines or cheek hollowing is concomitantly present.

Nasolabial folds are the creases that extend obliquely from the alar groove located lateral to the ala nasi down to the outer corners of the lips. They are formed along the border between the malar fat pad and the respective insertion points of the various upper lip elevators and zygomaticus major muscle into the skin surface. Significantly, similar to how the infraorbital crease running horizontally below the pretarsal roll does *not* constitute a facial wrinkle associated with aging, the nasolabial folds represent one of the primary arcs which naturally make up the three-dimensional human face as a gradient between the tall cheeks and the lips. Consequently, even young people in their teens have nasolabial folds, though the folds may deepen and elongate with age as the skin loses elasticity and the malar fat pad begins to droop and bulge inferiorly. As such, complete eradication of the alar groove during a nasolabial fold treatment with HA filler should not be attempted, as the fusing of injected volume with the malar fat pad located immediately above removes three-dimensionality from the face, blows the malar cheeks out of proportion, and ultimately confers an unnatural simian appearance to the face. It bears noting the *absence* of this vital structure on the face of a monkey in this regard.

Depending on the underlying cause, nasolabial folds which warrant aesthetic improvement with HA filler consist of deep static folds visible even at rest and dynamic folds which appear only upon facial animation such as talking and smiling due to the activity of relevant musculature including the upper lip elevators and the zygomaticus major m. Loss of skin elasticity with aging can exacerbate the appearance of the dynamic folds, while repeated wrinkling in the nasolabial area over time eventually causes these dynamic folds to deepen and elongate into static folds. Treatment of deep static nasolabial folds involves placement of HA filler directly into the folds (Fig. 4.81). In contrast, dynamic nasolabial folds are treated using the fern technique aimed to enhance the

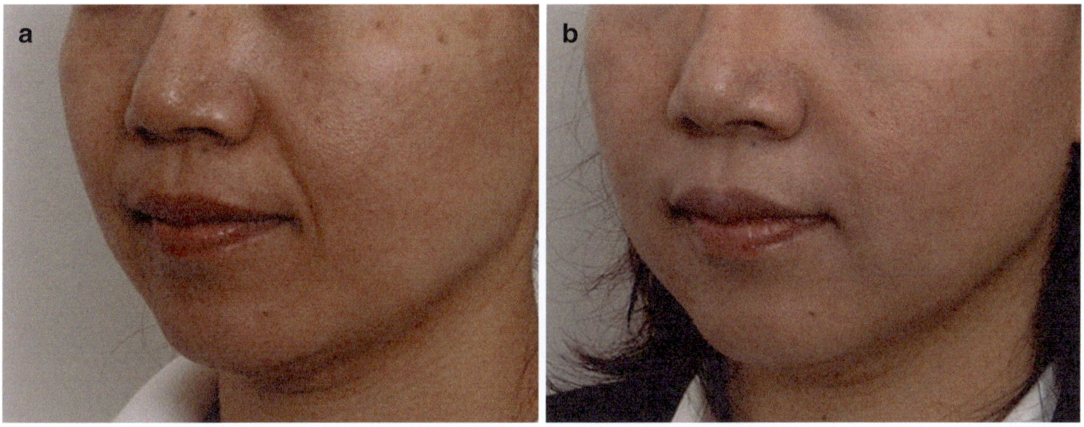

Fig. 4.81 (**a**) Before and (**b**) after treatment of deep static nasolabial folds

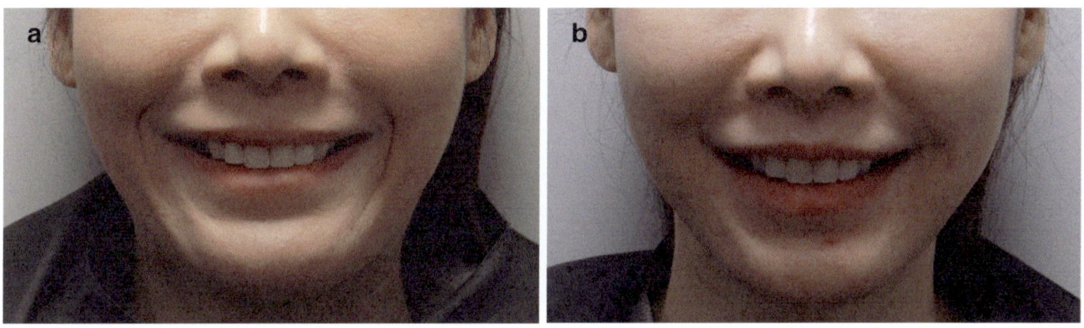

Fig. 4.82 (**a**) Before and (**b**) after treatment of dynamic nasolabial folds using the fern technique

overall elasticity and resilience of the surrounding skin (Fig. 4.82) [26].

4.11.1 Anatomical Considerations

The upper lip elevators including the LLSAN (levator labii superioris alaeque nasi), LLS (levator labii superioris), zygomaticus minor m., and some muscle fibers of zygomaticus major m. attach directly into the skin overlying the nasolabial folds (Fig. 4.83) [27]. Insertion of these muscles into the skin where the nasolabial folds form gives rise to the prominence of nasolabial folds upon smiling due to relevant muscle contracture (i.e., dynamic nasolabial folds), and delineates a boundary that keeps the malar fat pad lying above the fold from descending further. The deepening of this demarcation over time eventually leads to static nasolabial folds that are obvious at rest. Considering the origin, insertion, and vector of each of these mimetic muscles, it can be postulated that the medial one-third of the nasolabial fold is formed by the LLSAN and LLS, the middle one-third by the zygomaticus minor m., and the lateral one-third by the zygomaticus major m.

The use of a cannula is preferred over a needle to avoid injuring the facial artery running parallel if not along the nasolabial fold. Vigilance must be exercised not to rupture the facial artery, as it may cause extensive hematoma (Fig. 4.76).

The facial artery branches from the external carotid artery, loops around the antegonial notch from which it reemerges, and passes the masseter muscle anteriorly before coursing tortuously up to the nasion. Along the path, it is known to give off the branches of the inferior labial a., the superior labial a. and the lateral nasal a. before terminating as the angular a. Given that the superior labial a. typically arises from the facial artery within an area 15 mm superolateral to the mouth corner, particular care must be practiced not to injure the relevant vasculature when using a needle in this region [27]. Note also that while the

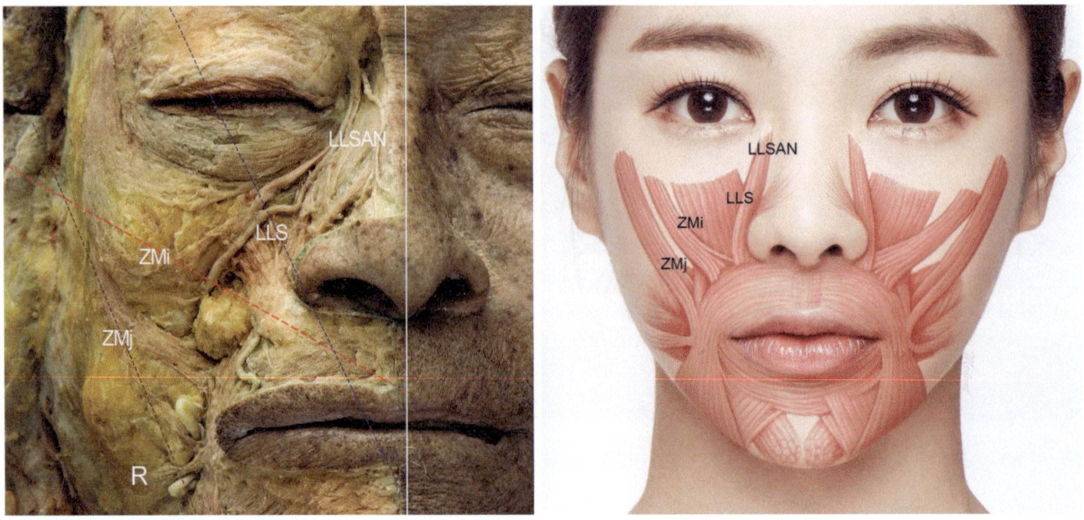

Fig. 4.83 The upper lip elevators including the LLSAN (levator labii superioris alaque nasi), LLS (levator labii superioris), zygomaticus minor m., and some muscle fibers of zygomaticus major m. attach directly into the skin overlying the nasolabial folds. (Photo: courtesy from Professor Hee-Jin Kim)

facial artery mostly runs deep to mimetic muscles during its course, it is afforded no such protection in the spaces immediately above and below the risorius m. by the overlying musculature. Hence, caution is required when injecting this segment with a needle as the facial artery runs superficially beneath the skin without any cover. Likewise, when puncturing the cannula entry point with a needle, care should be taken to insert the needle very slowly, at an angle almost horizontal to the skin with the bevel facing down so as not to traumatize the facial artery running superficially in this area. A sudden swelling occurring within seconds of injection followed by a palpable hematoma indicates that the facial artery has been transected upon.

4.11.2 Pretreatment Assessment

Establish the type of nasolabial fold the patient wishes to improve, that is, whether it is the deep static nasolabial folds visible at rest or the prominent dynamic nasolabial folds formed upon smiling and tailor the approach accordingly. Identify the presence of any sunken cheeks, marionette lines, saggy jowls or prominent nasolabial fat pads in the adjacent regions to ensure overall facial balance and harmony. Sunken cheeks should be restored in conjunction with the nasolabial folds, as correction to the nasolabial folds alone may result in an unbalanced facial appearance. Where the nasolabial folds extend into the marionette lines, concurrent correction of the marionette lines is advised. Meanwhile, excess volume in the nasolabial fat pad contributes to the deepening of the nasolabial folds as the upper cheeks sag and fold over across the nasolabial crease. In such case, results can be optimized with adjuvant fat-reducing injections or liposuction, which should ideally precede the nasolabial fold correction with HA filler. Likewise, saggy jowls shouild be better treated with concominant fat-reducing injections, liposuction or thread lifting.

4.11.3 Injection Method (Table 4.13)

4.11.3.1 Deep Static Nasolabial Folds

Both biphasic HA fillers with large particle size and monophasic HA fillers with high viscoelasticity are acceptable for treating deep static nasolabial folds. A23-G 5-cm cannula is used for injection. A25-G or 27-G cannula may also be employed to perform double layering in the superficial subcutaneous fatty layer.

Note that the nasolabial fold should never be effaced completely, as it constitutes an essential curvilinear structure of a three-dimensional human face. This applies particularly to the alar groove located lateral to the ala nasi. Full leveling of the alar groove removes dimensionality from the face, makes the face appear doughy and pillowy, and overinflates the nasolabial fat pad hanging above the nasolabial fold. Moreover, repeated movement of the upper lip elevators which attach to the skin can tug and displace the product into the nasolabial fat pad located above the nasolabial fold, further exaggerating the upper cheek volume. Correction of the alar groove should, therefore, be reserved only for severe cases and performed only to the minimum necessary extent. Hence, it is often the case that the alar groove is intentionally left untreated, while enhancement is directed only at the lower two-thirds of the nasolabial fold.

Table 4.13 Summary of nasolabial fold treatment technique

Item	Contents
Needle vs. Cannula	23-G 5-cm cannula
HA filler	Biphasic HA filer with large particle size or monophasic HA filler with high viscoelasticity
Amount of HA filler	0.5–2 mL per side
Depth of injection	Deep subcutaneous layer above the muscle layer Superficial subcutaneous layer if necessary
Entry point for cannula	1–1.5 cm lateral and 1 cm inferior to the mouth corner
Target area	Lower 2/3 of nasolabial fold
Anesthetics	Topical anesthetics
Nondominant hand	Hold the skin inferiorly in order to maintain skin tension

The cannula entry point is made 1–1.5 cm lateral and 1 cm inferior to the mouth corner. Typically, this should put the cannula entry point along the continuum of the nasolabial fold. Where concurrent correction of sunken cheeks is desired, the relevant cannula entry point can be made slightly lateral to this point (Fig. 4.84). The desired depth of injection depends on the relevant indication. Where cor-

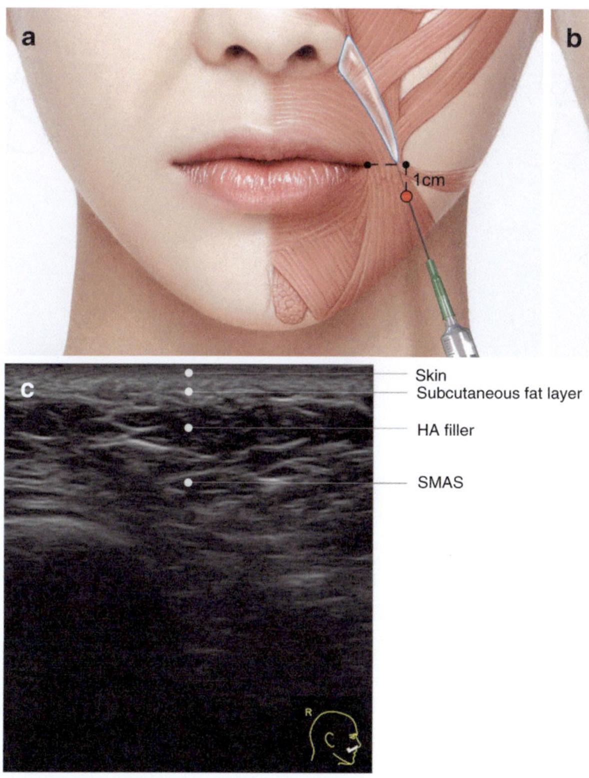

Fig. 4.84 The cannula entry point and appropriate location for the volume restoration of the nasolabial fold. (**a**) Correction of the alar groove should, be reserved only for severe cases, and (**b**) correction performed only to the lower two-thirds of the nasolabial fold (**c**) Sonographic image displaying HA filler placed in subcutaneous layer at nasolabial fold

rection of the alar groove is required, deep injection into the supraperiosteal plane of the canine fossa is performed, while to address volume in the lower two-thirds of the nasolabial fold, volume is placed in the superficial subcutaneous fat lying superficial to the orbicularis oris m. (Fig. 4.85). Utilizing the double-layering technique, additional volume may be administered in the subdermal layer. Where necessary, HA filler may be injected intradermally to address any surface wrinkles.

Using the retrograde linear threading technique, place the HA filler to fill out the deep static groove as needed. A parallel injection of HA is then delivered medially to the nasolabial fold to achieve a smooth gradation in contour. The volume range is 1–2 mL per side, depending on the depth of the fold. For anesthesia, application of topical numbing cream should suffice. The nondominant hand should be used to stretch the skin taut both inferiorly and laterally during the injection to facilitate cannula advancement.

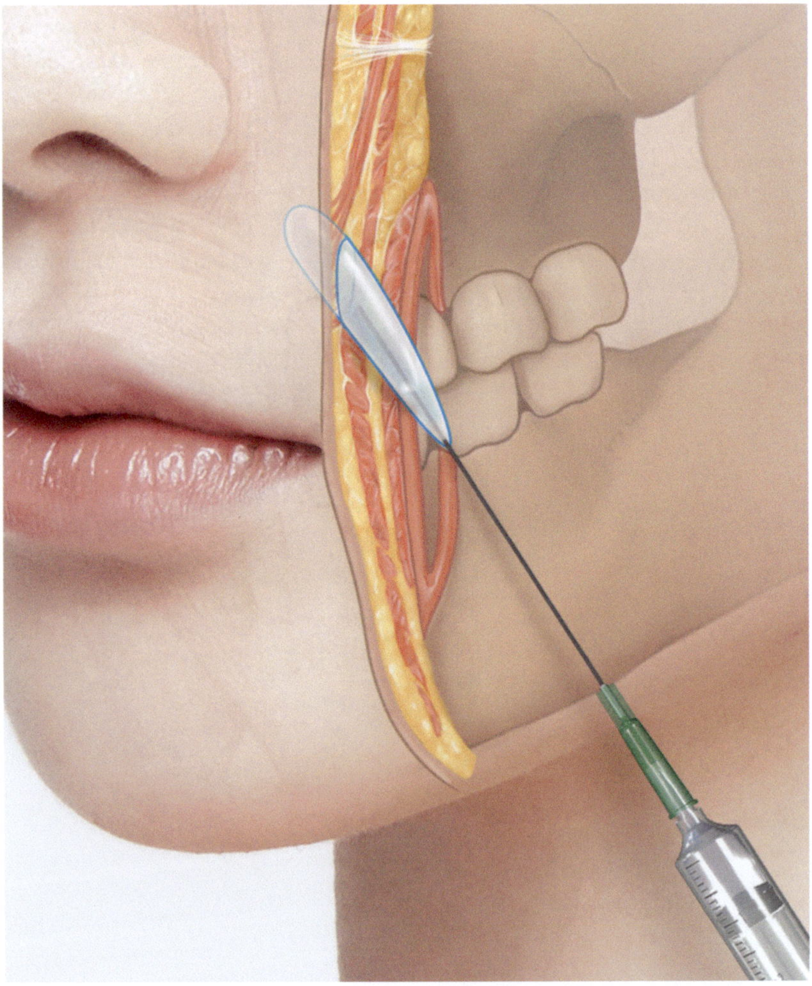

Fig. 4.85 The depth of injection for the nasolabial fold

4.11.3.2 Dynamic Nasolabial Folds

For improving the prominence of dynamic nasolabial folds upon smiling (Fig. 4.82), HA filler is placed perpendicularly in a fern pattern technique by depositing numerous aliquots of HA filler perpendicular to the direction of the nasolabial fold in the dermal plane (Fig. 3.11a). A monophasic HA filler with medium viscoelasticity is typically selected for treating dynamic nasolabial folds. Injection is performed with a 30-G needle and 0.25–0.5 mL of HA filler is dispensed per side in the dermal plane. Application of topical numbing cream for more than 30 min is advised to minimize pain.

4.11.3.3 Combination Treatment

Concurrent correction of the labio mandibular folds or marionette lines is recommended where applicable, as the presence of these lines contributes to an elongated appearance of the nasolabial folds. Meanwhile, depressions in the cheeks should preferably be addressed concomitantly for a more fluid transition to the nasolabial folds. In patients with prominent nasolabial fat pads, it is advisable to undertake 2–3 rounds of corticosteroid fat-reducing injections to achieve a more natural and toned appearance.

4.11.4 Complications

Bruising: Care should be taken to avoid the facial a. running along the nasolabial fold, the damage to which can cause severe bruising such as hematoma when a needle is used for the nasolabial fold correction instead of a cannula or when puncturing the cannula entry point with a needle.

Vascular Insufficiency: Compression of the lateral nasal a. caused by injection of too much filler at the canine fossa may bring about vascular insufficiency in the nasal region in patients whose vascular circulation has already been compromised by a previous nose surgery involving injury to the columella a., etc. Meanwhile, filler embolization from inadvertent injection of filler into the facial artery may bring about vascular complications including necrosis of the nose, glabella, and forehead due to the broad anastomosis present at the nasal dorsum between the lateral nasal artery as a branch of facial artery and the dorsal nasal artery, a branch of supratrochlear artery (see Sect. 5.1).

Irregularity: Injection of too much filler too superficially in the superficial dermis may result in surface irregularities. Meanwhile, treating only the nasolabial folds in isolation without considering the balance with the rest of the face may also bring about contour irregularities. For example, correcting the nasolabial folds only without concomitant treatment of the hollow cheeks may accentuate the prominence of the cheek hollowness. Likewise, in patients with prominent nasolabial fat pads, filling out the alar groove may contribute to a more pronounced appearance of the nasolabial fat.

Sagging Jowls: In patients in their mid-40s and above with preexisting saggy jowls or bulging buccal fat, cheek augmentation can result in the exacerbation of jowl descent (Fig. 4.86). Accordingly, care must be taken to augment nasolabial fold only in minimum amounts in patients with preexisting jowls. Concominant steriod fat reducing injection, liposuction or thread lifting for the sagging jowl should be considered.

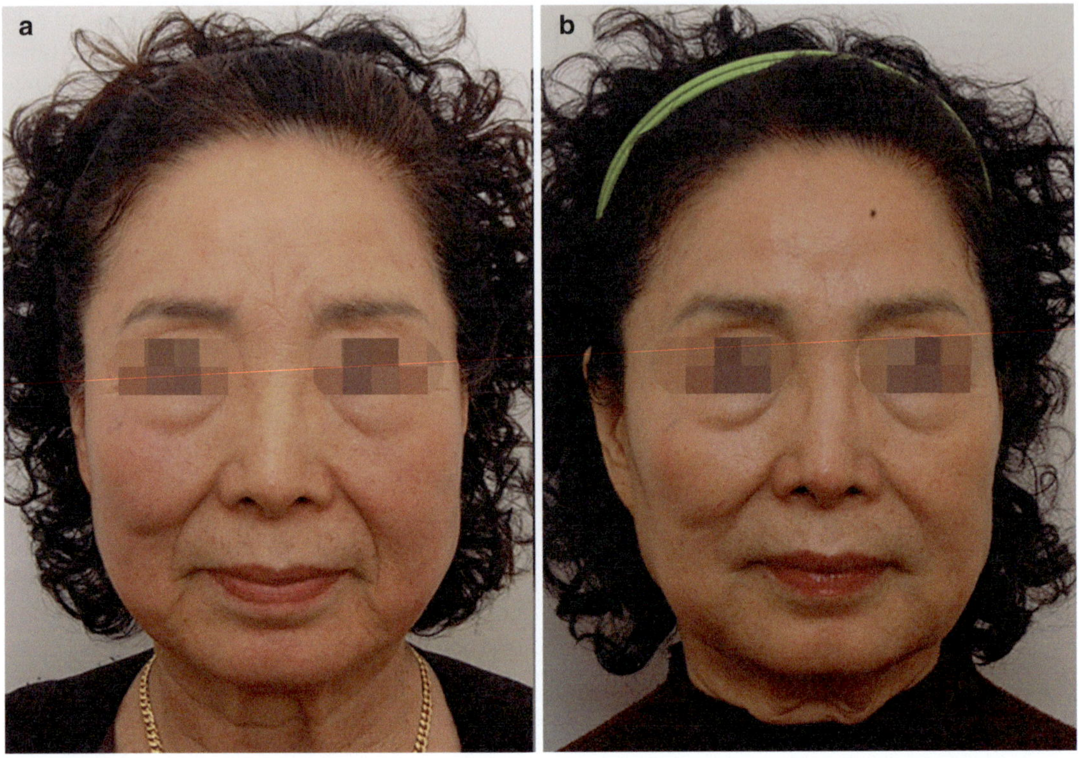

Fig. 4.86 (**a**) Before and (**b**) after anterior sunken cheek augmentation for the nasolabial fold improvement in 68-year-old-patient with preexisting sagging jowls or bulging buccal fat. She also received concominant steriod fat reducing injection and butulinum toxin injection for the masseteric reduction

4.12 Lip Filler

Difficulty Level: B, Effectiveness: A, Complications: B

Summary 1: Inject using a 27-G 3-cm cannula or 30-G needle. The target plane of injection is either the subdermal or the submucosal layer of dry mucosa. The cannula insertion point is created 0.3 cm lateral to the oral commissure. Use only monophasic HA fillers.

Summary 2: The lips consist not of a single long unit but of a sum of different anatomical subunits, including the central tubercle and lateral tubercles, which must be respected during the augmentation with HA filler.

Summary 3: Age-related changes in the lips include the thinning of the lips, elongation of the philtrum, and loss of prominence in the vermillion border. With age, the lower lip progressively rolls inward, the mouth corners invert downwards, and multiple fine lines develop in the perioral area.

Summary 4: It is important to assess the lips from the lateral view before the injection, to check for any over-projection of the upper lip. Patients with a protruded upper lip require HA placement in the lower lips only. Inject no more than 2 mL per session to avoid an overdone appearance.

Lips represent an essential focal point in the face, as it constitutes the only part of the face that appears red in color. In Asia, the expression "*red lips and white teeth*" has been used traditionally to capture the ideals of female facial beauty.

Adequately full voluptuous lips are associated with youth and beauty in both men and women. By contrast, thinning of the lips is considered an aging feature which also creates the perception of coldness and apathy. Lip augmentation is instrumental not only to adding fullness to the lip but also to creating balance between the upper and lower lips or between the left and right lips. In brief, lip enhancement serves not only as a beautification tool for plumping and refining lips in a young patient but also as a rejuvenation tool in older patients for addressing lip thinning as well as counteracting other morphological changes that occur in the lips with age (Fig. 4.87).

4.12.1 Anthropometry of the Lips

Anatomically speaking, the lips are not confined only to the red mucosal region, but instead consist of the red portion, or the vermillion body, and the white part, or areas of cutaneous skin surrounding the circumference of the red lip. Underlying the white lips is the musculature that enables the mouth to perform such functional aspects as the puckering and closure of the lips. In reference to the relevant facial landmarks, the lips extend from the subnasale superiorly down to the pogonion inferiorly and to the nasolabial folds laterally. The boundary between the red and

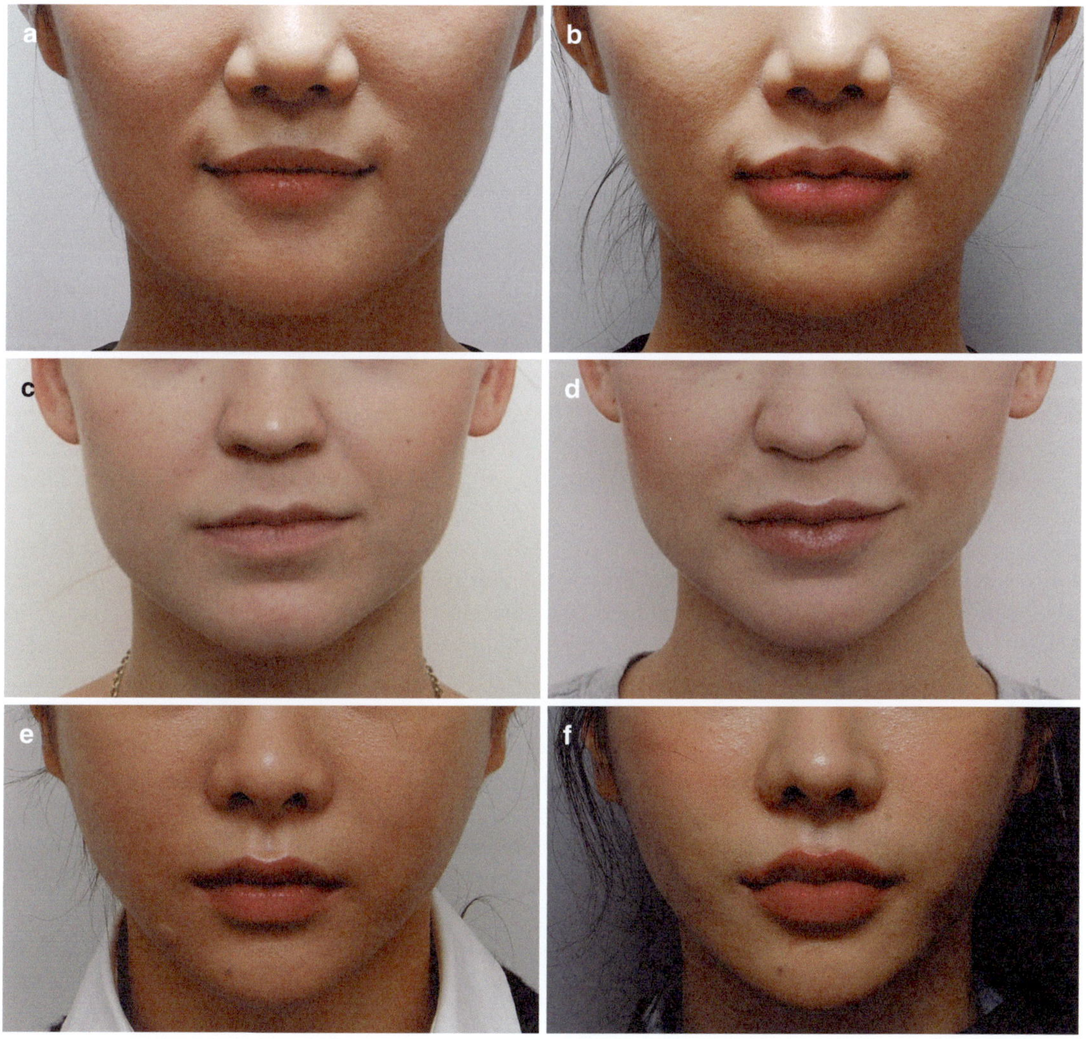

Fig. 4.87 (**a**, **c**, **e**) Before and (**b**, **d**, **f**) after volumization of the lips

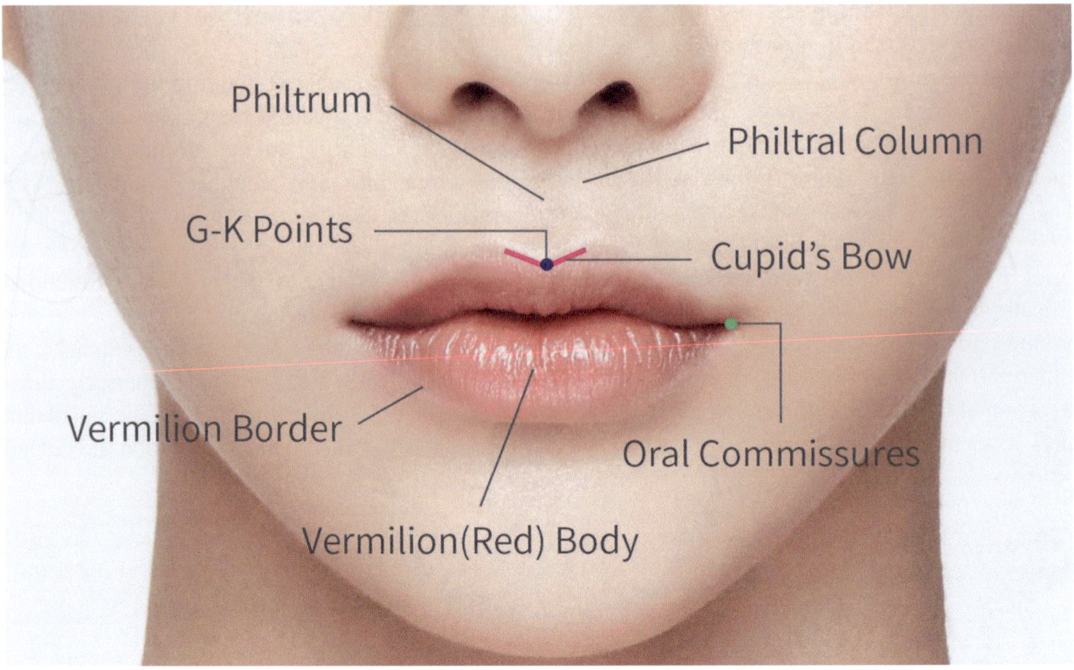

Fig. 4.88 Anatomic landmarks of lips

white lips is demarcated by the vermillion border. The red lip is further divided into the dry mucosa on the outside and the wet mucosa on the inside (Fig. 4.88).

Knowledge of aesthetic facial proportions is a prerequisite to defining the ideal shape and size of the lips and their balance with the rest of the face. The ideal proportion between the upper, middle, and the lower face, extending respectively from hairline to glabella, from glabella to subnasale, and from subnasale to gnathion is described as 1:1:1 [28] (Fig. 4.89). It should be noted, however, that in aesthetic Asians, the lower third of the face is known to be smaller with the ideal facial ratio approaching 1:1:0.8 [29]. The lower face is further divided into equal thirds, with the ideal ratio between the distance from subnasale to stomion relative to the distance from stomion to gnathion described as 1:2. In aesthetic lips, the lower lip should also be slightly thicker than the upper lip, with the ideal vertical height ratio between the upper and lower lip described as 2:3 or 1:1.6 (π). The ideal lip width is where each oral commissure is aligned precisely with a line dropped vertically from the medial pupil. On profile, a number of facial analysis have been described, which aid in the evaluation of the relative prominence of the upper an lower lips to the facial profile, especially to the nose and chin. The upper lip should ideally project slightly over the lower lip from the provile view. Accordingly, based on a straight line connecting the subnasale (Sn) and the pogonion, the upper lip should protrude 3.5 mm and the lower lip 2 mm anterior to this line (Sn-Pog' line by Burston) (Fig. 4.90). Based on the different anthropometric analyses which exclude the influence of the chin protrusion, the upper lip should be 1–2 mm anterior to the true vertical line from the Sn (SnV) while the lower lip should be on or 1 mm in front of this SnV (to exclude the influence of the chin protrusion). The Pog' should be on a line drawn tangent to the upper and lower lips (Riedel line). The lips should also fall behind the line connecting Pog' and nasal tip (Pronasale, Prn) (Ricketts line). In Caucasians, the upper lip should be 4–6 mm behind the Ricketts line with the lower lip 2–4 mm behind; while this should be to a lesser degree in Asians. However, in Black individuals, the lips tend to protrude beyond this line due to the greater soft tissue thickness of the lips and a greater tendency

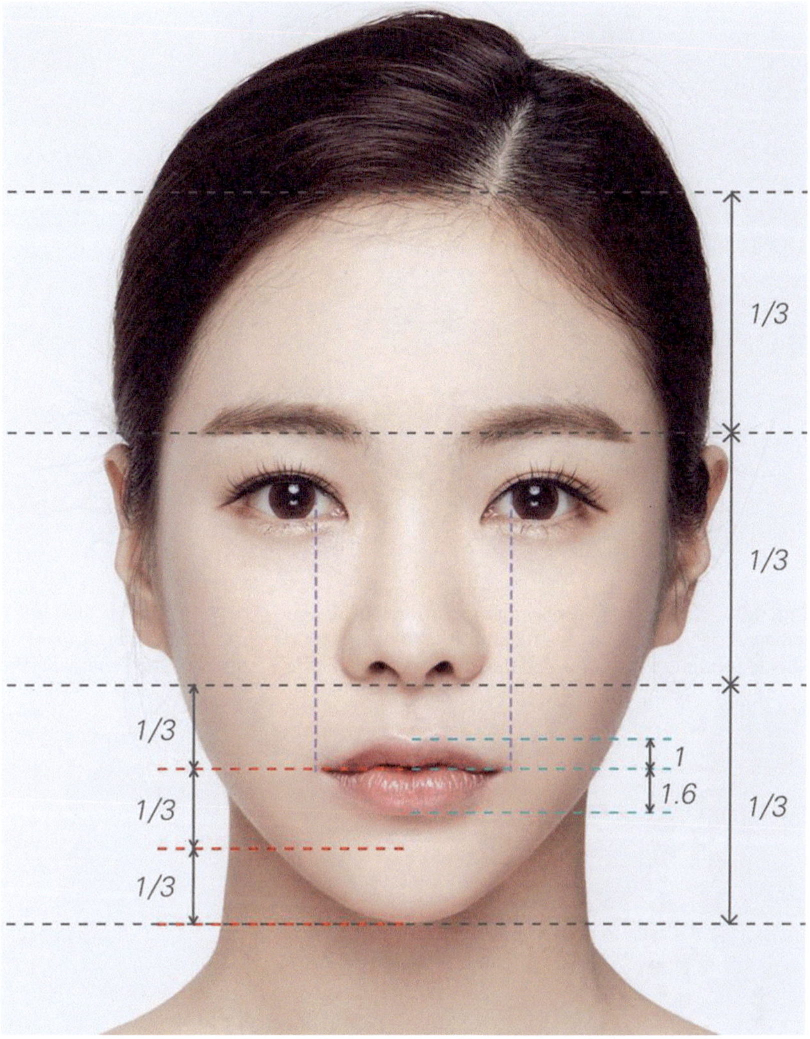

Fig. 4.89 Facial proportions relevant to the lips

for bimaxillary dentoalveolar protrusion as well as the reduced prominence of the nose and the chin compared with Caucasians. Intermediate and Southern type Asians also show a tendency for the lips to protrude beyond the Ricketts line due to the reduced prominence of the nose and the chin. Meanwhile, the philtrum lies immediately superior to the upper lip and is flanked by two raised vertical philtral columns extending respectively from the bilateral peaks of the cupid's bow. The lowest point of the cupid's bow on the midline of the philtrum is referred to as the GK point.

The lip anatomy is highly detailed as the lips consist not of a single long uniform entity, but as a sum of various different anatomical subcomponents, which should be appraised and volumized as such (Fig. 4.91). On the upper lip, there is one central tubercle below the cupid's bow with two lateral tubercles sitting on either side. Meanwhile, the lower lip features a central depression with two lateral tubercles formed on either side. The two tubercles on the lower lip should fit neatly into the relative recesses of the upper lip, while the three upper lip tubercles should rest comfortably on the corresponding flatter regions of the lower lip. Accordingly, in beautiful lips, the presence of these structures should create a smooth waveform along the oral fissure when the mouth is closed with alternating convexities and convexities undulating from one end of the mouth corner to the other (Fig. 4.91).

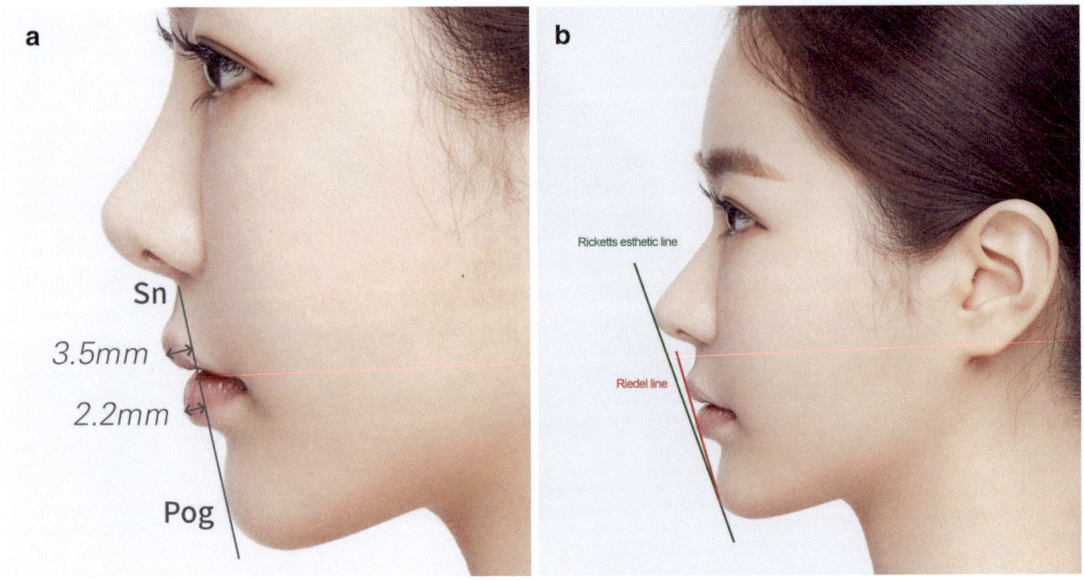

Fig. 4.90 Lateral view of ideally proportioned lips (Sn: subnasale, Pog': soft tissue pogoniion). (**a**) The upper lip should protrude slightly beyond the lower lip from porfile view. (**b**) Pog' is on a line tangent to the upper and lower lips (Riedel line). Lips should be behind the line connecting Pog' and Pronasale (Prn) (Ricketts line)

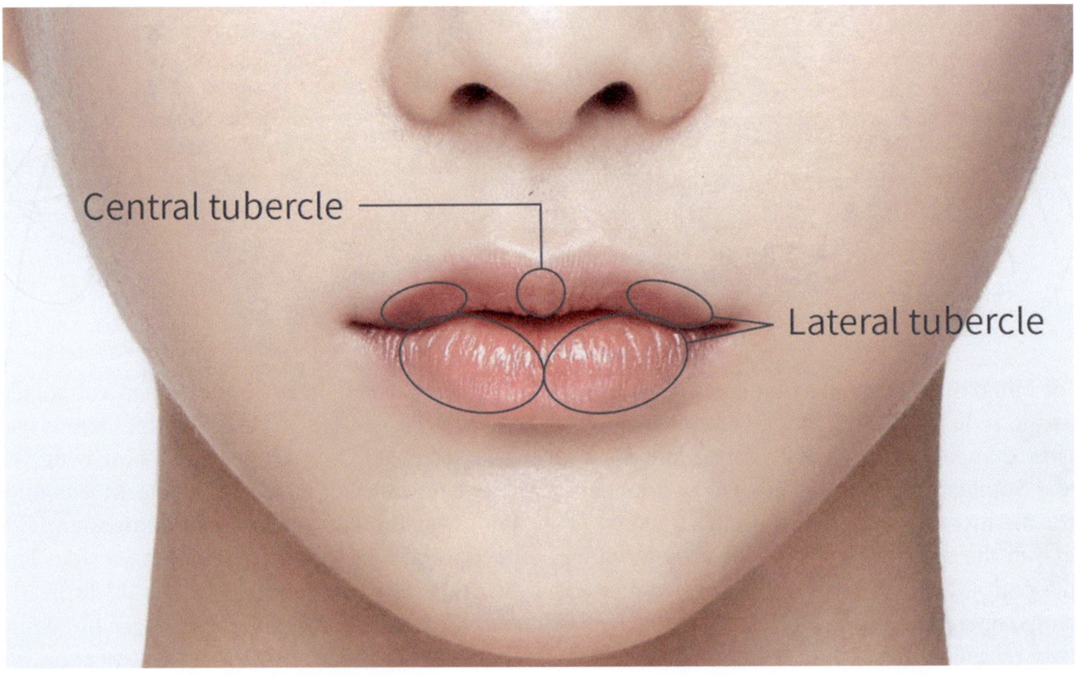

Fig. 4.91 Subunits of the lip anatomy

4.12.2 Anatomical Considerations

4.12.2.1 Sagittal View of the Lips

In the sagittal view, the anatomical layers of the lips from the outer to the innermost layers are comprised as follows: the skin or the dry mocosa of lips—subdermal or submucosal layer—orbicularis oris m.—submucosa—wet mucosa in oral cavity. The lip mucosa can be divided into the dry mucosa on the outside

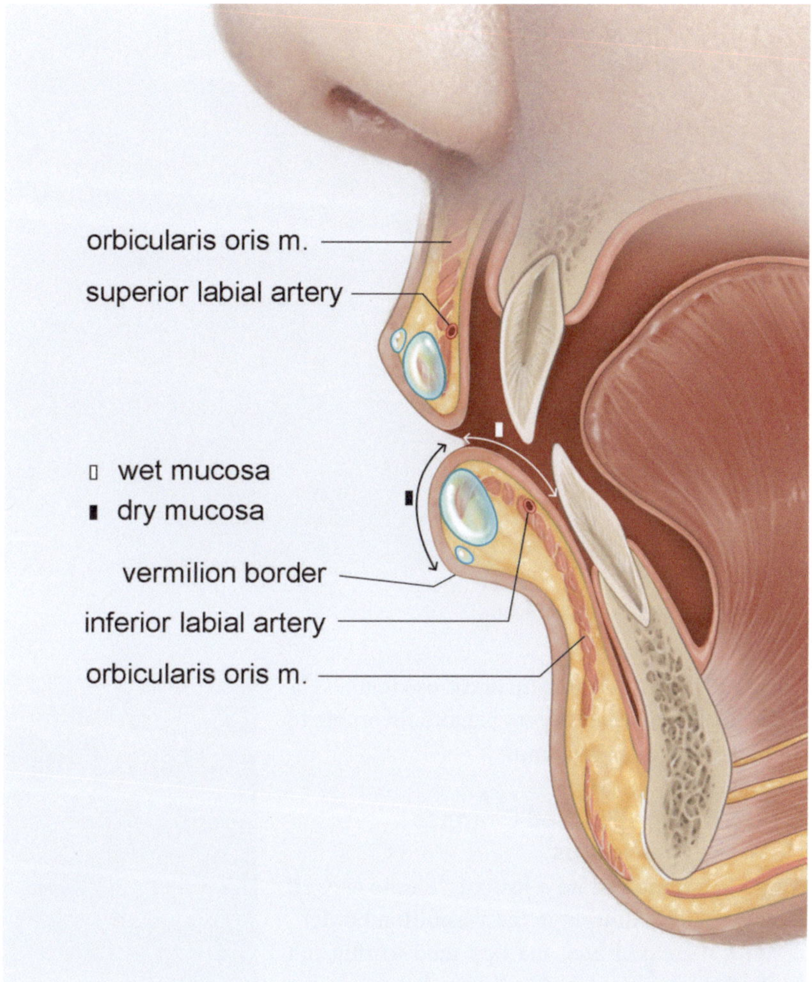

Fig. 4.92 Depth of injection for lip augmentation is submucosal (body) or subdermal (vermillion bordore) layer

and the wet mucosa in the oral cavity. The submucosa on the oral cavity side lies deep to the orbicularis oris m. and is supplied by the labial artery, the labial glands, and the branches of the mental nerve (Fig. 4.92).

4.12.2.2 The Labial Artery

The superior labial artery branches from the facial artery within the perimeters of a square drawn 15 mm lateral and 15 mm superior to the oral commissure and courses along the vermillion border of the upper lip within the substance of the orbicularis oris m., if not at the depth between the orbicularis oris m. and mucosa [29]. Before reaching the peak of the cupid's bow, it descends from the vermillion border into the red lip and runs medially toward the midline of the upper lip, where it either terminates as the columellar artery superiorly or anastomoses with the contralateral superior labial artery approaching from the opposite side. Unlike the superior labial artery, the inferior labial artery seldom traverses along the vermillion border and shows individual variations in its distribution pattern. Branching from the facial artery, it often traverses between the lower lip and the chin within the substance of the depressor anguli oris (DAO) and the depressor labii inferioris (DLI) before ascending superiorly and terminating at the lower lip mucosa (Fig. 4.93).

Both the superior and inferior labial arteries lie close to the wet mucosa of the inner lip, with the superior labial artery located at a depth of 5.3 mm from the vermillion border and the inferior labial artery at a distance of 4.2 mm [30]. Since both labial arteries routinely run deep to the orbicularis oris m., injection of HA superfi-

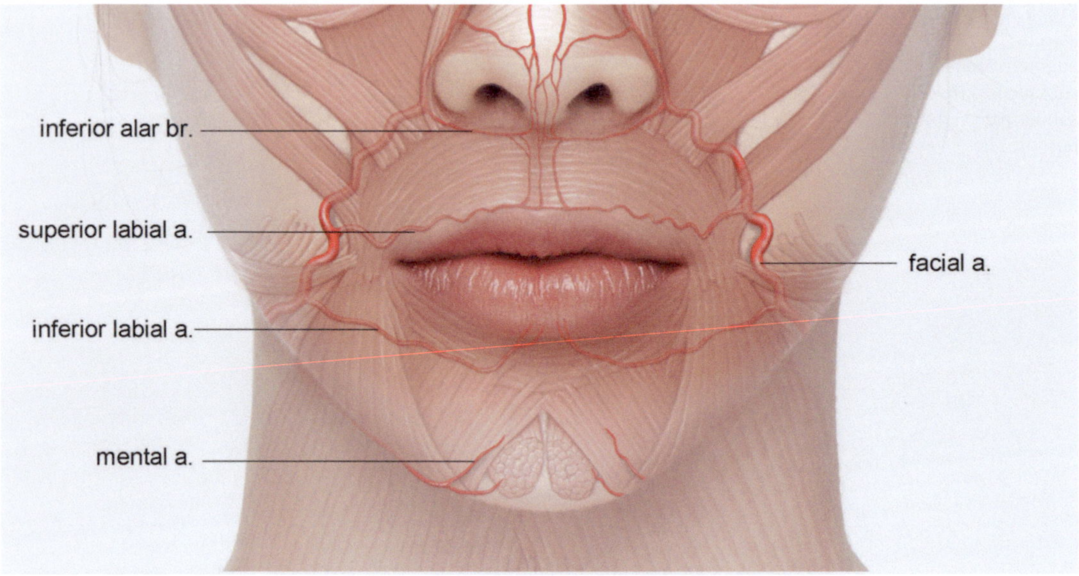

Fig. 4.93 Vascular supply of the lip

cial to the orbicularis oris m. and close to the subdermal or submucosal layers is more favorable to avoid the risk of arterial injury.

4.12.2.3 Age-Related Changes in the Lips

Aging lips demonstrate a loss of volume as well as the loss of definition in the vermillion border.

With increased age, the lips tend to thin out while the vermillion border loses definition due to volume deflation. Aging upper lips demonstrate a loss of volume, elongation of the philtrum, and loss of definition in the philtral columns, the cupid's bow, and the vermilion border. The lower lip also becomes progressively thinner and starts to rotate inwards. Multiple perioral lines begin developing around the periphery of the lips while the mouth corners start to invert downwards (Fig. 4.94).

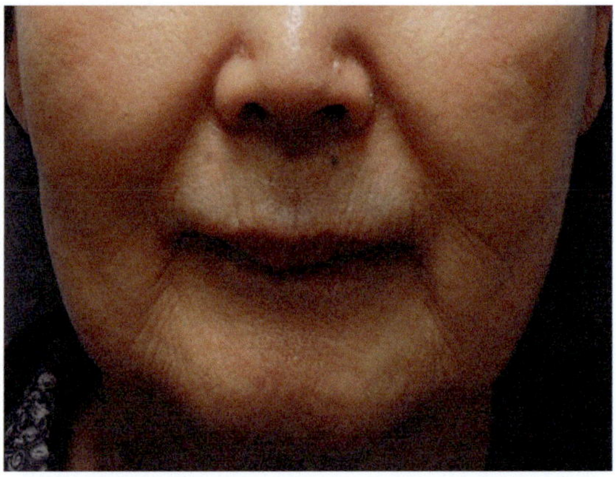

Fig. 4.94 Aging of the lips

4.12.3 Pretreatment Assessment

Assessments should be made of the proportion between the upper and lower lips as well as the presence of any asymmetry between the left and right lips on the frontal view prior to treatment. While no consensus has been reached on what constitutes the ideal lip volume, thin lips are generally considered aesthetically unfavorable, as they tend to impart a lack of warmth and callousness and are typically associated with an aging face. It is important to consult with the patient regarding the desired lip volume, since the adequacy of injected volume hinges significantly on the specific aesthetic preferences and desires of the individual.

Generally speaking, younger patients tend to favor augmenting their natural lip size and fullness while the main aesthetic goal in older patients is the restoration of age-related lip volume loss. The patient's ethnicity must also be considered since ethnic differences exist with respect to desired lip volume. Asians tend to prefer relatively smaller lips compared to Caucasians [31]. Blacks prefer the biggest lip size, followed by Caucasians and Asians. Arabs whose facial bone structure bears a close resemblance to Caucasians also tend to show a preference for fuller and more voluptuous lips as wearing a hijab serves to draw more attention to the aesthetics of individual facial features. It is also essential to examine the lips from the profile view to determine the presence of any bimaxillary protrusion or over-projection of the upper or the lower lip. Note that lip augmentation with HA is not recommended in patients presenting with a protruded mouth, or bimaxillary protrusion, while an over projected upper lip can be balanced out with the placement of HA filler in the lower lips only. In case the patient has a visibly prominent central tubercle on the upper lip, the volume should preferably be added only in the lateral tubercles without further augmenting the central tubercle.

In older patients in their fifth decade and beyond seeking lip rejuvenation with HA fillers, it may be worthwhile to also identify opportunities for rejuvenation in other parts of the perioral complex which manifest signs of aging. For instance, the appearance of deep perioral rhytids is an indication for the combined use of BoNT-A and HA filler for the treatment of fine lines. Placement of HA filler additionally in the marionette lines can produce a more synergistic outcome in everting the downturned mouth corners.

4.12.4 Injection Technique (Table 4.14)

Inject using only soft monophasic HA fillers. The injection tool is primarily a 27-G × 3-cm cannula. However, a 30-G needle can be used (see Sect. 4.12.4.3). The target depth of injection varies depending on the specific indication. Inject subdermally to enhance the vermillion border and into the submucosal layer of the dry mocosa to plump the body of the lips. The entry point of cannula insertion is created 0.3 cm lateral to the oral commissure (Fig. 4.95). When creating the

Table 4.14 Summary of lip filler injection technique

Item	Contents
Needle vs. Cannula	27-G 3-cm, or 30-G needle can be used
HA filler	Monophasic HA filler
Amount of HA filler	1–2 mL per session
Depth of injection	Subdermal layer for the vermilion border Submucosal layer of the dry mucosa for the body of the red lip
Entry point for cannula	0.3 cm lateral to the oral commissure
Target area	Vermilion border Central tubercle and lateral tubercles Philtral columns if necessary
Anesthetics	Topical anesthetics and local anesthetics at entry point Infraorbital and mental nerve block may be required in patients sensitive to pain
Nondominant hand	Used to press the midline of the lower lip and medial one-third of the upper lip

lateral tubercles of the upper and lower lips respectively, the nondominant hand should be used to press the medial one-third of the upper lip or the midline of the lower lip as the case may be to prevent the spread of HA filler into areas of relative concavity.

Regarding the injection volume, first place 1–1.5 mL of HA across the lips for overall volume and assess the interim result with the patient using a mirror before deciding if additional HA filler may be appropriate. Note, however, that lips can appear larger immediately following the injection due to the surplus volume of the anesthetics mixed with the HA filler as well as the immediate postprocedure swelling of tissue. Where practicable, make sure to inject no more than 2 mL per session to avoid the appearance of "duck lips" due to overfilling.

For anesthesia, application of topical numbing cream and local anesthetic injection at the cannula entry point should suffice. The use of infraorbital and mental nerve blocks may be considered in patients highly sensitive to pain, but generally not advised since the temporary drooping of the lips from the nerve block

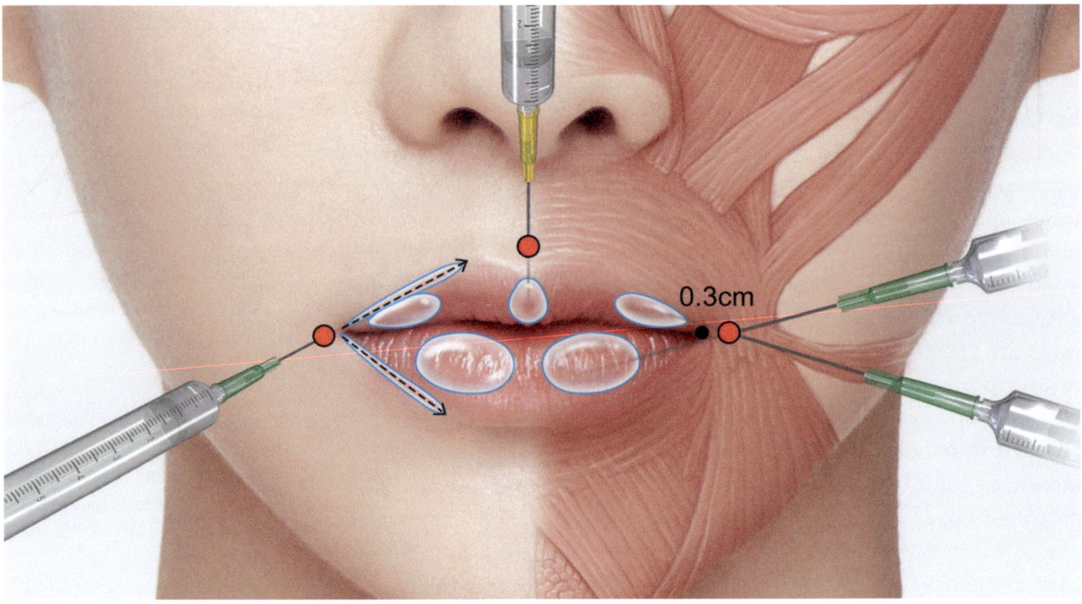

Fig. 4.95 Injection technique for lip augmentation using cannula

may hinder proper postinjection assessment of the lip volume.

4.12.4.1 The Upper Lip

Advance the cannula subdermally along the vermillion border toward the peak of the cupid's bow. Place HA filler using the retrograde linear thread technique to enhance the vermillion border. Next, proceed to augment the lateral tubercles of the upper lip by redirecting the cannula toward the red lip lying below the vermilion border and placing HA filler in the submucosal layer. This gives a slightly upturned appearance to the oral commissures when the mouth is closed as the inferior border of the upper lip curls up into a relative concavity at the mouth corners. Note, however, that no more than 0.2–0.3 mL should be injected into each upper lateral tubercle as overfilling the tubercles to achieve this perceived eversion might lead to the appearance of unnatural lumps. Where accentuation of the central tubercle is desired, introduce a 30-G sharp needle through the midpoint of the cupid's bow, a.k.a. the GK point, and advance inferiorly toward the central tubercle. 0.1 mL of HA is appropriate for enhancing the central tubercle. The use of the 30-G needle is also employed to define and enhance the cupid's bow and the philtral columns in case they are either congenitally weak or have flattened with age. To enhance the philtral columns, insert the 30-G needle at the peak of the cupid's bow and advance superiorly to deliver 0.1 mL of HA at the dermal and subdermal layer.

4.12.4.2 The Lower Lip

The same method can be applied for lower lip augmentation. First, HA filler is injected along the vermillion border to define and enhance the lower lip contour. Once the outline has been treated, volumize the body of the lips by augmenting the lateral tubercles. The nondominant hand should be used to press down the midline of the lower lip to prevent the spreading of HA filler into the midline. The presence of two distinct bumps resembling "cherries" formed on either side of the midline culminates in the appearance of aesthetically pleasing *cherry lips*. It is also worth pointing out that lower lip volumization is usually performed only at the medial two-thirds of the lip, and that the lateral edges are rarely addressed, as the flattening of the lip volume toward the lateral edges provides a more natural appearance. However, when treating patients presenting a horizontally short lower lip, volume can also be placed in the lateral one-third of the lower lip to elongate the lip width. Typically, 0.3–0.4 mL of HA is placed into each lateral tubercle. To fill out the remaining lateral edges of the bottom lip, however, more than 0.5 mL of HA is required per side of the lower lip.

4.12.4.3 The Needle Technique

A 30-G needle can be used instead of a cannula by placing several short retrograde linear threads of HA filler sequentially along the border (Fig. 4.96). Alternatively, merely pushing in the product at the mouth corner into the subdermal layer of the vermillion border allows the product to track along the ridges, even without advancing the needle, toward the medial aspect of the lips. From this, it can be inferred that a particular path of least resistance exists within the anatomy of the vermillion border. When augmenting the body of the lips with a needle, the injection should be made at the submucosal level superficial to the muscular layer as the labial arteries run deep to the orbicularis oris m. As with all needle injections, aspiration before each injection is critical to prevent inadvertent intravascular filler injection.

4.12.4.4 Combination Treatments

Lip enhancement can include the use of BoNT-A for the treatment of perioral rhytids. For severe perioral rhytids, intradermal or subdermal placement of HA filler into the cutaneous part of the lips following the restoration of the vermillion border can provide direct wrinkle improvement as well as overall enhancement in skin elasticity in the perioral region. Meanwhile, downturned mouth corners can be addressed by placing 0.2–0.5 mL of HA filler immediately below the oral commissure, either intradermally or subdermally, to provide upward structural support. Volume restoration in the marionette lines may also produce more synergistic results (Fig. 4.96). The adjunctive use of BoNT-A injections in the depressor anguli oris (DAO) is also commonly performed to relax its downward pull on the mouth corners (Fig. 4.97).

4.12.5 Complications

Duck Lips: Overcorrection of lip volume should be avoided as it may result in the so-called "duck lip" appearance (Fig. 4.98).

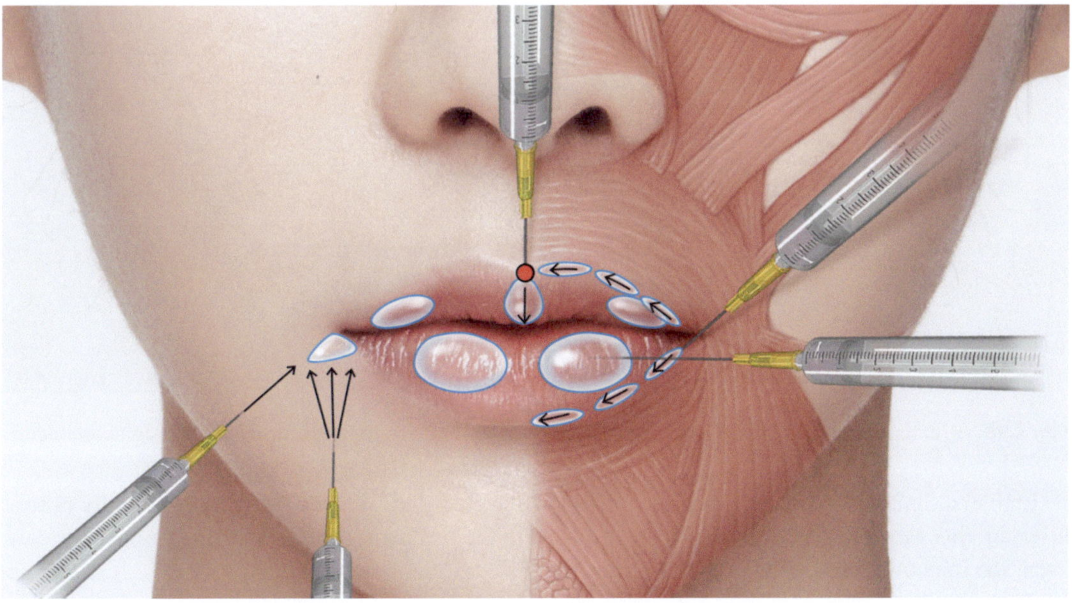

Fig. 4.96 Injection technique for the lip augmentation using needle (left lip) and mouth corner elevation (right mouth corner)

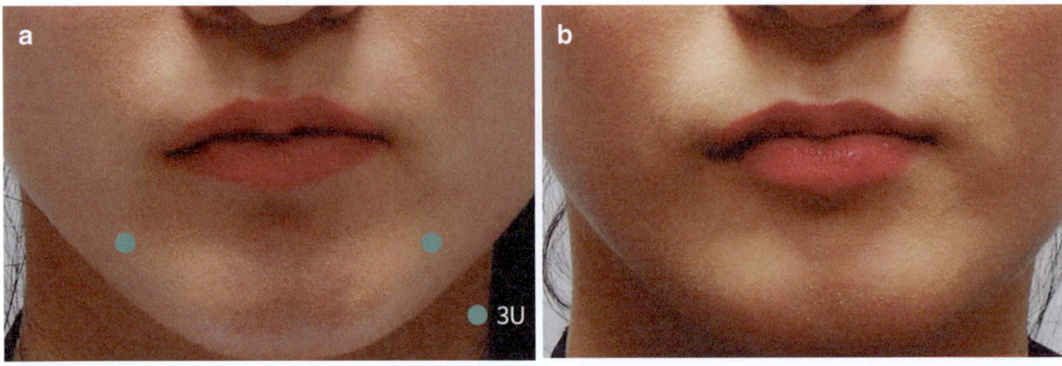

Fig. 4.97 (**a**) Before and (**b**) after Botulinum toxin injections 3U per side in the depressor angularis oris (DAO) for mouth corner elevation

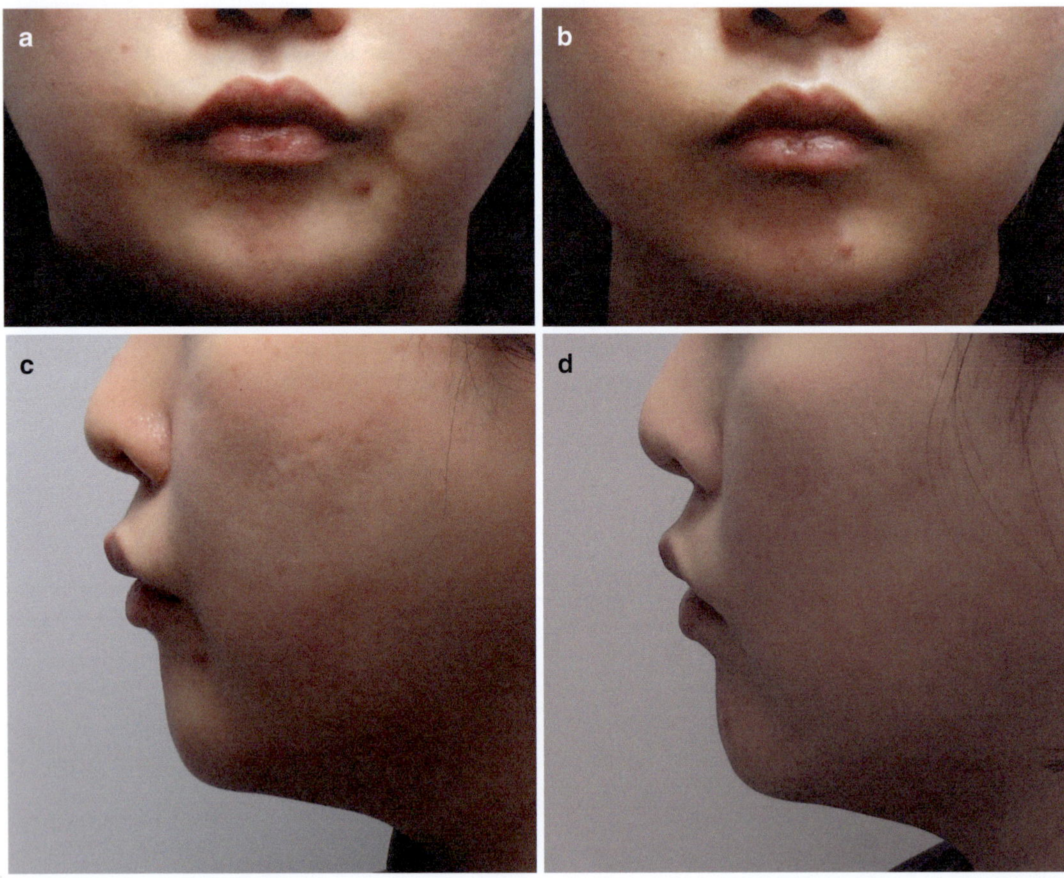

Fig. 4.98 (**a**, **c**) Before and (**b**, **d**) after hyaluronidase injection at upper lip for the treatment of "duck-lip" from overfilling

Embolization: Intra-arterial injection of HA filler in the labial arteries may occur in the event the injection was performed with a needle. Violaceous discoloration of lips following HA filler injection is highly indicative of an embolic event which requires immediate dissolution of the HA filler. While tissue necrosis hardly occurs in the lips owing to its extensive vascularity, care is advised nonetheless.

Bumps and Lumps: On occasion, the injection pressure may cause the HA filler to shift within the soft and loose matrix of the wet mucosa and

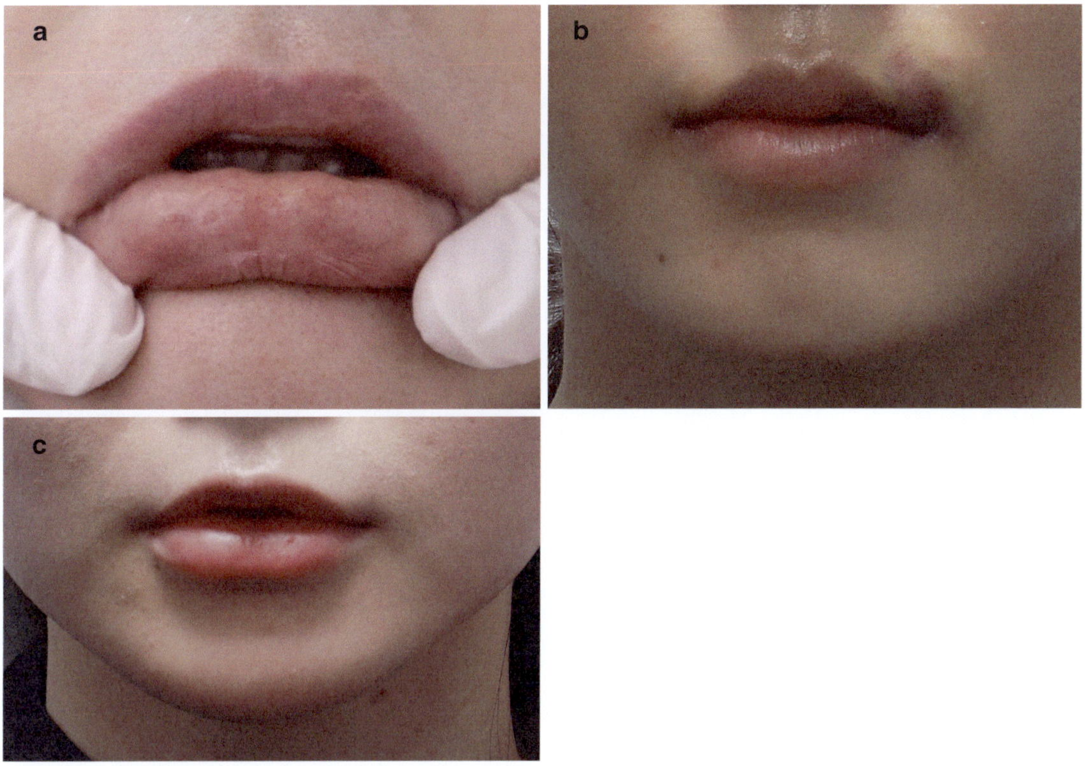

Fig. 4.99 (**a**) Frog egg-lke protrusion at wet mucosa, (**b**) Bruising due to rupture of the superior labial artery, (**c**) Asymmetry of lower lip after lip filler

protrude like frog eggs from inside of the lips. This appearance can be disfiguring and requires dissolution (Fig. 4.99).

Bruising: Rupture of the superior labial artery must be avoided as it may result in a significant hematoma (Fig. 4.99).

Asymmetry: Asymmetric volume change may occur after lip filler.

Herpes Simplex: Outbreak of herpes simplex following HA filler injection has been reported, if only rarely.

Episode: Beautiful Red Lips, the Eternal Symbol of Beauty.

Traditionally, a wide variety of idiomatic expressions have been used in Asia to refer to exceptionally beautiful women. Women with unrivaled beauty have been exalted as possessing *"out of this world beauty," "beauty that only exists at the edge of the world,"* or *"beauty to match the heaven."* Indeed, history is replete with examples of ancient kings and emperors who have led their kingdoms to doom due to their blind infatuation with lethally beautiful women. Examples include *King Zhou of Shang* and his consort *Daji*, *King You* of *West Zhou* dynasty and *Baosi*, *King Fuchai* of *Wu kingdom* and *Xi Shi*, *Emperor Xuan Zibg* of *Tang* and *Yang Guifei*. Hence, expressions such as "*beauty capable of overthrowing a dynasty*" or "be*auty that could precipitate the downfall of a kingdom*" have been used to glamorize women possessing an almost dangerously stunning charm. Other traditional descriptors used to praise exquisite female beauty include *"face like a flower and posture resembling the moon," "lucent irises and lustrous teeth"* (from the poem *Lament by the River* by renowned poet *Du*

Fu during the Tang dynasty) and *"red lips and white teeth*." Among these, the origins of *"red lips and white teeth"* can be traced to the Chinese historical text *"Records of the Three Kingdoms" (Sanguozhi)*. According to the narrative, *Cao Cao*, one of the key figures of the book and portrayed as a master strategist, defeats Yuan Shao in the battle of Ye (present-day Handan, Heibei) in 204. Upon conquering Ye, Cao Cao's son Cao Pi (187–226) kills Yuan Shao's second son Yuan Xi and claims Yuan Xi's wife, lady Zen (182–221) as his own. Lady Zen was a woman of sublime beauty. Indeed, her gorgeousness was such that Cao Cao lamented that the battle of Ye might have been fought ultimately to acquire lady Zen. Even Cao Pi's 13-year-old baby brother Cao Zhi secretly kept amorous feelings for his sister-in-law. In 220, Cao Pi succeeded Cao Cao as the king of Wei and took in the two daughters of the dethroned emperor Xian of the Han dynasty as his concubines. Cao Pi was a king of violent and ruthless temperament, and when he suspected lady Zen of being jealous of the young concubines, he mercilessly ordered his first wife of many years to be executed. While many stifled their grief of lady Zen's death for fear of inviting Cao Pi's wrath, only his younger brother Cao Zhi dared to dedicate a poem in memory of his once beloved sister-in-law, entitled *"Ode to the goddess of the Luo River*." A passage from the poem reads, "your red lips luminesce outwards while your white teeth gleam from within" from which the expression "red lips and white teeth" originates and has been used almost as a byword for female beauty.

In my general perception, the expression "red lips and white teeth" applies not only to describing beautiful *Asian* women. "Tess" (1979) directed by Roman Polanski based on Thomas Hardy's classic novel, is a film I saw as a young boy and one that introduced me to the irresistible allure of Nastassja Kinski. As is the case with many old movies, the film is only remembered in odd snippets of scenes. One scene, however, remains engraved into my mind like a still image; the one where Alec d' Urberville with a penchant for beautiful women tries to seduce Tess with strawberries. The tight close-up shot of Nastassja Kinski's luscious red lips and brilliantly white teeth as she bites into the freshly picked strawberry was mesmerizing to the point of being intoxicating. Spellbound by the pure, pristine, almost wild beauty of Nastassja Kinski captured in the scene at her innocent age of 18, my tender teenage heart longed to be the strawberry she was devouring. Without doubt, it can be said that the allure of full red lips transcends both time and space as the eternal hallmark of youthful beauty. Having said that, it should come as no surprise that Nastassja Kinski was the goddess whose picture adorned the plastic writing board that I kept between the notebooks in my school bag.

Episode: Origin of the Term "Vermillion"

Vermilion (otherwise spelled vermillion) refers to a bright red, almost scarlet-colored pigment (Fig. 4.100), obtained from a red mineral called cinnabar. The name vermilion is originally derived from the term *vermeillon*, meaning worm, as in Ancient times, red dye was extracted from scale insects or *cochineal* insects. That said, the production of vermillion today bears no relation to insects and is extracted instead from minerals.

Fig. 4.100 The color of Vermillion

4.13 Marionette Lines

Difficulty Level: B, Effectiveness: B, Complications: B

Summary 1: Injection is performed using 23-G × 5-cm/27-G × 3-cm cannulas and monophasic HA fillers with high viscoelasticity.

Summary 2: The marionette fold is not simply an indented line or wrinkle but represents a three-dimensional curvilinear structure produced by the sagging of the jowls. While the fold itself may be filled in with HA filler, the inferior descent and protrusion of the cheek fat giving rise to the fold must be addressed using the appropriate adjunct treatment modality.

Summary 3: HA filler is deposited along the depressed area under the mouth corner along the marionette line. Considering that the depression is the deepest at the area immediately under the mouth corner as well as along the depth of the fold itself, augmentation should be directed primarily at these areas, with a gradual decrease in injection volume toward the medial and inferior aspects of the marionette line. The relevant plane of injection lies above (superficial to) the DAO (depressor anguli oris m.).

Summary 4: Concurrent volume restoration is recommended if any volume deficiency is present in the cheeks, nasolabial folds, prejowl sulcus, or the labiomandibular folds.

Marionette lines are the oblique creases that extend from the oral commissures to the mandibular border. They take their name from the marionette string puppets featured in European puppet shows with visible crevices running down the mouth corners to allow animation of the jaws. Similar to the nasolabial fold, the marionette fold is not simply an indented crease or line but represents a three-dimensional structure produced by the sagging of the jowls precipitated by the laxity of cheek skin and the clumping and descent of the jowl fat pad. The repeated contraction of the DAO (depressor anguli oris m.) and the platysma m. which pull the mouth corners downwards also cements the static marionette lines in place. In sum, marionette lines result from several contributing causes; hence, each cause should be approached individually to achieve the most effective outcome (Fig. 4.101).

4.13.1 Anatomical Considerations

The marionette line is caused by the suspension of the superficial jowl fat and the deep buccal fat pad over the boundary against the modiolus, the risorius m. and the mandibular ligament, which anchors and restricts these overhanging structures from further descent. The downward displacement of the redundant cheek skin and underlying

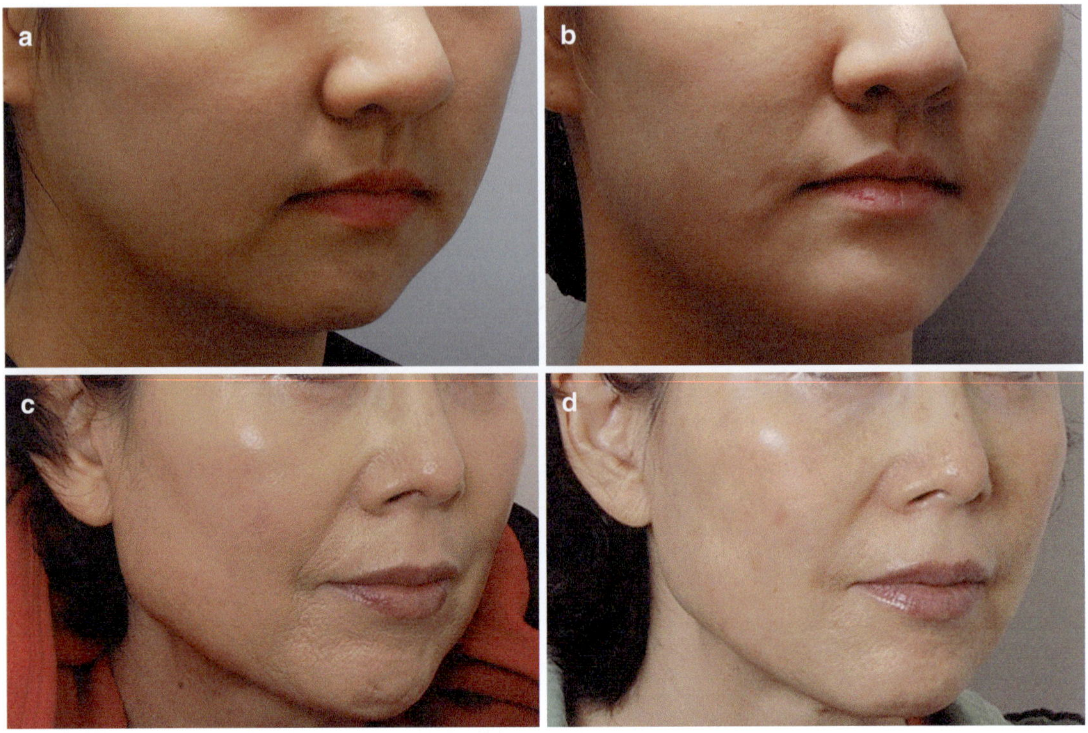

Fig. 4.101 (**a**, **c**) Before and (**b**, **d**) after the treatment of marionette line

fat pads with age leads to the elongation and deepening of the marionette lines as well as the formation of jowls and the pre-jowl sulcus, a dip in the jawline appearing anterior to the jowl. Another cause of the marionette lines is the repeated contraction of the DAO and the platysma m. which continuously pulls the mouth corners downwards and outwards, causing the static marionette lines to deepen with time. When treating the marionette lines, the use of a cannula is preferred over a needle as the facial artery advancing superomedially toward the nasolabial fold gives off the inferior labial artery under the lower lip medial to the marionette line (Fig. 4.92) [32].

Modiolus and Marionette Lines

The term modiolus is derived from Latin and means the "hub of a wheel." Histologically, the modiolus is a small, thick, and dense structure. As the name aptly suggests, it represents a point of convergence for various facial expression muscles which insert near the angle of the mouth [33] (Fig. 4.102). The insertion of the zygomaticus major m., depressor anguli oris m., levator anguli oris m., depressor labii inferioris m., orbicular oris m., risorius m., and the buccinator m into the modiolus plays a pivotal role not only in the development of nasolabial folds and marionette lines but also in the animation of facial expressions in the perioral region for communicating various emotions such as joy and sorrow. Whereas the modiolus is more commonly located above the intercheilion horizontal line in Caucasians (66%), the modiolus in Asians is more commonly located below this line (58.4%) and is visible to the naked eye in up to 21.4% of the population [34] (Fig. 4.103). Presumably, this explains why a semblance of marionette lines can be seen in Asians even as early as their teens and twenties. Loss of volume in the cheek contributes to the increased prominence of the modiolus. As a tendinous nodule with dense collagen fibers, the visibility of the modiolus can overage the face in patients exhibiting even the slightest degree of jowl fullness by giving the appearance of age-related jowl descent and accentuating the marionette lines.

4.13.2 Pretreatment Assessment

Presence of any cheek depressions, nasolabial folds, or prominent buccal fat pad in the adjacent regions must be identified to ensure overall facial balance and harmony. Sunken cheeks should preferably be restored in conjunction with the marionette lines, as

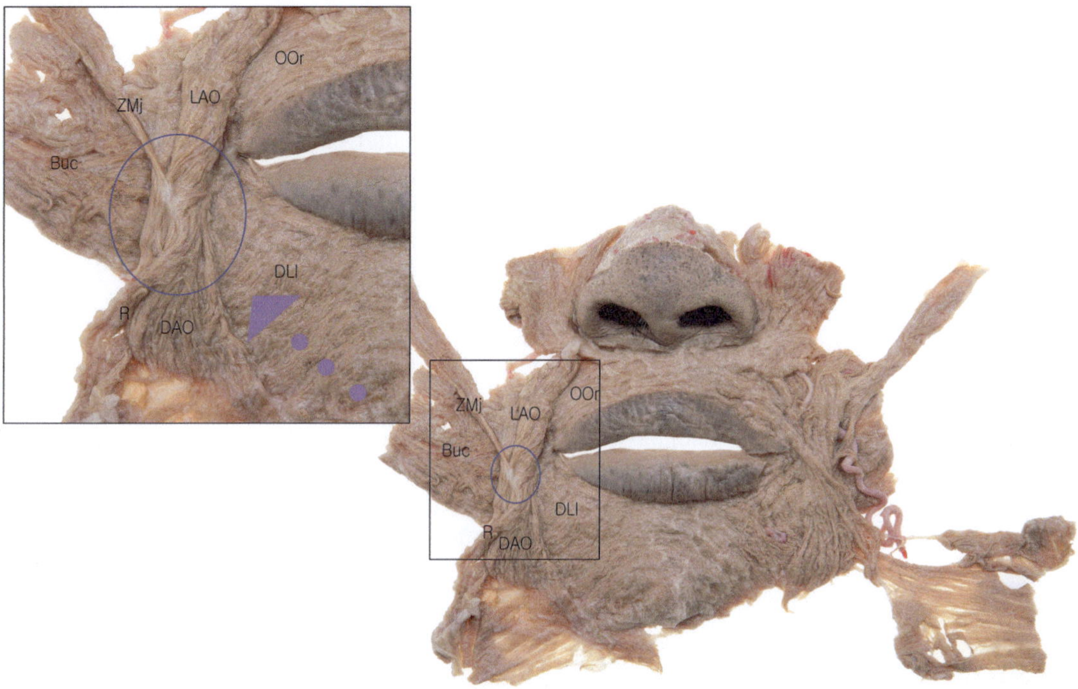

Fig. 4.102 The modiolus. The structure in the blue circle represents the tendinous nodule located in the center of the modiolus. To clearly demonstrate the tendinous nodule, the LAO and the risorius were folded open to the medial side. (*OOr* orbicularis oris, *Zmj* zygomaticus major, *Buc* buccinators, *R* risorius, *LAO* levator anguli oris, *DAO* depressor anguli oris, *DLI* depressor labii inferioris) (photo: courtesy of Professor Hee-Jin Kim)

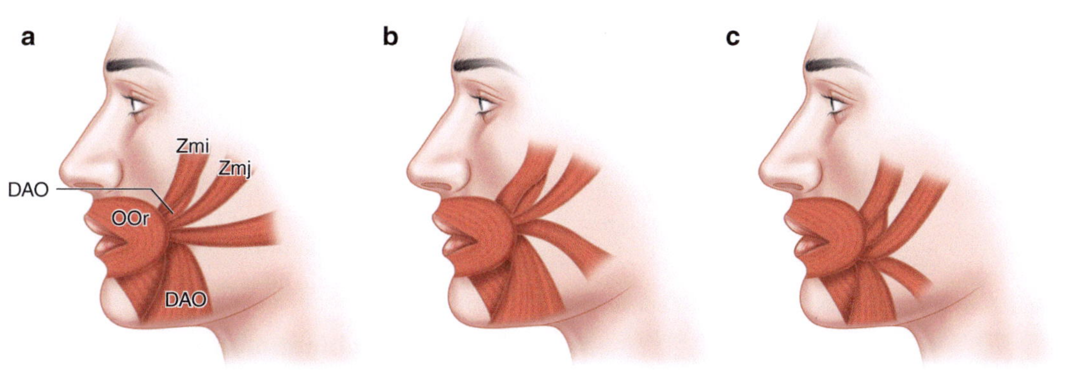

Fig. 4.103 Position of the modiolus by reference to the intercheilion horizontal line. Type A—Modiolus is located lateral to the cheilion on the intercheilion horizontal line. Type B —Modiolus is located above the intercheilion horizontal line. Type C —Modiolus is located below the intercheilion horizontal line (*OOr* orbicularis oculi, *DAO* depressor anguli oris, *R* risorius, *Zmj* zygomaticus major, *Zmi* zygomaticus minor, *LAO* levator anguli oris) (Modified from Ref. [32])

correction to the marionette lines alone can serve to highlight the cheek hollows. Concurrent correction of the nasolabial folds is recommended where the marionette lines merge with the said folds. In patients with a severe pre-jowl sulcus, it is advisable to also place HA filler along the mandibular line on either side of the chin to mask the pre-jowl concavity and straighten the jawline.

Concurrent correction of the sagging jowl fat using other treatment modalities such as fat-reducing injections or liposculpture should also be considered as well as energy devices such as high-intensity-focused ultrasound (HIFU) or thread lifting to provide contraction and suspension to a sagging face.

4.13.3 Injection Technique (Table 4.15)

4.13.3.1 Deep Static Marionette Lines

Correction is performed using monophasic HA filler with high viscoelasticity and a 23-G 5-cm cannula. A25-G or 27-G cannula may also be employed to perform double layering in the superficial subcutaneous fat layer. The 30-G needle can also be used for subdermal or intradermal injection of HA filler just inferior to the oral commissures to concurrently lift the downturned mouth corners (Fig. 4.96). It is useful to envisage a three-dimensional space in the shape of a triangular pyramid with the base at the marionette line and with the lower vertex at the point where the marionette line meets the inferior mandibular border (Fig. 4.104).

Table 4.15 Summary of marionette line injection technique

Item	Contents
Needle vs. Cannula	23-G 5-cm cannula 27-G 3-cm cannula for superficial correction 30-G needle for correction of the oral commissure
HA filler	Monophasic HA filler with high viscoelasticity Monophasic HA filler with moderate viscoelasticity for superficial correction and oral commissure correction
Amount of HA filler	0.5–2 mL per side
Depth of injection	Deep subcutaneous layer above the DAO muscle Superficial subcutaneous layer if necessary
Entry point for cannula	Point where the marionette line meets the mandibular border
Target area	The depressed area under mouth corner along the marionette line
Anesthetics	Topical anesthetics
Nondominant hand	Hold the skin inferiorly and posteriorly in order to maintain tension on the skin

The cannula entry point is created at the vertex of the pyramid (Fig. 4.104). The HA filler is deposited in the depressed area under the mouth corner along the marionette line using linear threading and fanning in the deep subcutaneous plane above the DAO (Fig. 4.105). Since the depression is the severest at the top end of the marionette line just below the mouth corner and along the length of the line itself, volume augmentation should be directed primarily in these areas with a gradual tapering off toward the medial and inferior aspects of the marionette line. In patients with severe jowls, the goal should be to soften the appearance of the deep-set marionette line rather than its obliteration as full leveling of the depression can exacerbate the appearance of jowl ptosis and reinforce the perception of a perpetual frown in these individuals.

The deep-set part of the marionette line should be filled to 80–90% using a 23-G cannula. Superficial refinements can then be made in the subdermal layer with a 27-G cannula to complete the correction. A 30G needle can be used for mouth corner elevation.

The standard amount of HA filler injected is 0.5–1.5 mL per side, depending on the depth of the marionette line. The use of topical anesthetic cream is sufficient for numbing the treatment area. The nondominant hand should be used to stretch the skin both inferiorly and laterally during the injection to maintain tension on the skin and facilitate cannula advancement.

4.13.3.2 Combination Treatment

Concurrent correction is recommended where volume deficiency exists in adjacent regions, including the labiomandibular folds, pre-jowl sulcus, or the nasolabial folds. Note, however, that in patients with extremely heavy jowls, treatment of the pre-

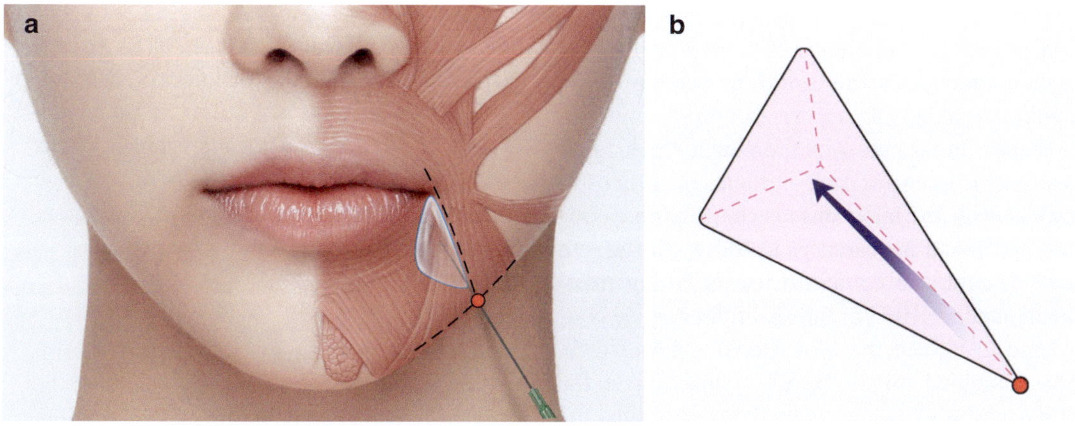

Fig. 4.104 (**a**) The cannula entry point for the treatment of marionette line (**b**) Schematic diagram of the volume augmentation for marionette line conceptualized as filling the three-dimensional space in the shape of a triangular pyramid

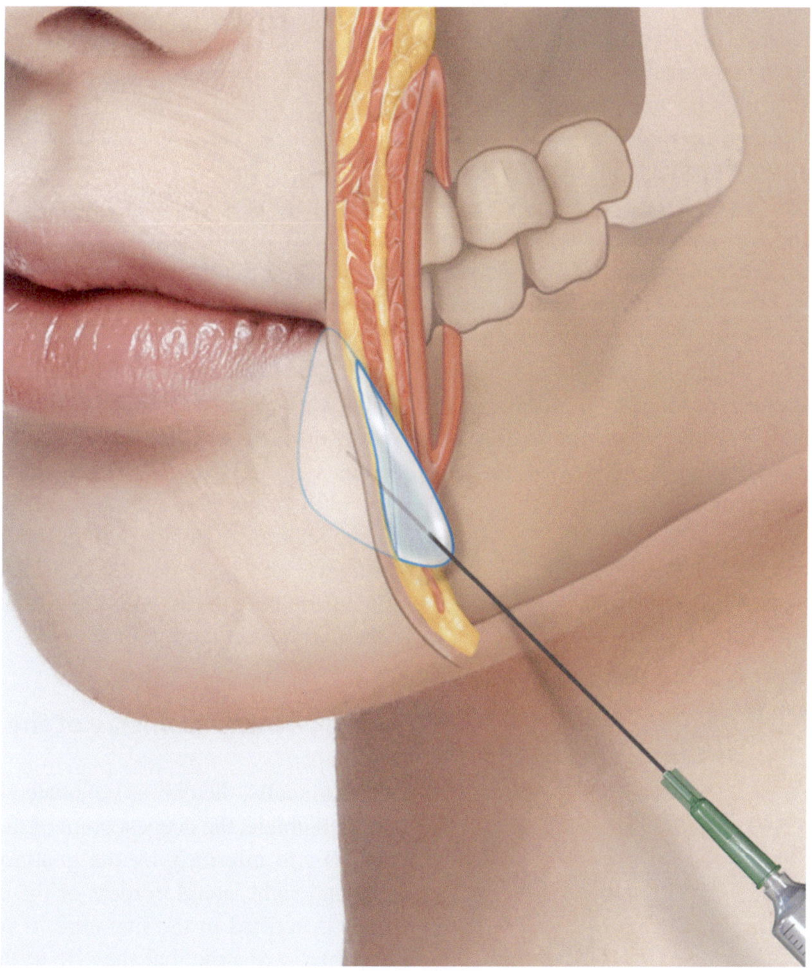

Fig. 4.105 The depth of injection for the treatment of marionette line

jowl sulcus should aim for a slight under-correction, as excessive plumping of the pre-jowl sulcus in these individuals can distort the contour of the jawline, making it appear bottom-heavy and U-shaped. In patients with prominent cheek fat, it is advisable to undertake 2–3 rounds of corticosteroid fat-reducing injections to achieve a more optimal and toned appearance. In those with severe jowl descent, the combined use of lifting treatments such as HIFU or thread-lifting may be considered to tighten the heavy-looking lower face. The combined use of BoNT-A injection in the DAO may also be considered for elevating the downturned mouth corners.

4.13.4 Complications

Irregularities: Disfiguring bumps in the form of round buttons may occur over time under the mouth corners where perioral muscle movements are active, in case too much volume had been initially placed or where the injected HA filler subsequently expanded in volume due to water absorption.

Note that the area under the modiolus is characterized by significant perioral muscle activity. The rigorous contraction of the perioral musculature and the occasional presence of cheek dimples in the region may affect the injected HA filler in such a way to clump it together or split it apart. Meanwhile, full correction of the marionette folds in those with pronounced jowl fat may exacerbate the heaviness of the jowls.

4.14 Chin Augmentation

Difficulty Level: A, Effectiveness: A, Complications: B

Summary 1: Four key factors to consider before augmenting the chin include the height and width of the chin relative to the entire face, the presence of chin retrusion and chin asymmetry.

Summary 2: Treat using a 23-G 5-cm cannula. The target plane of injection is either the supraperiosteal or the mentalis layer and additionally in the superficial subcutaneous adipose layer where necessary. Monophasic HA fillers with high viscoelasticity is generally used for augmenting the chin.

Summary 3: For improvement of anterior projection, HA filler should be placed at the central protuberance (soft tissue pogonion, Pog') of the chin conceptualized as an 'ellipsoidal dome'.

Summary 4: HA filler is injected below the soft tissue *gnathion (Gn')* as opposed to the Pog' for elongation of the chin, while augmenting the left and right lateral aspects of the chin results in widening of the chin.

Reshaping a small or receded chin with HA filler can significantly contribute to a more refined and sculpted appearance by enhancing the overall balance and proportionality of the entire face, as is the case with filler rhinoplasty. Indications for chin augmentation include the elongation of a short chin, widening of a narrow chin, projecting a retruded chin, and balancing chin asymmetry (Fig. 4.106). Notably, improving the chin projection with HA can help diminish the appearance of an over-projected mouth in patients who have normal chin size and dental occlusion but present with bimaxillary protrusion due to other orthodontal factors.

4.14.1 Anthropometry of the Chin

Anatomically, the chin is delineated superiorly by the sublabiale, the deepest point of the labiomental sulcus and inferiorly by the gnathion. While the left and right lateral borders of the chin have not been described in the literature, it would be reasonable to assume that they lie at the marionette lines. Significantly, the vertical length of the chin

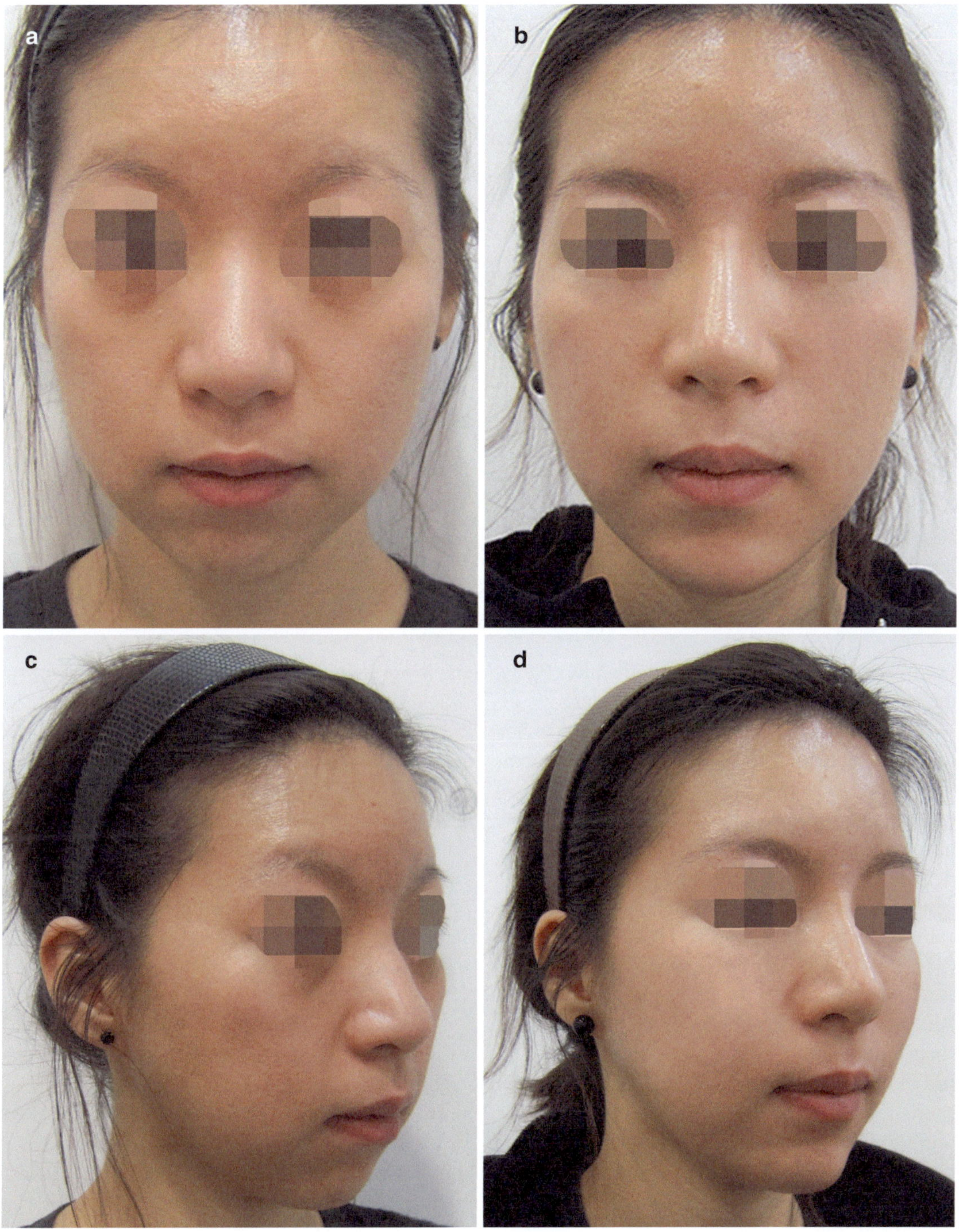

Fig. 4.106 (**a**, **c**) Before and (**b**, **d**) after chin augmentation

tends to be shorter in Asians than in Caucasians. Accordingly, while the ideal facial proportion from hairline to glabella, glabella to subnasale, and subnasale to gnathion is generally described as 1:1:1, the preferred ratio approaches 1:1:0.8 in Asians on account of their smaller [35]. Likewise, while a 1:2 ratio should exist ideally between the distance from subnasale to stomion and the dis-

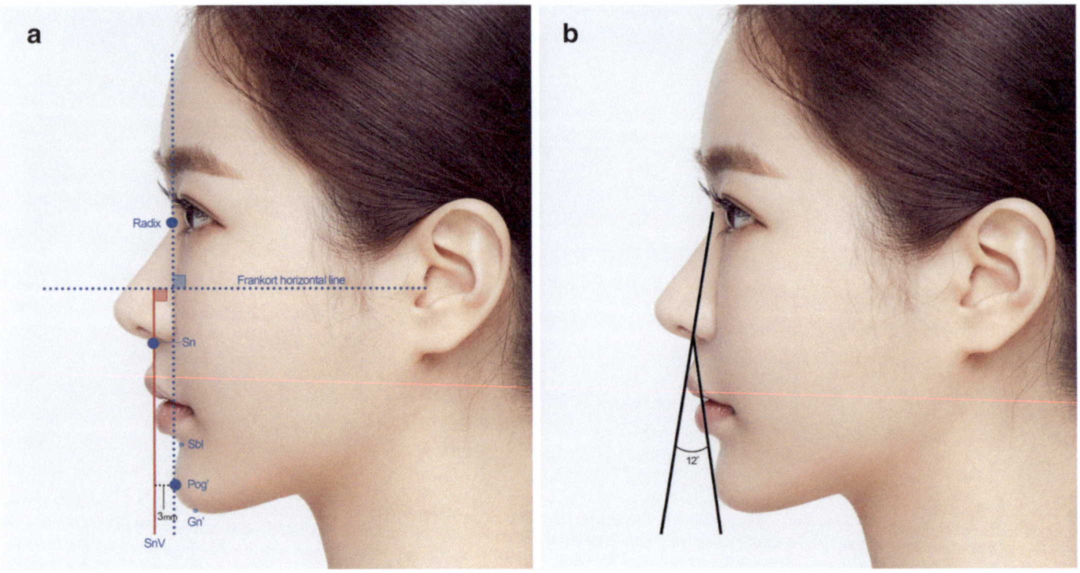

Fig. 4.107 Lateral view of an ideally proportioned chin. (**a**) the Pog' (soft tissue pogonion) should be located approximately 3 mm posterior to a perpendicular line (SnV) drawn from the Frankfort horizontal through the subnasale (Sn). (**b**) the angle formed between the line from the radix to the Sn and the line connecting the Sn to the Pog' should correspond to 12 ± 41°

tance from stomion to soft tissue gnathion (Gn'), the latter distance is also shorter in Asians.

Assessment should be made not only of the height of the chin but also of its width. A congenitally weak chin tends to lack not only vertical height but also horizontal width. Males tend to have wider chins, while females have characteristically narrower chins. According to a study of the gender difference in chin morphology, men typically presented with bi-lobed (33%) or square (58%) chins, while the shape of the chin in women was more pointed (55%) than square (45%) [36]. An aesthetic chin features a central protuberance shaped like an ellipsoidal dome, with the horizontal width of the said dome being similar to or shorter than the width of the lips. Ideally, the most prominent point of the chin, or the soft tissue pogonion (Pog'), should lie adjacent to the inferior one-third point of the stomion-to-gnathion line. On profile, the Pog' should be located approximately 3 mm posterior to a perpendicular line (SnV) drawn from the Frankfort horizontal through the subnasale (Sn) (Fig. 4.107) [37]. Generally Pog' should never protrude beyond the lower lip on the profile view. If Pog' lies anterior to the SnV, the chin is protrusive and is described as showing prognathia or progenia or the bulging of the lower jaw vis-a-vis the upper jaw. Conversely, where the Pog' falls more than 10mm behind the SnV, the chin is retrusive otherwise described as retorgnathia or retrogenia, where the lower jaw is set back behind the upper jaw. It is also suggested that, ideally, the angle formed between the line from the radix to the subnasale and the line connecting the subnasale to the Pog' should correspond to 12 ± 4° [37]. An angle greater than 12° is indicative of a retrognathic or receded chin. Conversely, where this angle is narrower than 12°, it suggests prognathia.

For reference, the notions of retrognathia and prognathia were defined and classified by Angle in 1899 [37]. According to Angle's classification, normal occlusion is where the teeth are aligned properly with the first molar of the maxilla aligned with the mandibular first molar. Class 2 malocclusion represents retrognathia where the mandibular first molar lies posterior to the maxillary first molar, while Class 3 malocclusion constitutes prognathia where the mandibular first molar lies anterior to the maxillary first molar. By comparison, a Class 1 malocclusion occurs where a normal relationship between the molars exists, but there is a protrusion of the mouth due to an overbite or bucked teeth, etc.

Retrognathia or a receded chin manifests as a lack of anterior projection of the chin. A deficient chin projection gives rise to the appearance of an over-projected mouth, making the face appear dull, goofy, and washed-out on profile. According to established guidelines, the lower lip vermilion in Caucasians should ideally fall behind a line from the nose tip to the pogonion, defined as the Ricketts' esthetic line. In Asians, the lower lip vermillion should preferably touch this line. (Fig. 4.107).

4.14.2 Anatomical Considerations

In the sagittal view, the anatomical layers of the chin from the outer to the innermost layers are comprised as follows; the skin-subcutaneous fat-mentalis m.-mandible. The mentalis originates from the mandible and inserts to the skin of the chin. Its medial fibers intersect and overlap each other as they insert to the skin at the median plane, resulting in a dome-shaped prominence at the center of the anterior chin (Fig. 4.108).

The vessels of the chin include the mental a., inferior labial a., and submental a. The mental a. originates from the maxillary artery and exits the mental foramen. The inferior labial artery extends from the facial artery and courses between the lower lip and the chin within the substance of the depressor anguliorís (DAO) and the depressor labii inferioris (DLI) before ascending superiorly and terminating at the lower lip mucosa. The submental artery may also provide branches that rise superiorly from under the chin (Fig. 4.92).

4.14.3 Pretreatment Assessment

Four key factors to consider before augmenting the chin include the height and width of the chin relative to the entire face, as well as the presence of chin retrusion or asymmetry. The chin should be examined frontally for the adequacy of its vertical height and horizontal width, as well as symmetry. A blunt U-shaped chin with adequate width but lacking sufficient height should be distinguished from a congenitally weak chin which

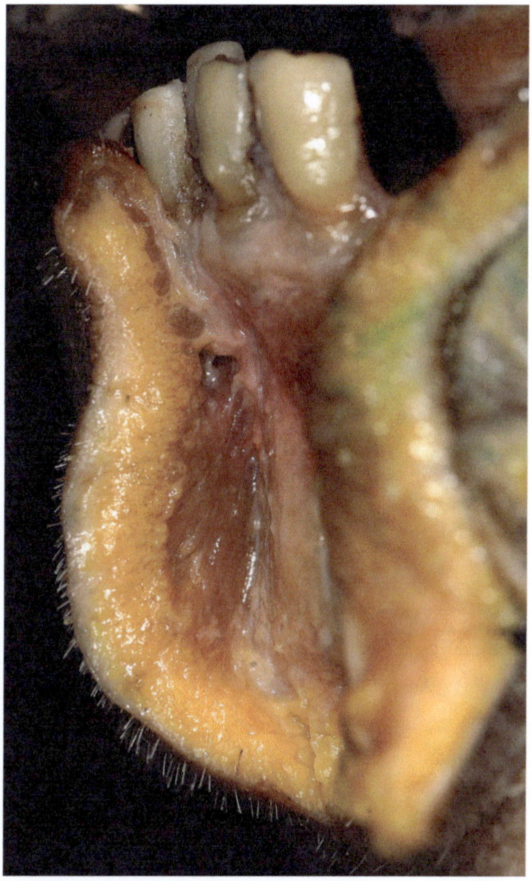

Fig. 4.108 Sagittal section of the chin (photo: courtesy of Professor Hee-Jin Kim)

manifests both the lack of width and height. Asymmetry of the chin may appear from a disparity in the size of the left and right chin or due to the deviation of the underlying maxilla or mandible. Chin asymmetry can be improved to an extent by enhancing the smaller side of the chin with HA filler.

From the lateral view, the chin should be assessed for the presence of any retrusion (retrognathia), protrusion (prognathia), or a protrusive mouth. Consideration must also be given to the patient's gender as the ideal chin shape varies between males and females. Ethnic differences should also be taken into account as the presence of a small receded chin is more prevalent in Asians than in Caucasians. In particular, a round face with a relatively small chin is a defining characteristic of the intermediate type Asian face, found typically in those from Hong Kong, Taiwan, and

Southern China [18]. The use of HA filler to elongate the chin in these populations serves not only to visually narrow their round faces by increasing the overall facial length but also to add definition and dimensionality to their undefined chin.

4.14.4 Injection Technique (Table 4.16)

Table 4.16 Summary of chin filler injection technique

Item	Contents
Needle vs. Cannula	23-G 5-cm
HA filler	Monophasic HA fillers with high viscoelasticity
Amount of HA filler	1–2 mL for chin projection 0.5–1 mL for chin elongation 1 mL per side for chin widening
Depth of injection	Intramuscular and supraperiosteal layer Subcutaneous layer if necessary
Entry point for cannula	The intersection between a vertical line from the oral commissure and the horizontal line which would pass through the repositioned Pog posttreatment
Target area	Pog' for chin projection Gn' for chin elongation Left and right sides of the chin
Anesthetics	Topical anesthetics Mental nerve block if necessary
Nondominant hand	Press the opposite side of the dome and Gn' Press the chin from under the Gn'

While biphasic HA filler is generally used for augmenting the chin, monophasic HA fillers with high elasticity can also be applied. A 23-G × 5-cm cannula is used to deposit HA filler first into the supraperiosteum and the mentalis layer and additionally in the superficial subcutaneous adipose layer where necessary (Fig. 4.109).

While the use of topical anesthetic cream is sufficient for local numbing, a mental nerve block may be administered in patients with a low pain threshold. Note, however, that in this case, the procedure should begin at least 20 mins after administering the nerve block following sufficient massage to avoid superfluous creation of volume by the local anesthetic agent.

4.14.5 Improvement of Anterior Projection

This technique is indicated in patients presenting a retrusive chin (retrognathia) on profile (Fig. 4.110). The labiomental sulcus on the chin should be preserved to create a horizontally long ellipsoidal dome when viewed from the front. Care should be taken to ensure symmetry during the procedure as even the slightest asymmetry in the chin can become patently obvious due to its central location along the facial midline. Accordingly, the injection volume should be controlled so that most of the HA filler is located at the very center of the ellipsoidal dome. Further, the nondominant hand should be used to press the area opposite the cannula entry point during the injection to prevent excess HA filler from diffus-

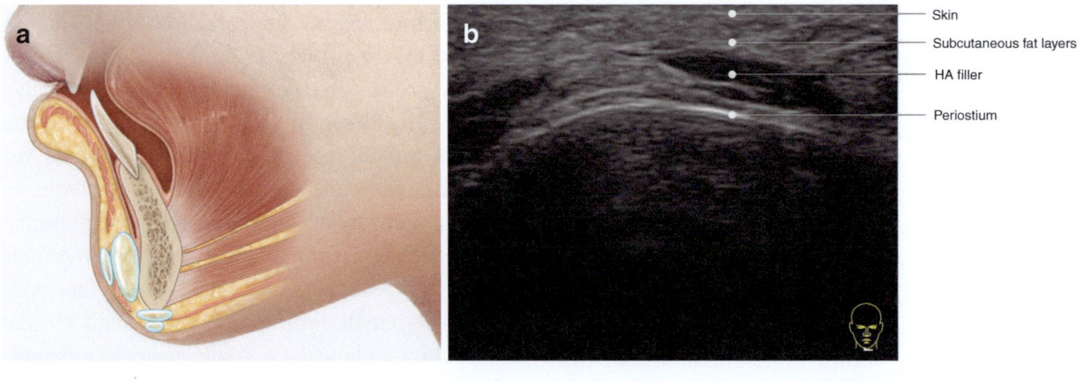

Fig. 4.109 (**a**) The depth of injection for chin augmentation. (**b**) Proper placement of HA filler in the chin confirmed by sonography evaluation

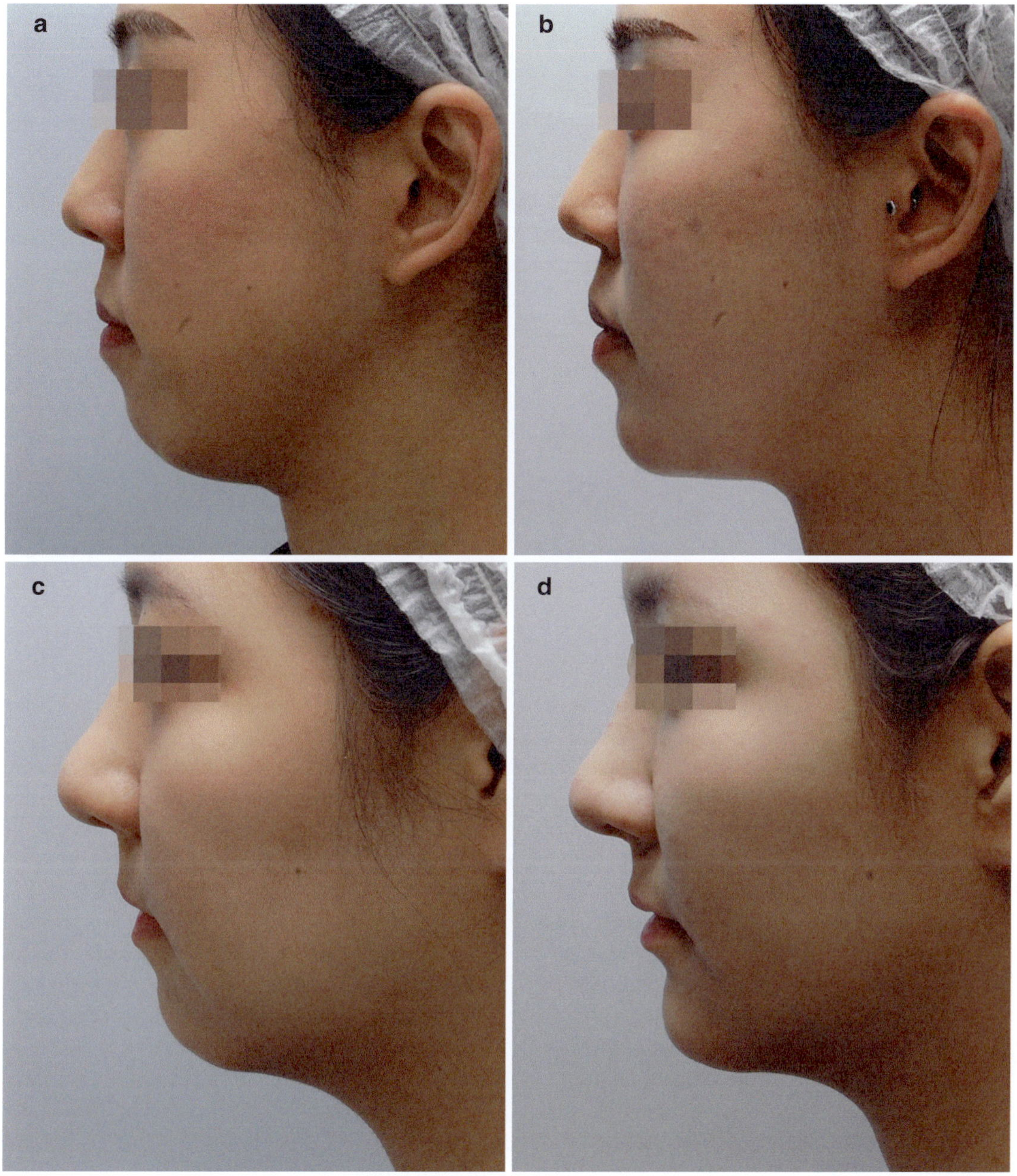

Fig. 4.110 (**a**, **c**) Before and (**b**, **d**) after improvement of anterior projection

ing into the opposite side of the said dome. Note that projecting the chin forward has the incidental effect of elongating the chin downward as the injected HA filler tends to push not only anteriorly but also inferiorly due to gravity and pressure. This implies that the relevant cannula insertion point in a patient with a short, receded chin should be made at the junction where a vertical line from the oral commissure meets the horizontal line passing through *the anticipated* location of the Pog' *after* treatment, which should be closer to the patient's Gn' at baseline (Fig. 4.111). This is because elongating the chin causes the soft tissue Gn' to drop more inferiorly,

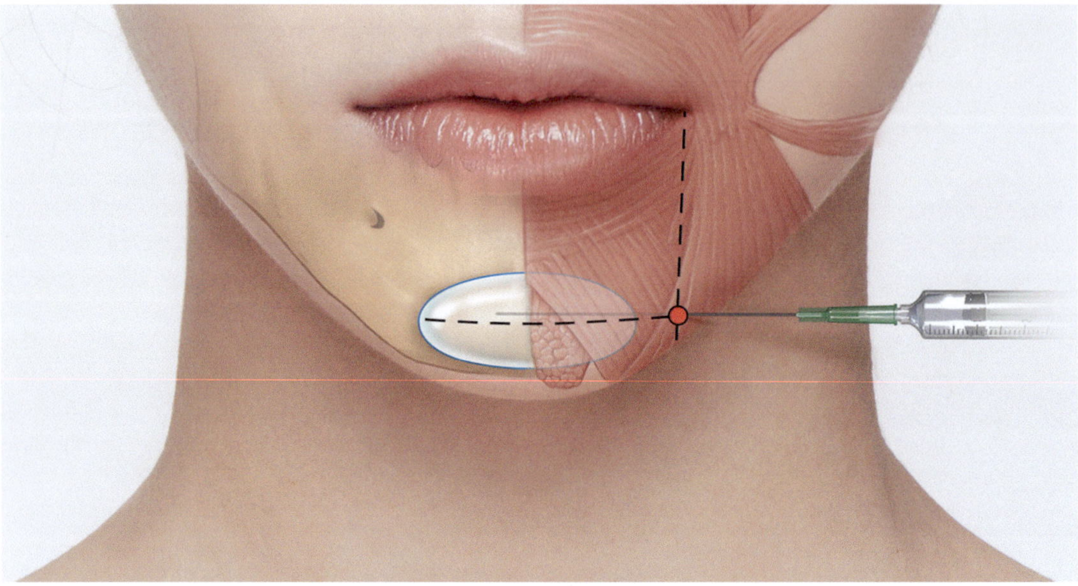

Fig. 4.111 The cannula entry point for the improvement of anterior projection

and given that the ideal position of the Pog' is at a point marking the inferior one-third of the stomion-to-Gn' line, it logically follows that the repositioned Pog' should also shift more inferiorly, sitting more closer to the patient's existing Gn'. On the other hand, where anterior projection of the chin is desired *without* the accompanying increase in the chin length, injection should be made instead at the patient's current Pog'. Here, the nondominant hand should be engaged to compress the Gn' from the base of the chin to prevent the HA filler from migrating inferiorly down the platysma due to the injection pressure. Meanwhile, the width of the ellipsoidal dome at the chin should be shorter than the width of the lip, corresponding preferably to two-thirds of the lip width. In general, 1–2 mL of HA filler is required to achieve anterior projection of the chin.

4.14.6 Lengthening of Chin Height (Elongation of the Chin)

In patients who have decent chin width and projection but present a blunt U-shaped chin due to the lack of chin height, simply extending the chin vertically along the midline can create the perception of a narrower, more oval face with a sharp v-shaped jawline (Fig. 4.112). Here, the HA filler is injected below the *Gn*' as opposed to the *Pog.* The entry point is created 1 cm superior to the intersection between a vertical line dropped from the oral commissure and the inferior margin of the mandible (Fig. 4.113). To create the appearance of a distinctly sharp pointy chin, inject first into the deep supraperiosteal layer for primary volumization before adding a small top-up amount of HA at the superficial subcutaneous fat level. When injecting the Gn', the nondominant hand should be used to press the base of the chin to prevent the HA filler from migrating inferiorly down the platysma due to the injection pressure. A minimum of 0.5–1 mL of HA filler is needed for chin elongation.

4.14.7 Widening of the Chin Width

In patients with a congenitally weak chin (micrognathia), the chin lacks not only vertical length but also horizontal width, both of which must be addressed (Fig. 4.114). Extending the chin inferiorly without addressing the horizontal dimension in patients with a congenitally narrow chin can result in the appearance of a

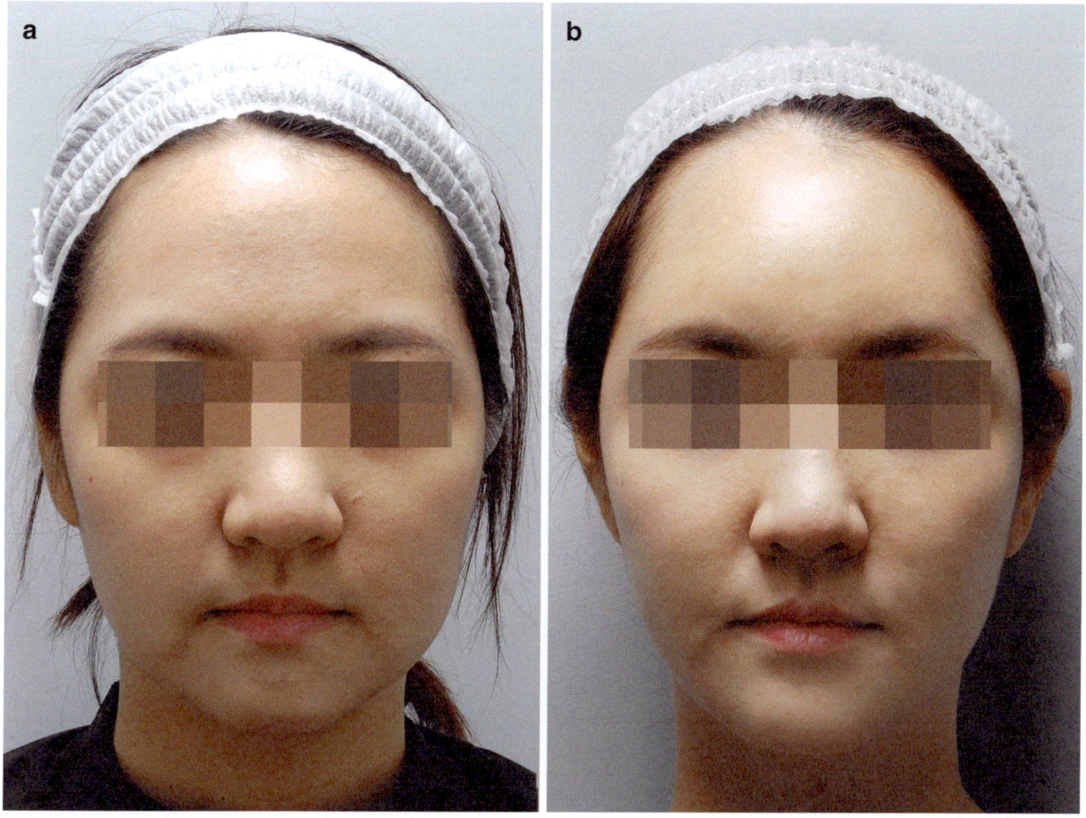

Fig. 4.112 (**a**) Before and (**b**) after chin elongation combined with widening of chin width

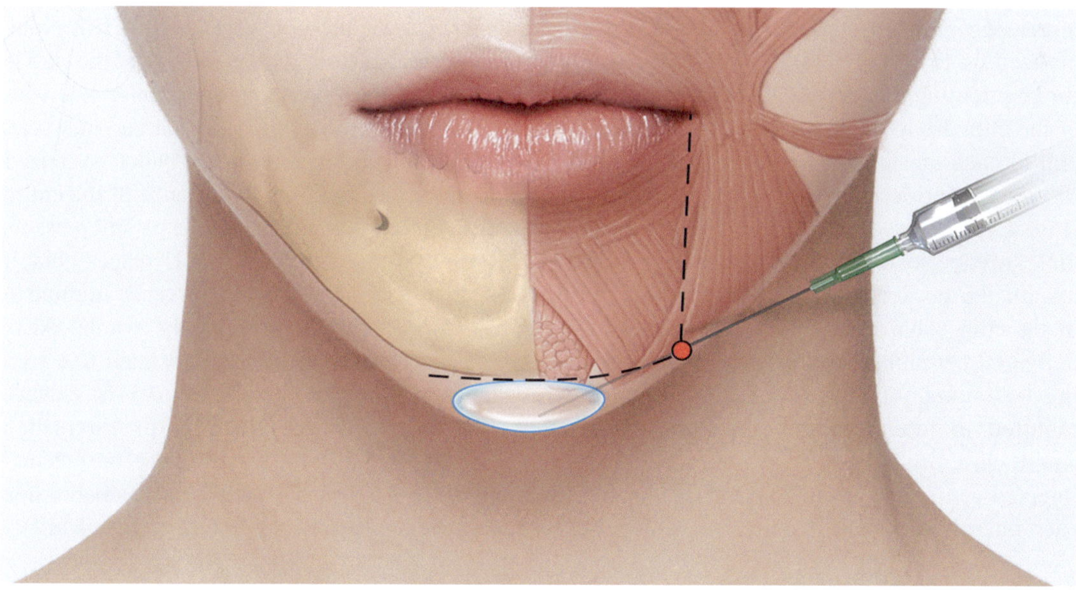

Fig. 4.113 The cannula entry point for chin elongation

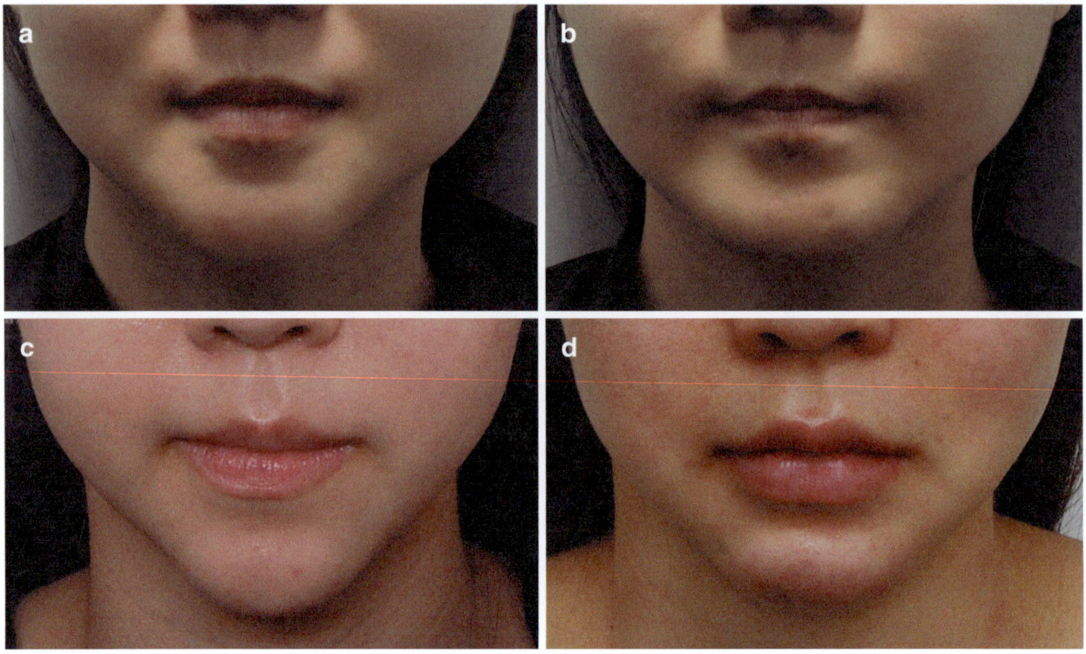

Fig. 4.114 (**a**) Before and (**b**) after widening of chin width. (**c**) A bizarre droopy chin resembling the mask of Tutankhamun and (**d**) after the hyaluronidase injection for this bizarre droopy condition

bizarre droopy chin resembling the mask of Tutankhamun (Fig. 4.114). The proper sequence of augmenting a deficient chin is to first extend the chin anteriorly as well as inferiorly using the aforementioned approaches for increasing chin projection and height, before proceeding to widen the chin. The entry points for augmenting the left and right lateral aspects of the chin are to be created at points 1 cm lateral to each marionette line and 1 cm superior to the inferior border of the mandible (Fig. 4.115). The cannula is inserted deep into the supraperiosteal level and approached toward the border of the central protuberance of the chin, where HA filler (at least 1 mL) is delivered per side using the retrograde threading technique. At least 4 mL of HA filler is required in total to augment a congenitally small chin, including a minimum of 2 mL injected centrally and at least 1 mL placed on each lateral aspect of the chin.

4.14.8 Correction of Chin Asymmetry

Where asymmetry exists between the left and right sides of the chin on the frontal view, balance can be restored by augmenting the lateral aspect of the smaller side of the chin (see Sect. 4.18). Note, however, that in cases where one side of the chin is overly large, overcorrecting the smaller side with the intention of matching the larger side can instead result in an excessively bulky, oversized chin that serves to throw the balance of the entire face. In this case, to the extent the patient presents an innately short chin or a blunt U-shaped chin, it helps to also elongate the chin along its midline to create a V-shaped jawline on the whole. Also, where the overall face appears slanted due to a deviated mandible or maxilla (Fig. 4.116), extending the length of the chin with HA filler to realign it with the midline of the upper face before enhancing the lateral aspect of the chin on the smaller side can provide moderate improvement (Fig. 4.117).

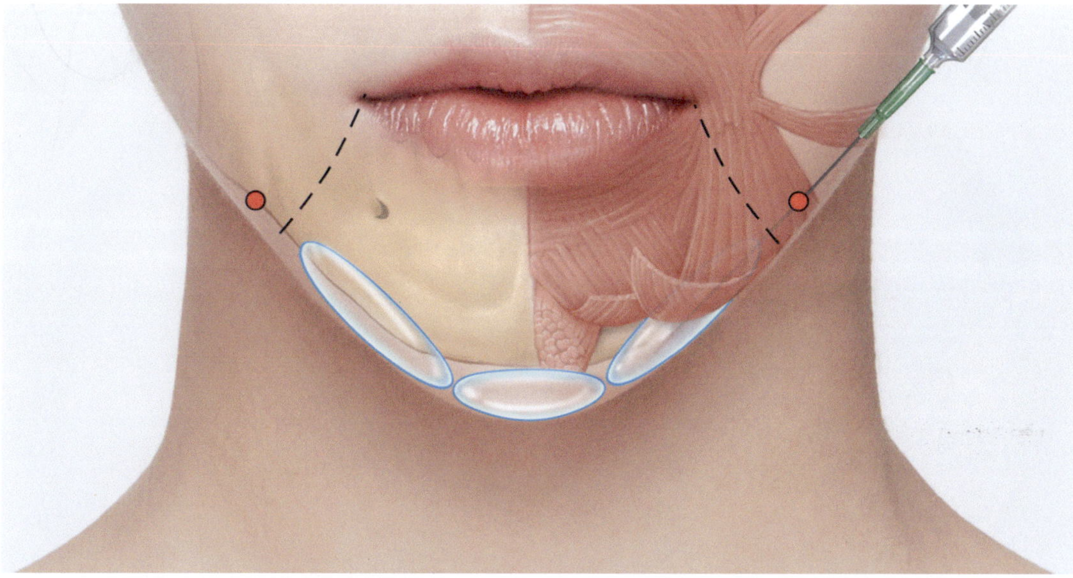

Fig. 4.115 Cannula entry point for widening of chin width

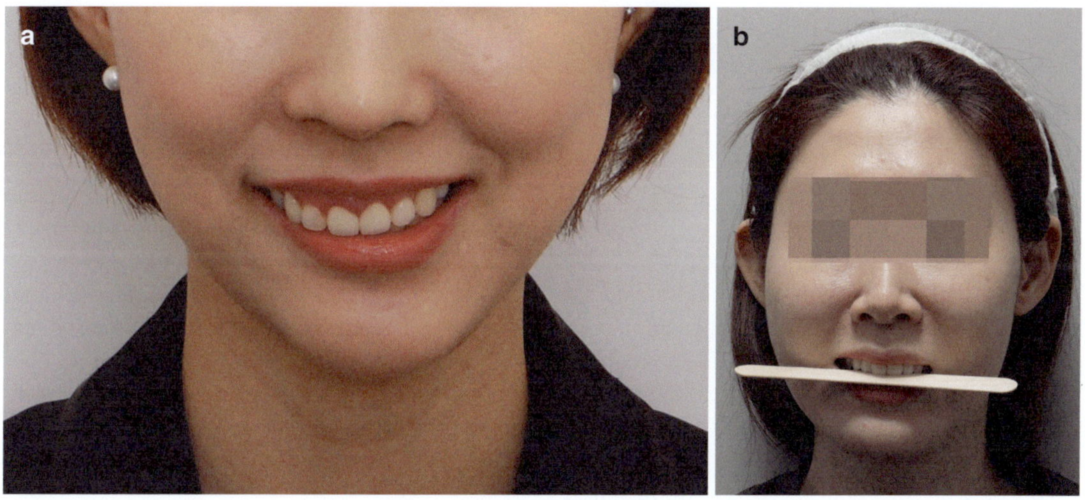

Fig. 4.116 Deviated maxilla (**a**) smile asymmetry, (**b**) tongue depressor bite test

4.14.9 Combination Treatment

The appearance of cobblestone chin or chin dimpling is not uncommon in Asians, as the bimaxillary protrusion prevalent in these populations often requires over-contraction of the mentalis to achieve a lip seal. Accordingly, synergistic use of BoNT-A to relax the mentalis strain can be beneficial when augmenting the Asian chin with HA. Also, where chin augmentation is performed to camouflage a bimaxillary protrusion, concurrent volume restoration in the buccal hollows and nasolabial folds can further help blend the prominence of the protrusive mouth by restoring and restructuring the perioral complex as a whole. In patients with an innately deficient chin or deep marionette lines from aging, filling the marionette lines can help optimize results.

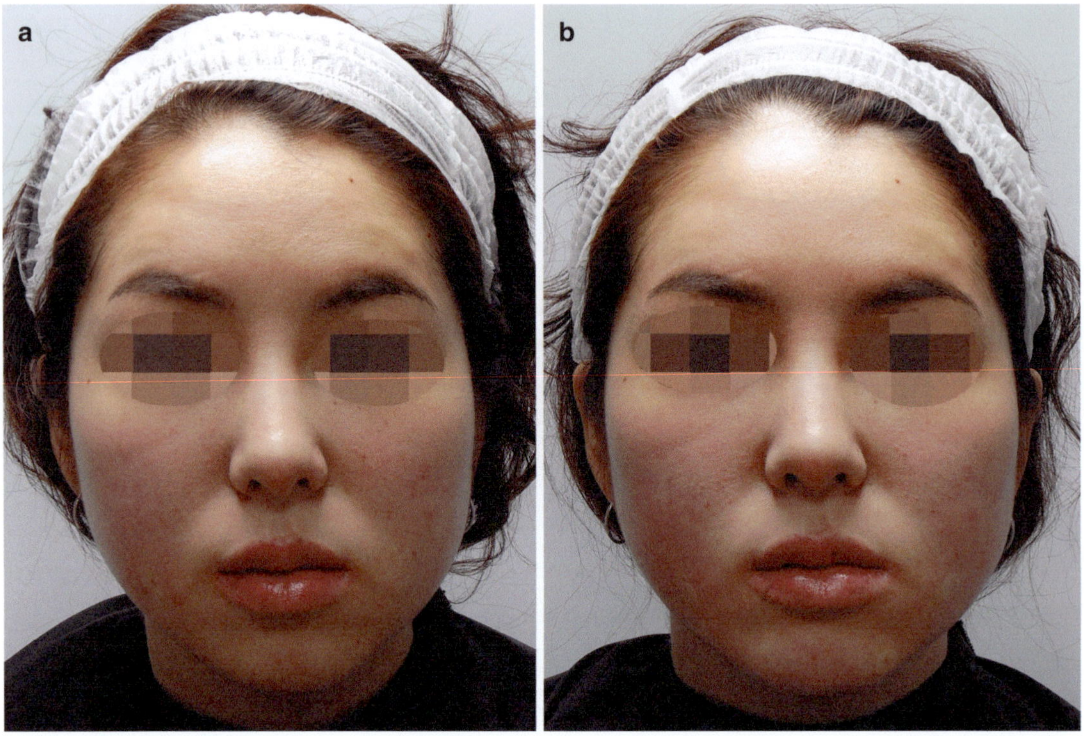

Fig. 4.117 (**a**) Before and (**b**) After correction of chin asymmetry

4.14.10 Complications

Tutankhamun's Chin: Augmenting a weak chin only in its central aspect without addressing the lateral dimensions can create the appearance of a ptotic chin similar to that of Tutankhamun. (Fig. 4.114c) Make sure to also treat the left and right lateral aspects of the chin.

Asymmetry: Note that even the slightest asymmetry in the chin becomes immediately noticeable due to its central position along the facial midline. Envisioning the chin as an ellipsoidal dome, make sure to locate most of the volume at the center of the said dome. The nondominant hand should be used to press the opposite end of the dome to prevent the spread of excess HA filler into the area.

Irregularities: When injecting the soft tissue Gn, the injection pressure may send HA filler traveling down the platysma band, causing it to collect under the chin. Pressing the base of the chin with the nondominant hand during the injection can prevent this from occurring.

Bruising: Be mindful of the inferior labial artery or the mental artery, as injury to these vessels may lead to significant bruising. Use of a cannula is advised in this regard together with gentle maneuvering.

4.15 Jawline Filler

Difficulty Level: A, Effectiveness: A, Complications: A

Summary 1: Inject using a 23-G 5-cm cannula and biphasic HA filler with large particle size.

Summary 2: The cannula entry point is created at the anterior one-third point of the mandible when viewed in profile, 0.5 cm superior to the mandibular lower border. The desired depth of injection is in the supraperiosteal and supramuscular layers (i.e., superficial to the masseter m). Augmentation of the jawline should start at the angle of the mandible and proceed along the jawline.

Summary 3: Gender-based differences should be taken into consideration, as men generally have wider jaws and more prominent mandibular angles than females. HA filler placement in the jawline and angle of the mandible is not recommended for brachycephalic northern facial type Asians with a relatively wide face and angulated jaws, as accentuating the mandible only serves to broaden their wide faces.

Summary 4: In Asians, jawline fillers can be used to recreate the bone volume lost at the angle of the mandible due to an overly aggressive mandibular angle reduction surgery.

Jawline augmentation is a procedure best suited for patients presenting a thin narrow face on the frontal view or aspiring to have a more angulated, square or pentagonal jawline. This makes the procedure particularly popular among Caucasians endowed with a dolichocephalic head that is long in the anteroposterior direction and narrow in the horizontal direction. Augmenting the jawline and mandibular angle with HA filler in this population can add definition and structure to an overly narrow or weak lower face. The presence of a robust, chiseled jawline is also considered a desirable feature in men which enhances male charisma and attractiveness. By extending the jawline laterally, jawline augmentation also creates the optical illusion of reducing the facial height in individuals with a long face. Conversely, jawline filler is seldom requested by Asian patients who already have a wide brachycephalic head, apart, perhaps, from when seeking to address the asymmetry between the left and right mandible. The procedure *may* be attempted in Asian patients with an overly narrow pointy jaw that visually elongates the face or in males who wish to enhance their charisma based on a stronger jawline. That said, there is a unique demand for jawline fillers within a subset of Asians to address the suboptimum result of a previous mandibular angle reduction surgery. Here, HA filler can be used to restore the angle of the mandible aggressively removed during the surgery, and thereby address the unnaturally steep linear jawline extending from under the ear down to the chin when observed from the lateral view (Fig. 4.118).

4.15.1 Anatomical Considerations

When seen from the profile view, the mandible is an L-shaped bony structure consisting of the body of the mandible on the inferior aspect and the ramus on its posterior aspect. The junction at which the body of the mandible meets the ramus is defined as the angle of the mandible. The masseter m. inserts into the mandible. The facial a. passes the anterior border of the antegonial notch located just in front of the masseter m. before running upwards and forwards to the nose. The use of a cannula is therefore preferred over a needle during jawline augmentation to avoid hitting the facial artery. Meanwhile, the male lower face is generally wider and more angulated than that of a female. Indeed, a comparison study of the differences between the male and female mandibles has found that both the bigonial width and lateral flaring of the mandibular angle were greater in men compared with women.

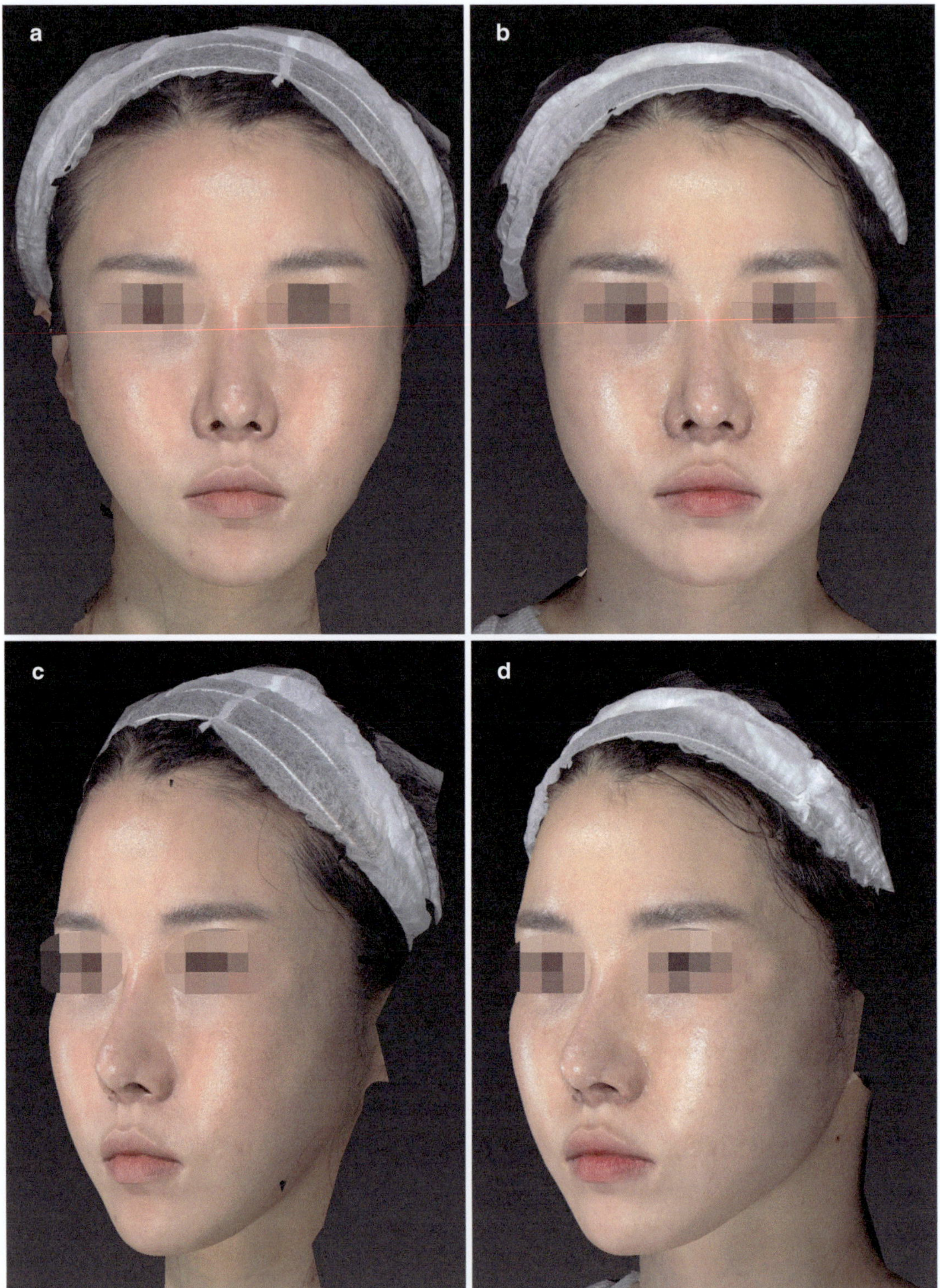

Fig. 4.118 (**a**, **c**) Before and (**b**, **d**) After jawline fillers. Jawline fillers can help to restore the angle of the mandible aggressively removed during a previous mandibular angle reduction surgery

4.15.2 Pretreatment Assessment

Prior to treatment, assessments should be made of the overall facial shape, width of the mandible relative to the entire face, position and prominence of the mandibular angle, and the presence of any asymmetry between the left and right mandible. Specifically, from the frontal view, it should be determined whether the face is horizontally wide or vertically long, whether the bigonial width is in adequate proportion with the overall face, and whether symmetry exists between the left and right mandible. On the lateral view, the position of the mandibular angle as well as any visible loss of mandibular angle due to a previous mandible resection surgery should be identified. Gender-based differences should also be taken into consideration, as men generally have wider mandibles and more prominent mandibular angles than females. Jawline filler is popularly requested by Caucasians demonstrating a thin narrow face but rarely sought by Asians, particularly Northern Facial Type Asians, with a relatively wide face and angulated jaws.

4.15.3 Injection Technique (Table 4.17)

Table 4.17 Summary of jawline filler injection technique

Item	Contents
Needle vs. Cannula	23-G 5-cm
HA filler	Biphasic HA filler with large particle size
Amount of HA filler	1–2 mL per side for jaw line augmentation >2 mL per side for mandibular angle augmentation
Depth of injection	Supramuscular and supraperiosteal layer Deep subcutaneous layer if necessary
Entry point for cannula	0.5 cm above the mandibular lower border at the anterior one third of mandible. (jaw line)
Target area	Jawline and mandibular angle
Anesthetics	Topical anesthetics
Nondominant hand	Hold the chin skin anteriorly

Injection is performed primarily using biphasic HA filler with large particle size and a 23-G 5-cm cannula, Regarding the desired depth of injection, injection is made first into the supraperiosteal layer and the supramuscular layer superficial to the masseter, before any further volume is added into the deep subcutaneous fat layer, where necessary. The use of local numbing cream should provide sufficient anesthesia.

4.15.3.1 Jawline Augmentation

The cannula entry point is made at the anterior one-third of the mandible in the profile view, 0.5 cm superior to the inferior border of the mandible (Fig. 4.119). Using the retrograde thread technique, deposit HA filler starting at the angle of the mandible and along the jawline. Where concavities are concurrently present in the adjacent cheeks, volume should also be restored in the cheek to allow a smooth transition down to the jawline. A minimum of 1–2 mL of HA is required per side.

4.15.3.2 Mandibular Angle Augmentation

Where too much bone has been resected at the mandibular angle during a angle reduction surgery, measures must be taken to recreate the lost bone volume. According to the study of mandibular shape by Hu et al., in a vast majority of cases, the mandibular ramus consist of "slanted types" (74.5%) when viewed in profile. As such, the angle of the mandible should be recreated such that the gonion (the outermost point of the mandibular angle at which body of the mandible angles upward and becomes the ramus) lies 1 cm inferior to the lower margin of the current jawline on a vertical line dropped from a point 1–2 cm anterior to the ear canal (Fig. 4.120). Using the same cannula entry point created for jawline augmentation, dispense a bolus of HA filler at the angle of the mandible. Connect the reshaped mandibular angle to the jawline by delivering HA filler in the retrograde linear thread technique along the jawline. When viewed in profile, the angle of the mandible should reside anywhere between a horizontal line extending from the mouth corner (i.e., the intercheilion horizontal line) and the

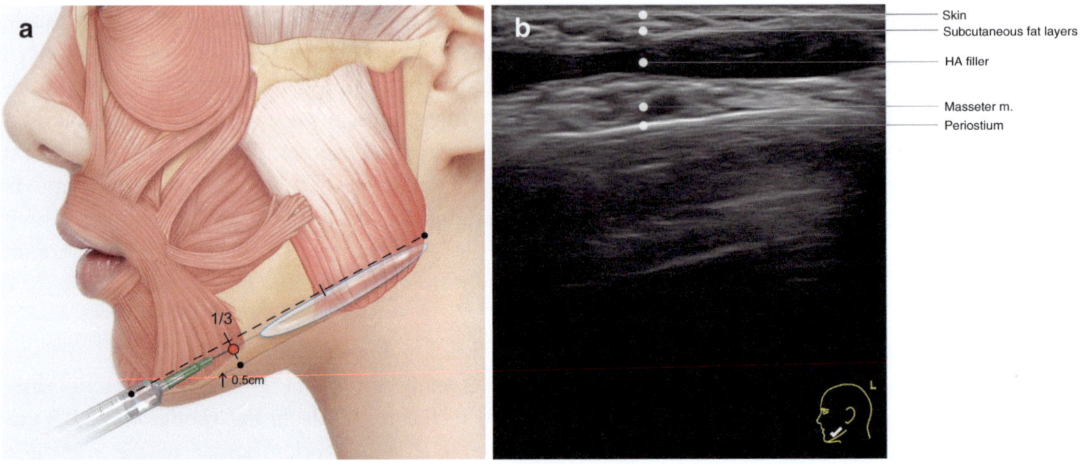

Fig. 4.119 (**a**) The cannula entry point for jawline augmentation (**b**) Sonographic image displaying HA filler properly placed in the supramuscular layer superficial to the masseter m

Fig. 4.120 The appropriate location for the mandibular angle augmentation

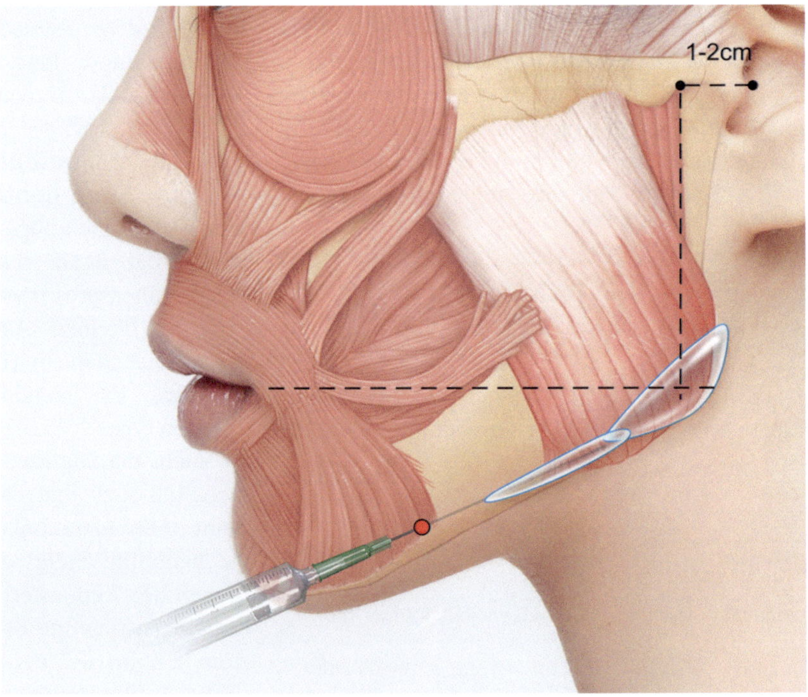

soft tissue Gn. The closer the mandibular angle sits to the intercheilion horizontal line, the slimmer to face appears when viewed from the front. Consequently, where a slim, tapered jawline is desired on the frontal view, the practitioner should ensure the mandibular angle, as it appears on profile, does not descend below intercheilion horizontal line (Fig. 4.118). In contrast, the mandibular angle in a male patient should ideally fall below this line (on the profile view) for the jawline to appear more angulated and masculine on the frontal view. It is preferable to also add volume to any concurrent cheek hollows to ensure a smooth transition toward the mandibular angle. A minimum 2 mL of HA is required per side.

4.15.3.3 Correction of Asymmetry

Where asymmetry exists in the size of the left and right mandible, augmentation should be made to the jawline, mandibular angle, and the cheek of the smaller side in a way that best suits each individual face. Concurrent HA filler placement is advised in the sunken cheeks, where applicable, to ensure a natural tapering of volume toward the jawline.

4.15.4 Complications

Irregularity: Care must be taken to distribute volume evenly across the treatment area to avoid irregularities. Concurrent restoration is required in the deflated cheeks to ensure a smooth transition to the jawline.

4.16 Earlobe Filler

Difficulty Level: A, Effectiveness: A, Complications: A

> *Summary 1*: Treatment is performed using a 23-G cannula and a monophasic HA filler with moderate viscoelasticity.

> *Summary 2*: A bolus of 0.3–0.6 mL is injected per side at the center of the lateral half of the earlobe.

> *Summary 3*: Where the patient desires extra-large-sized earlobes, it is advisable to repeat the treatment over 2–3 sessions at 2–3 month intervals.

The earlobe represents the most inferior part of the ear consisting entirely of soft tissue and skin without containing any cartilage. To many, large ears with long stretched earlobes is one of the first images that come to mind on hearing the word "Buddha." In Korea, where Buddhism has held strong cultural influence, a large ear is positively associated with wealth, good societal standing, familial bliss, health, and overall good fortune according to the traditional physiognomy. To this extent, patients may, on occasion, request augmentation of the earlobe to increase their ear size (Fig. 4.121).

4.16.1 Anatomy of the Outer Ear

The outer ear is an intricate structure consisting of delicate elastic cartilage covered by thin skin. Elements of the outer ears include, the helix, root (or limb) of helix, antihelix, scapha or scaphoid fossa, tragus, antitragus, inter-tragic notch, ear meatus, and earlobe (Fig. 4.122). The earlobe represents the noncartilaginous portion of the ear consisting only of fibrofatty tissue. At birth, the earlobe represents 66% of the ear length and 73% of the ear width. The ear reaches 80% of its mature size at age six, 90% at age 9, 95% at age 14, and continues its gradual growth into adulthood [38]. The ear is believed to continue increasing in size beyond the third and fourth decade, and to undergo a marked elongation after the sixth decade. Some scholars attribute this elongation of the ears with aging to the gravity-induced descent of tissue.

4.16.2 Injection Technique

Augmentation is performed using a 27-G cannula inserted through an entry point created 0.5 cm superior to the earlobe at the helix (Fig. 4.123). Using a soft monophasic HA filler with medium viscoelasticity, a bolus of 0.3–0.6 mL is injected per side at the center of the lateral half of earlobe. The desired depth of injection is the subcutaneous layer interposed between the skin of the earlobe. Care must be taken not to inject more than 1 mL of HA filler per each earlobe as it may impede the vascular circulation of the ear, possibly leading to severe pain and even necrosis of the skin. Postinjection molding is advised to prevent any irregularities. Should there be any hardness or blanching due to impaired blood circulation following an over-injection of HA filler, the patient should preferably be monitored

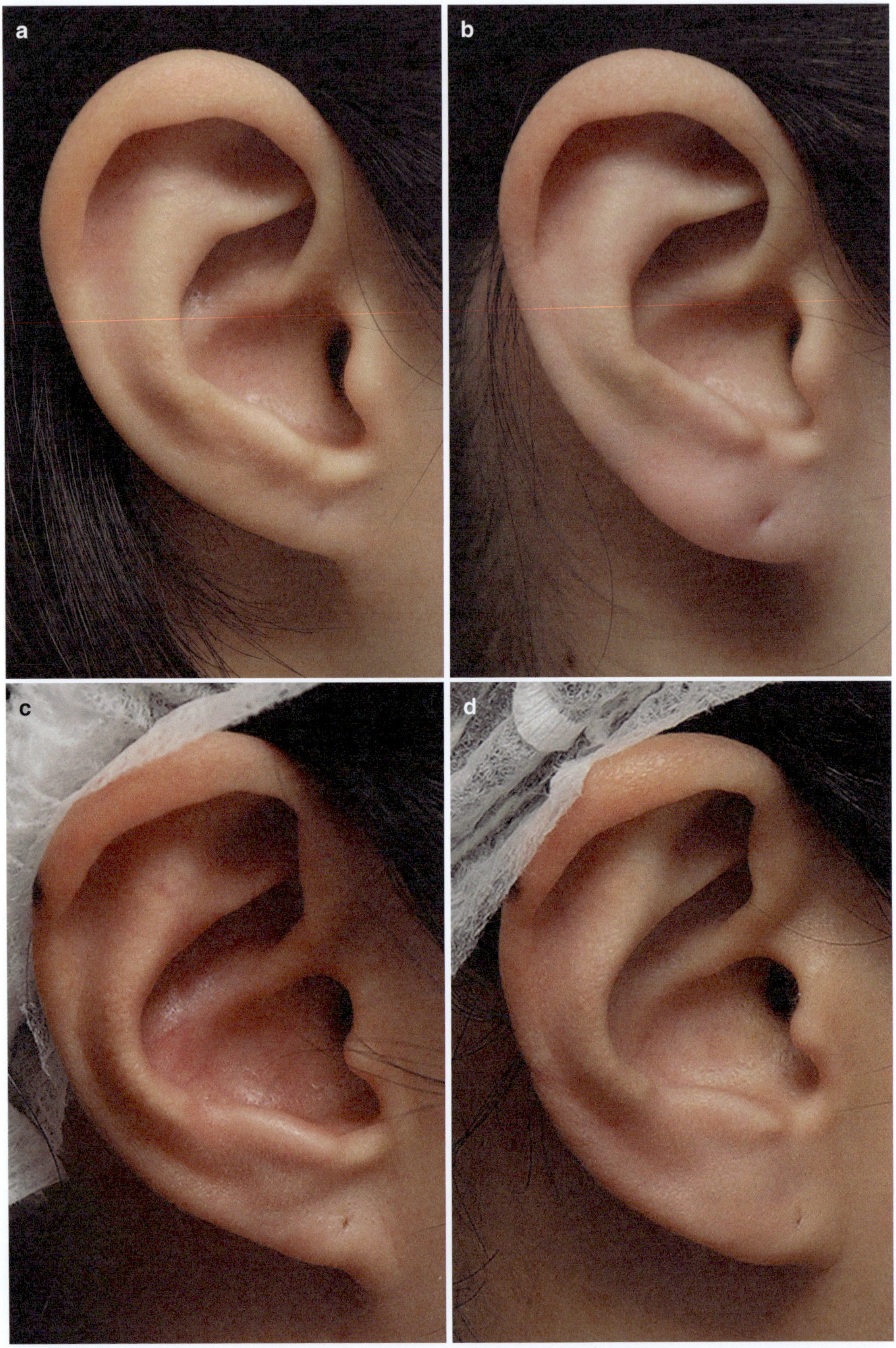

Fig. 4.121 (**a**, **c**) Before and (**b**, **d**) after earlobe augmentation

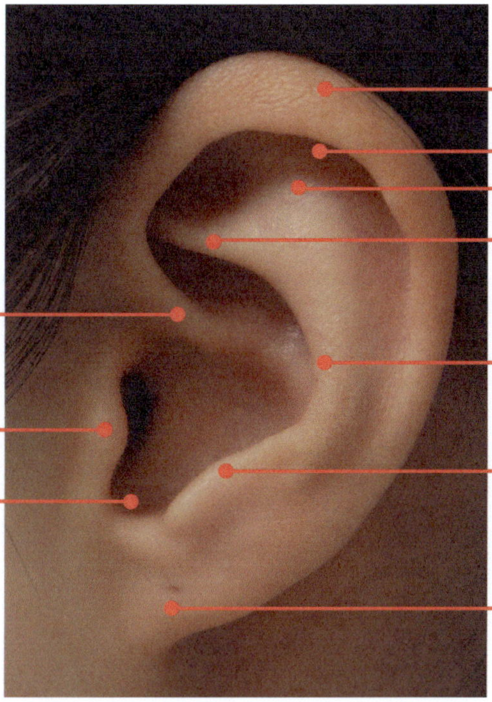

Fig. 4.122 Anatomy of the outer ear

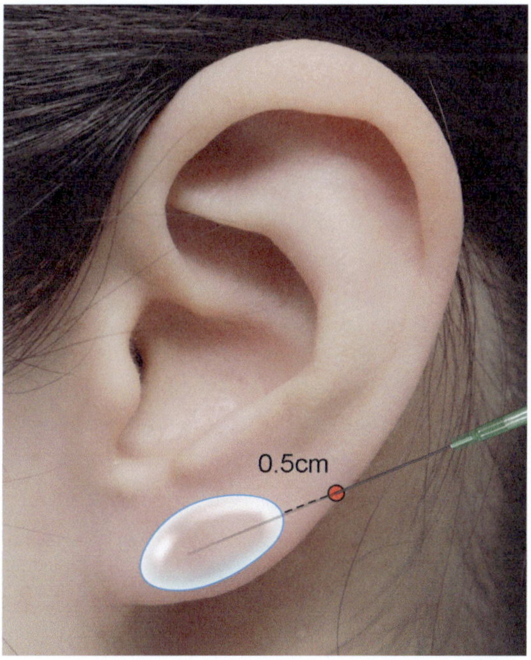

Fig. 4.123 The cannula entry point for earlobe augmentation

in-clinic for 20–30 min. In this regard, where the patient desires extra-large-sized earlobes, it is advisable to repeat the treatment over 2–3 sessions at 2–3 month intervals rather than attempting to inject an overly large amount in a single session. Injection of too much HA filler in the earlobe may also result in the complication of the Tyndall effect.

Episode: Where Are the Other Nine?

In Luke 17:17 of the Holy Bible, Jesus crosses the border between Galilee and Samaria en route to Jerusalem. Along the way, he enters a village where he is met by ten lepers who cry, "Jesus, Master, have pity on us!" Upon this, Jesus responds, "Go and show yourselves to the priests. You would have been cleansed." As the lepers set forth to meet the priests, they find they are miraculously cured of their leprosy just as Jesus had foretold. One of them turns back upon realizing he has been healed and falls on his face at Jesus' feet exclaiming, "Praise God!" As it happened, he was a Samaritan, not a Jew. To this, Jesus lamented, "Were not ten cleansed? Where are the other nine? How come nobody returned to give glory to God except for this foreigner?"

Leprosy is an infectious disease caused by the bacteria *Mycobacterium leprae*, which spreads throughout the body, primarily affecting the skin, the respiratory organs, and the peripheral nerves. It causes disfiguring rashes or nodules on the skin and undermines the person's ability to feel pain, leading to the necrosis of the skin or the loss of extremities, including the fingers and toes due to unnoticed wounds. Unsightly to the eyes and deemed highly infectious, those afflicted with leprosy during the ancient times were treated as sinners and shunned from the rest of the society as outcasts. With no effective cure at the time, leprosy patients were condemned to live with hideous deformities for the rest of their lives until their eventual death. So it was, in fact, a pretty big deal when Jesus gratuitously cured those ten lepers of their terrifying disease with his words alone. Yet, none of them even bothered to thank Jesus except for one, a foreigner from Samaria despised by the Jewish community at large at the time. It is not difficult then to appreciate Jesus' amazement when he asks where the other nine were.

According to the Roman philosopher Cicero, "Gratitude is the greatest of all virtues." Yet all too often, we find cases where an act of kindness instead backfires on those who bestowed it. "Save a drowning man only to be accused of missing his bag" as we say in Korean, I am reminded of a case 2 years ago where a young woman died due to an anaphylactic shock after receiving bee venom acupuncture from an oriental medicine clinic. Amazingly, the bereaved family proceeded to sue for damages not only against the oriental medicine doctor who performed the acupuncture but also the family medicine doctor practicing out of the same building who undertook the emergency treatment. The basis of their claim was that patient had passed away due in part to the inadequacy of the emergency treatment undertaken, throwing a major curveball at the family medicine doctor who simply acted in good faith to resuscitate the patient. Mercifully enough, the court ultimately found the family medicine doctor not liable for the patient's death.

I also had a similar experience once when I was visited by a female patient who complained of irregular contours in the forehead from a HA filler treatment received elsewhere, which she wanted dissolving. The HA filler was successfully removed as per her request, and smoothness was restored to the forehead within a week. This time, however, the patient took issue with "the descent of the cheeks" and "the thinning of the skin" she purportedly experienced following the removal of HA filler in the forehead even though the cheeks were never even treated with hyaluronidase in the first place. Of course, no difference could be noted in the cheeks between the pre- and posttreatment photos. Yet, the patient was adamant, insisting that she knew best when it came to her face and that I was somehow responsible for these problems. The situation escalated to the point where, following a prolonged attempt to reason with the unreasonable, the police had to be called in to deal with the patient's temper tantrums.

In contrast, I have patients who have received HA filler treatment at my clinic and are only too happy to show their appreciation for a job well done. With filler treatments, whether used for filling deep grooves or creases, smoothening irregular facial contours, or improving under eye dark circles, results are obtained instantly and can be checked in the mirror immediately posttreatment. While most of my patients are too busy scrutinizing for defects or imperfections, some are quite exuberant in expressing their pleasure, exclaiming how much they love their new look and describing the transformation as magical. Compliments such as these are inspiring as they are addictive and are enough to touch the heart.

The novel coronavirus pandemic (COVID-19) continues to set tragic new records as it rages on, with the U.S. COVID-19 death toll now topping a staggering 70,000 per day. In Korea, we seem to have turned a corner, with the government relaxing the social distancing standards and replacing it with the "lifestyle quarantine system," allowing the public to resume their normal economic activities while following the relevant health and hygiene guidelines. This achievement is in no short measure thanks to the passion and courage of the medical staff battling coronavirus on the front lines, clad in their stuffy, uncomfortable protective gear. The outpouring of support from the general public for the '#Thanks to You Challenge' on social media gesturing the word "respect" in sign language signifies the huge admiration they collectively feel for the unwavering dedication of the medical professionals. Though worlds apart in terms of the specialties we practice. I wish to join in the celebration of my fellow medical professionals and their splendid work in helping COVID-19 patients. "It is # thanks to you, my colleagues, I can provide filler treatment to my patients. Deepest kudos to you all." (Jul 17th, 2020)

4.17 Atrophic Scar volumization for Soft Tissue Depressions from Autoimmune Diseases

Difficulty Level: B, Effectiveness: B, Complications: B

Summary 1: To an extent, HA fillers can play a role in the revision of soft tissue depressions caused by localized scleroderma, linear scleroderma, progressive hemifacial atrophy, lupus panniculitis, and discoid lupus erythematosus.

Summary 2: Treatment is performed using a 23-G cannula and a firm monophasic or biphasic HA with high viscoelasticity.

Summary 3: Subdermal filling may be combined with the subcision technique to release the tissue adhesions prior to the placement of HA filler underneath.

To a certain extent, HA fillers can play a role in the revision of depressed or atrophic scars left as a sequela of autoimmune diseases that cause soft tissue depression. A case in point is scleroderma, a type of connective tissue disease that involves the hardening of the skin. Localized scleroderma usually affects only the skin without affecting other internal organs and can be classified into morphea and linear scleroderma. Localized scleroderma initially starts with erythema and gradually progresses to the atrophy and fibrosis of the skin, subcutaneous tissue, muscles, and the bone, resulting in the depression and hardening of the skin [39]. Linear scleroderma restricted to the forehead region is referred to as "en coup de sabre" signifying its resemblance to "the stroke of a saber sword." En coup de sabre may also be accompanied by a progressive hemifacial atrophy referred to as the "Parry-Romberg syndrome." Meanwhile, soft tissue atrophy resulting from lupus profundus (also known as lupus panniculitis) or discoid lupus erythematosus area can also be corrected with HA filler (Fig. 4.124).

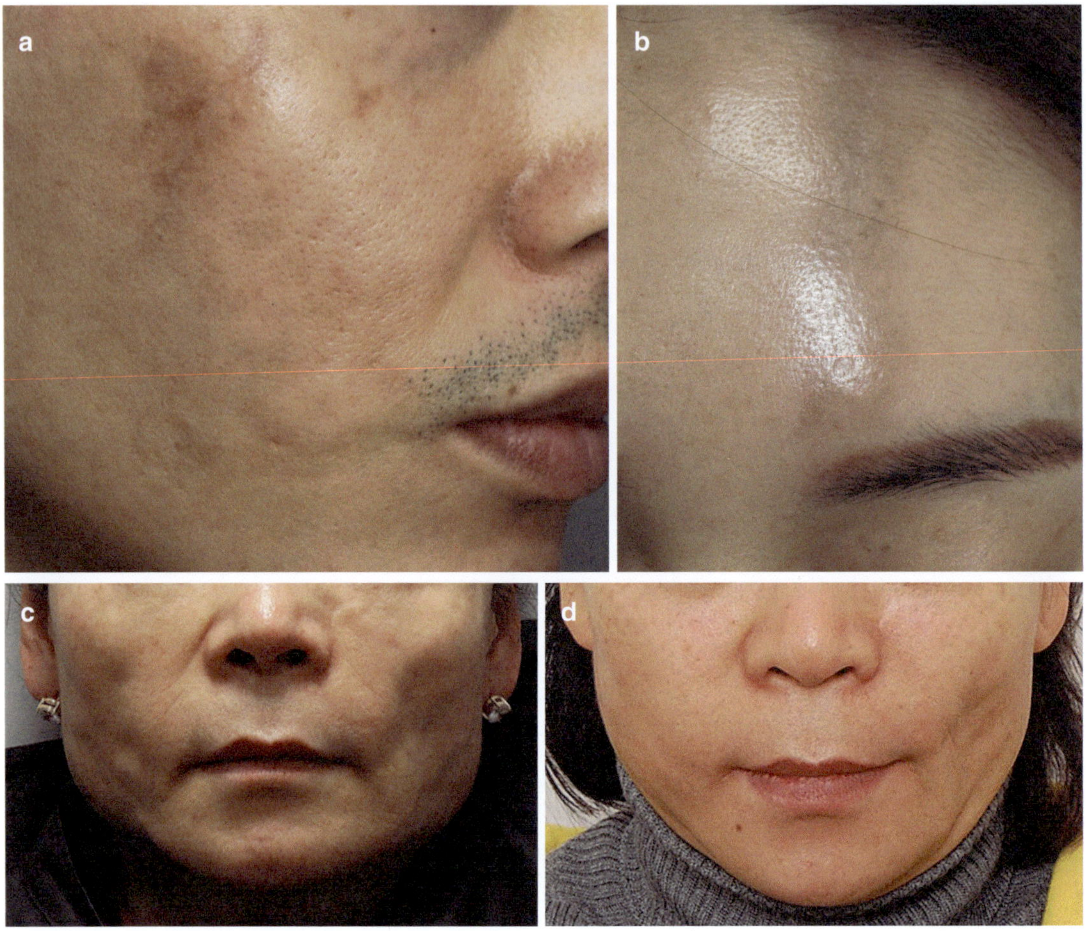

Fig. 4.124 (**a**) Morphea, (**b**) Linear scleroderma, (**c**) Before and (**d**) after filler volumization for morphea

4.17.1 Pretreatment Assessment

As a preliminary matter, it is essential first to ascertain whether the disease is still in progress or has been treated. Redness in the skin suggests ongoing inflammation, in which case treatment with HA filler should be postponed until a later time [40]. It is necessary to clarify whether the patient is still on medication or has completed the required drug therapy. To the extent the patient has undergone a complete course of acute-phase treatment, with no further progression of symptoms during the subsequent months, HA filler treatment may be attempted even where the patient is still undergoing maintenance procedures. Palpate the depression with the finger to estimate the degree of adhesion and the likely treatment outcome based on the hardness of the overlying tissue. Severely adhered or tethered down tissue can be very hard to treat, which should be clearly communicated to the patient in advance. Regarding the estimated injection volume; as a general rule of thumb, adhered or bound-down tissue requires a larger amount of HA filler compared with normal tissue to provide lifting. Areas such as the anterior cheek (buccal cheek) also tend to consume a larger-than-expected amount of product due to the absence of underlying bony structure to support the tissue from below.

4.17.2 Injection Technique

It is advisable to use monophasic or biphasic HA with good high viscoelasticity that can withstand the pressure exerted by the tough, hard scar tissues in the treatment area. The use of a cannula is advised over a needle to minimize inadvertent injection of HA filler into blood vessels adhered to the depressed tissue. It is also recommended to use cannulas sized 23G or thicker, as thinner cannulas can be too pliant and may bend under the force of the tough fibrous tethering. The cannula entry point is created 1 cm lateral to the border of the depressed scar along its longitudinal axis. Achieving full elevation of the depressed tissue with HA can be elusive where severe adhesions are present. In such case, another alternative is to combine subdermal filling with the subcision technique to release the tethered tissue away from the deeper layers before placing a layer of HA filler underneath [41].

The procedure can be highly painful, owing to the tight adhesions in the tissue. Accordingly, it is advisable to inject a small amount of lidocaine in the treatment area in advance, since numbing creams alone may be insufficient to provide necessary numbing. Sedation may be considered where soft tissue depressions are prevalent across broad areas of the face with tight adhesions to the deeper structures.

4.17.3 Complications

Elevating the tissue can be a challenge in areas where severe adhesions are present, as the tightly bound scar tissues would push the injected HA filler away into surrounding normal tissue, causing surface irregularities. Further, blood vessel perforation and bruising may occur even with the use of cannulas in areas with tissue adhesion. Bruising is a common occurrence, particularly where the subcision technique is used.

4.18 Facial Asymmetry Correction

Difficulty Level: A, Effectiveness: A, Complications: B

Summary 1: Moderate improvement in facial asymmetry can be achieved by balancing out the volume deficit on one side of the face and realigning the canted mandible leveraging the volumizing effect of HA filler.

Summary 2: The facial midline extending inferiorly from the upper face intersected by a horizontal line connecting the left and right pupils can be used to identify the presence of facial asymmetry and midline discrepancy on the frontal image.

Summary 3: To restore the facial summetry, it is necessary to create a new soft tissue gnathion (Gn') that is aligned with the midline of the upper face and to build volume on the smaller side of the chin.

Symmetry constitutes an essential element of a beautiful face. Facial symmetry can be disrupted, however, by a range of different factors, the correction of which requires orthodontic or even surgical interventions including upper and lower jaw surgery in severe cases. That said, moderate improvements in facial asymmetry can be achieved with HA fillers by building up volume on the weaker side of the face and restoring the alignment of the canted maxilla/mandible [42] (Fig. 4.125). Facial asymmetry can be either congenital or acquired, and can be broadly divided into those caused by skeletal discrepancies and those stemming from soft tissue problems between the left and right face. Skeletal discrepancies comprise hemifacial hypoplasia, hemifacial microsomia, hemifacial hyperplasia, maxillary canting, mandibular deviation, and hemimandibular hypoplasia. Soft tissue problems include imbalance of masseter muscles caused by the habit of chewing on only one side, asymmetrical sagging of the face with aging, discrepancy in the volume of malar fat pad or buccal fat pad on each side, or the rare incidence of progressive hemifacial atrophy also known as the Parry-Romberg syndrome [43]. Facial asymmetry may also be caused by injury or trauma or more recently by increased incidences of botched cosmetic procedures involving soft tissue fillers, autologous fat, liposuction or thread lifts. Successful correction of facial asymmetry with HA filler is premised on the proper pretreatment evaluation of the underlying cause and indication, as well as the feasibility of treatment with

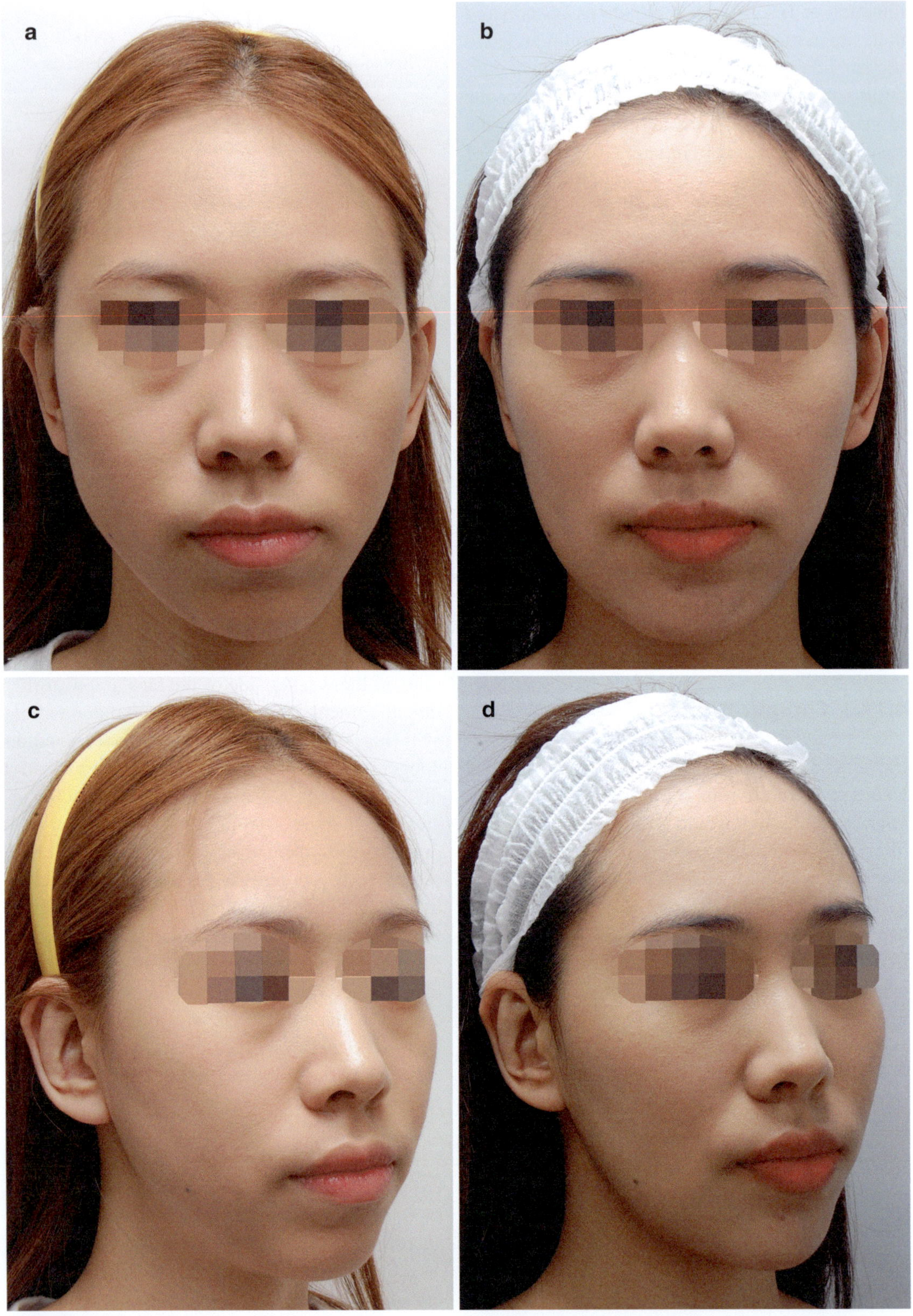

Fig. 4.125 (**a**, **c**, **e**) Before and (**b**, **d**, **f**) after correction of asymmetry with HA filler and botulinum toxin

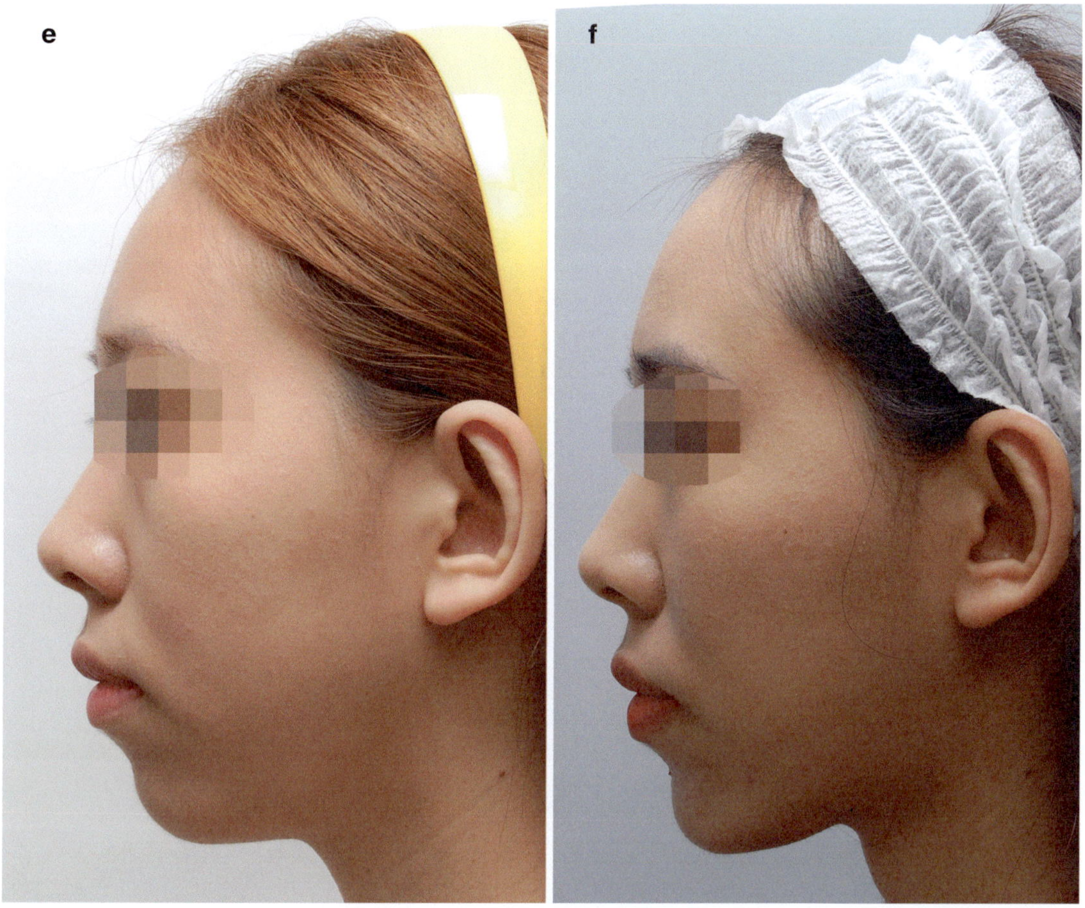

Fig. 4.125 (continued)

HA filler. Also, when volumizing the smaller side with HA to balance facial symmetry, it must be born in mind that simply mirroring the large side to achieve perfect symmetry can lead to an unnatural and overly large face or chin.

4.18.1 Pretreatment Assessment

While the use of medical imaging such as X-ray or CT of the underlying facial bony structure can offer a more accurate diagnosis, clinical photographs alone can be useful for determining facial asymmetry before treatment [44]. As a preliminary step, it is helpful to draw the facial midline on the patient's frontal face image extending inferiorly from the upper face, followed by a horizontal line connecting the left and right pupils (Fig. 4.126). Significantly, the interpupillary line is known to remain parallel to the floor even where facial asymmetry is present.

Using these lines as the reference, start by assessing the contour asymmetry between the left and right face in the upper, mid, and lower segments. Specifically, on the upper face, evaluate the bilateral symmetry in the frontal bone, recessed temples, superciliary arches, and brow height. On the mid-face, compare the size and height of the malar fat pad, malar eminence, and zygomatic arch on each side. On the lower face, examine the differences in buccal hollows, jowl sagging, masseter size and chin symmetry between the left and right face.

Next, assess whether or not the facial midline has been shifted to one side. More specifically, check for the presence of any nasal deviation in the midface or a chin deviation in the lower face. The nose is deviated if the glabella-subnasale line

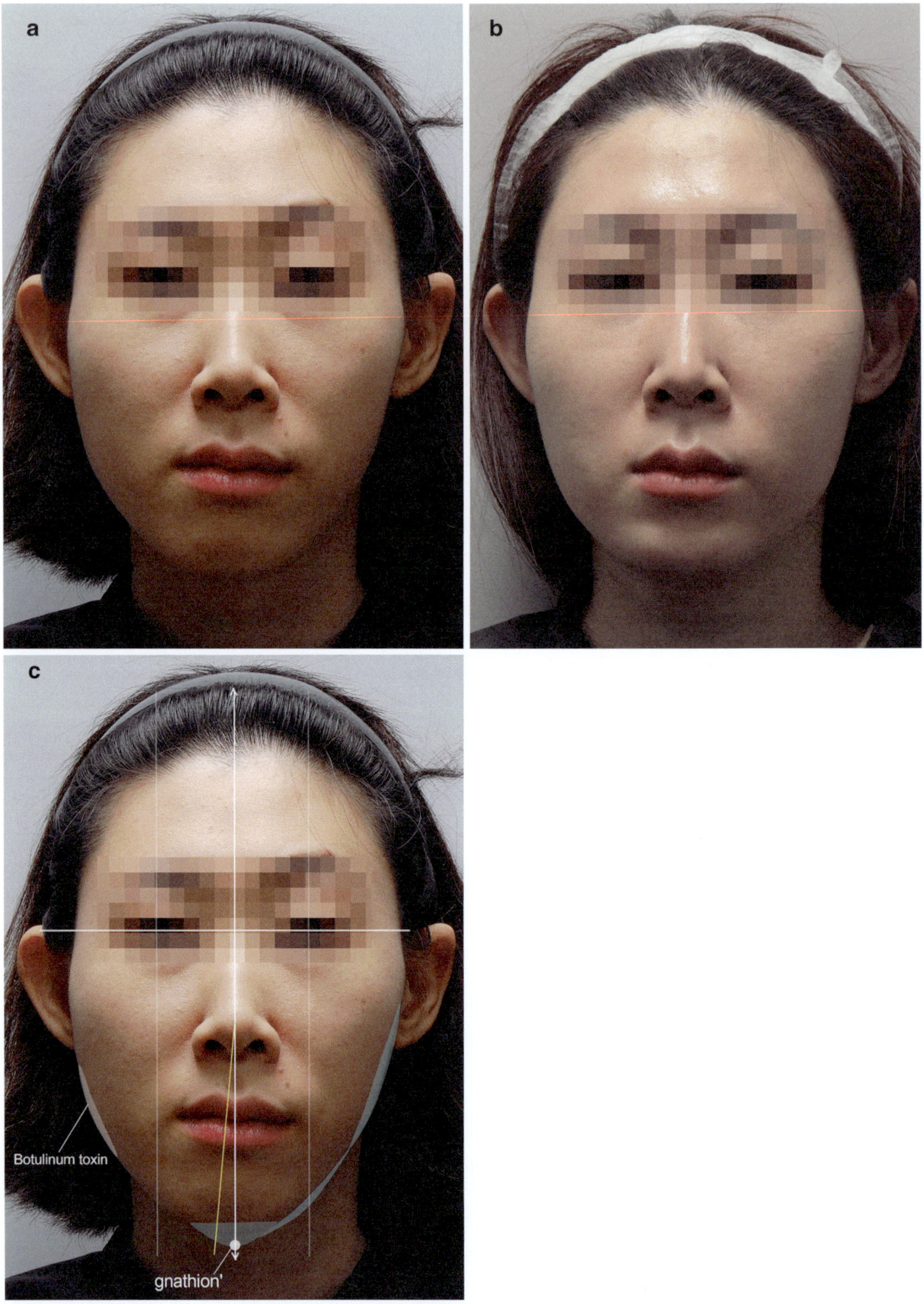

Fig. 4.126 Pretreatment assessment of facial asymmetry ((**a**) Before, (**b**) after treatment using fller and botulinum toxin and (**c**) assessment and treatment strategy for facial asymmetry)

is off to the midline of the upper face. This deviation to one side is caused primarily by a canted maxilla or hemifacial hypoplasia, that is, unilateral underdevelopment of one side of the maxilla. Patients with a maxillary cant tend to present not only a deviated nasal dorsum but also a tilted lip line. On smiling, they display an uneven show of upper teeth and gum between the left and right sides of the maxilla (Fig. 4.116). A maxillary cant is usually accompanied by chin deviation where the mandibular midline gravitates to one side. A chin deviation is identified when the subnasale-to-Gn' line is out-of-sync with the facial midline while the midline of the midface is in proper alignment. Patients with chin deviation demonstrate unilateral underdevelopment of the mandibular body or ramus on one side, with the Gn' tilted toward the smaller side of the mandible.

Meanwhile, facial depressions caused by traumatic injuries or facial asymmetries resulting from botched aesthetic procedures can also be improved moderately by adding HA filler to the side where volume is deficient. Note, however, that full correction of the depression/misalignment is elusive where scar tissue adhesions are present beneath the skin. Where the facial asymmetry is the result of an incorrect volume augmentation procedure where too much HA or fat was placed on one side resulting in an uneven outcome, hyaluronidase or fat reducing injection is required to reduce the excess volume.

4.18.2 Principles and Injection Technique for Facial Asymmetry Correction

The cardinal principle in correcting facial asymmetry with HA filler, regardless of the underlying cause, is to build up volume on the smaller side and to restore facial alignment, where necessary, by readjusting the midline of the chin (Fig. 4.127). Regarding the volume restoration, HA filler can be applied to improve asymmetry between the left and right forehead or temples by enhancing the volume on the smaller side in the upper face. In the midface, asymmetry between the bilateral malar eminence and zygomatic arches can be balanced out by augmenting volume on the smaller side. Note, however, that achieving perfect symmetry with the larger zygoma is neither necessary nor desirable in Asians who generally disfavor having a prominent zygoma. In the lower face, restoring the anterior (submalar) and posterior (subzygomatic) cheek and strengthening the jawline and chin of the smaller side can help resolve the asymmetry to some extent. In patients with a tilted lip line due to a maxillary cant, lip filler would be also helpful for restoring facial symmetry (Fig. 4.127).

Meanwhile, restoring facial symmetry through readjusting the midline of the deviated chin is a prerequisite process for facial asymmetry correction. In order to correct a chin deviation, it is necessary to create a new soft tissue Gn (Gn') that is aligned with the midline of the upper face, while enhancing volume on the smaller side of the chin to restore the facial symmetry. Caution must be taken against overfilling the smaller side of the chin to match the larger side as it may serve only to create a chin that is overly broad. In patients with a Class III malocclusion (prognathia) or a notably bulky chin, it may be preferable to forgo correction of chin deviation (see Sect. 4.14).

4.18.3 Combination Treatment

During the augmentation it is advisable to concurrently slim down the contralateral side of the face (i.e., the larger side) with BoNT-A injections in the masseter m. and fat-reducing injections in the sagging jowl. Meanwhile, in order to fix the bilateral difference in jowl sagging, it is necessary to undertake thread-lifting procedures on the areas concerned in addition to fat-reducing injections. In patients with an uneven gum display or a tilted lip line due to a maxillary cant, the treatment may be combined with injection of 3 U of BoNT-A for mouth corner elevation in the downward-tilting side (Fig. 4.128), or conversely with 1–2 U of BoNT-A in the zygomaticus minor muscle of the upward tilting side (Fig. 4.129).

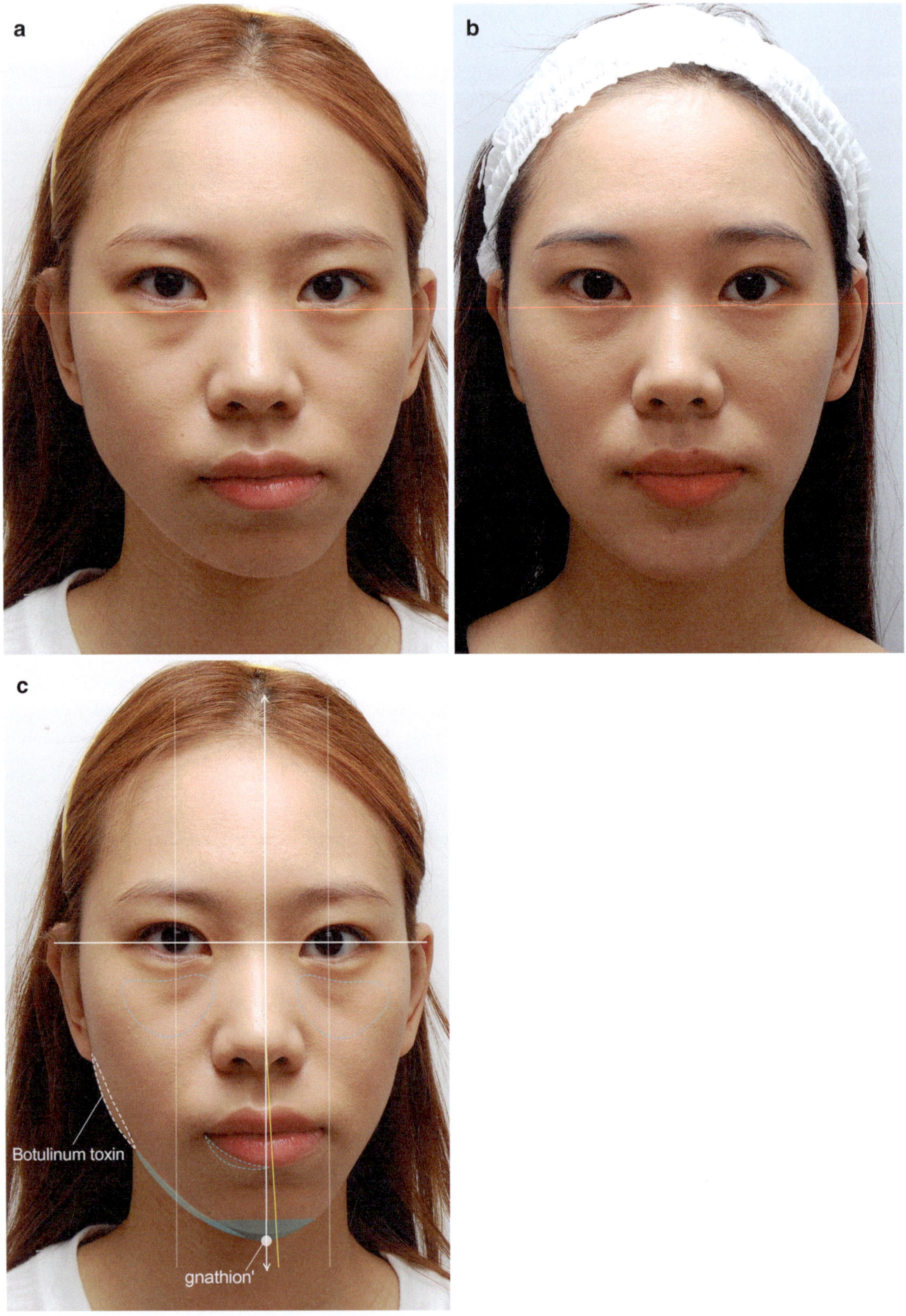

Fig. 4.127 Injection technique for the correction of facial asymmetry using filler and botulinum toxin ((**a**) Before, (**b**) after treatment, (**c**) assessment and treatment strategy for facial asymmetry)

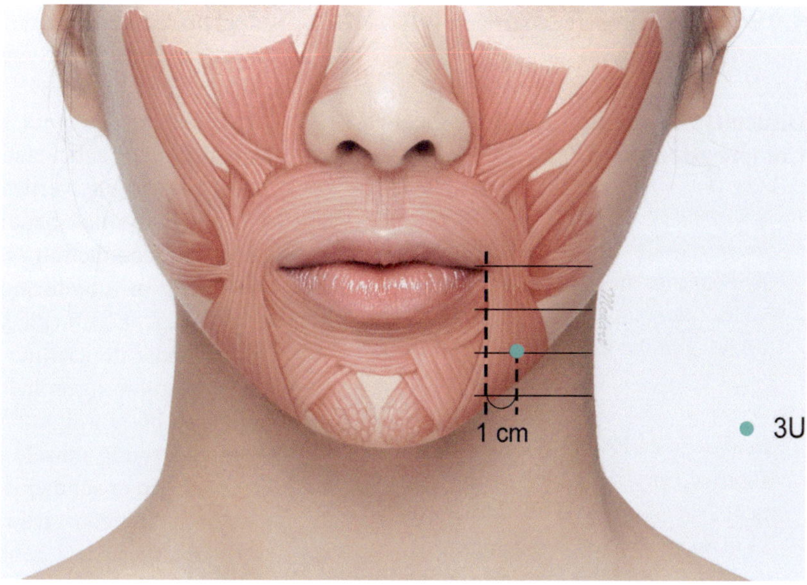

Fig. 4.128 Botulinum toxin (3U) injection point for mouth corner elevation

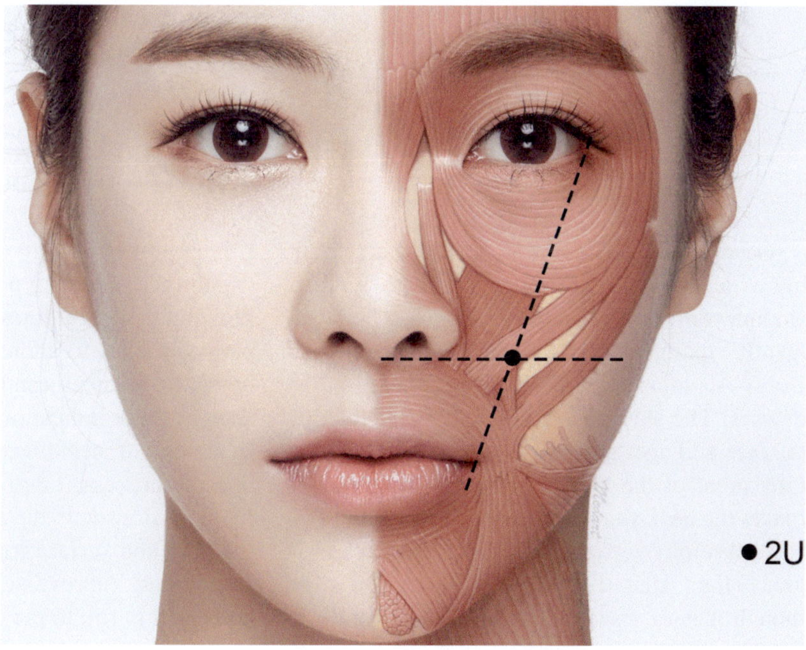

Fig. 4.129 Botulinum toxin injection point for relaxing the zygomaticus minor m

4.19 Neckline Treatment with HA Filler

Difficulty Level: B, Effectiveness: B, Complications: B

Summary 1: Necklines can largely be divided into horizontal necklines, vertical bands (platysma banding), and crépey fine wrinkles of the neck.

Summary 2: Horizontal necklines can be improved to some extent by filling the etched-in horizontal creases using 30-G, 33-G needle and a 27-G cannula. Soft monophasic HA fillers with high spreadability is recommended.

Summary 3: Crépey fine wrinkles of the neck can be improved to some extent with hydrolifting treatment using HA to restore skin elasticity and firmness in the neck.

Occasionally, people may present with a visibly wrinkled neck that is not congruent with their smooth youthful-looking faces that have been diligently maintained with the regular use of BoNT-A, injectable fillers, and energy-based devices. The skin of the neck is thinner than on the face and ages more easily, while the frequent movement of the platysma muscles in this area makes the neck skin more prone to wrinkling as it loses elasticity with age. Moreover, the neck is an area often missed with sun protection even though it is exposed to the sun as frequently as the face. It is for this reason that necklines are metaphorically referred to as "the tree rings of a woman," that reveal her age as does the dorsum of the hand.

Necklines can largely be divided into horizontal necklines, vertical bands (platysma banding), and crépey fine wrinkles of the neck. Horizontal necklines are a congenital feature present from birth together with other horizontal flexion creases of the body such as those found in the wrists and finger joints. Anatomically, the horizontal lines of the neck are formed by the attachment of the fibrous septa (underlying these rhytides) vertically to the muscles below. The rhytid depth progressively increases with age due to the increased deposition of subcutaneous fat in the adjacent tissue. Meanwhile, vertical necklines, often referred to as platysmal banding, develop due to the repeated contraction of platysma muscles during speaking or mobilization of the perioral muscles [45] (Fig. 4.130). Platysma bands run vertically from under the jawline to the clavicle and tend to appear more prominently in thin people with reduced body weight and little soft tissue to cover the underlying muscle contraction. Coupled with excess skin or submental fat under the chin, platysmal banding can give rise to the appearance of a "turkey neck" or "gobble neck deformity" commonly found in elderly Caucasians. Finally, crépey fine wrinkles of the neck occur due to the natural loss of skin elasticity with aging, and typically appear anterior to the thyroid cartilage or trachea during the swallowing of food or the movement of the neck (Fig. 4.130).

4.19.1 Pretreatment Assessment

It is important first to clarify precisely which of the three different types of neck wrinkles (i.e., horizontal/vertical lines, or crépey neck skin) the patient wishes to address [45]. To add a caveat, however, the neck can be a tricky area to treat in each of these indications. Unlike facial wrinkles, treatment of necklines is usually not a single, one-off process, often requiring multiple treatment sessions with the associated downtime from bruising and surface irregularities, while delivering modest improvements; such aspects must be conveyed in full to the patient before treatment.

4.19.2 Injection Technique

Horizontal necklines are congenital structures that cannot be eradicated completely. For what it is worth, however, moderate improvements can be achieved by filling the etched-in horizontal creases that deepen with age from the deposition of subcutaneous fat in the adjacent tissue [46] (Fig. 4.131). Regarding the choice of HA filler, it

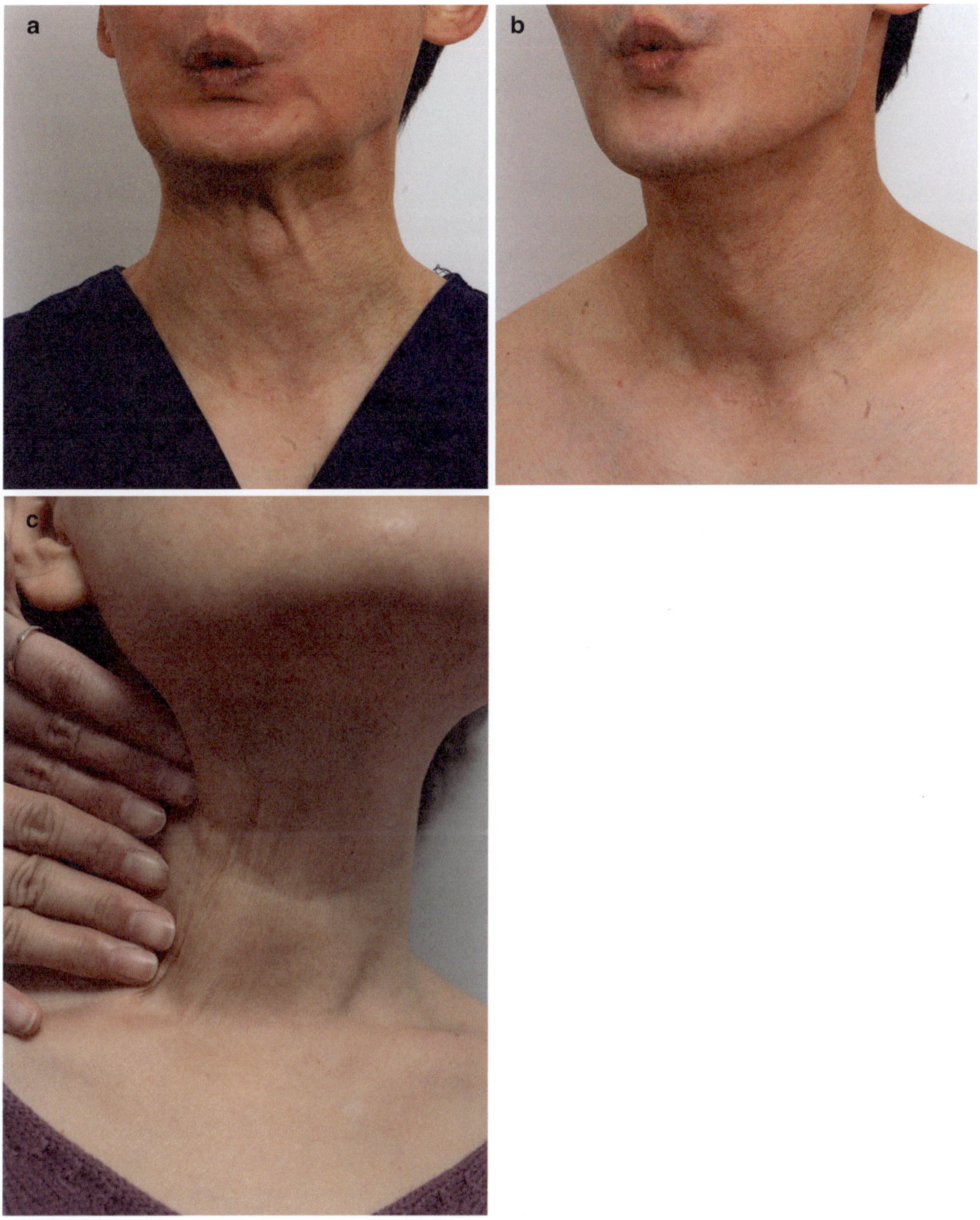

Fig. 4.130 Platysma bands (**a**) before and (**b**) 2 weeks after 50 U of botulinum toxin injection per side, (**c**) crépey fine wrinkles of the neck

is recommended to use soft flexible monophasic HA fillers such as Belotero® Soft with high spreadability (Table 4.18). In the author's experience, Restylane® Vital is effective for filling the creases due to its good elasticity while requiring much less amount of product but are more likely to leave the appearance of bumps on the surface; in contrast, thinner products such as Belotero® Soft cause much less irregularity owing to its more fluid and cohesive property but involve

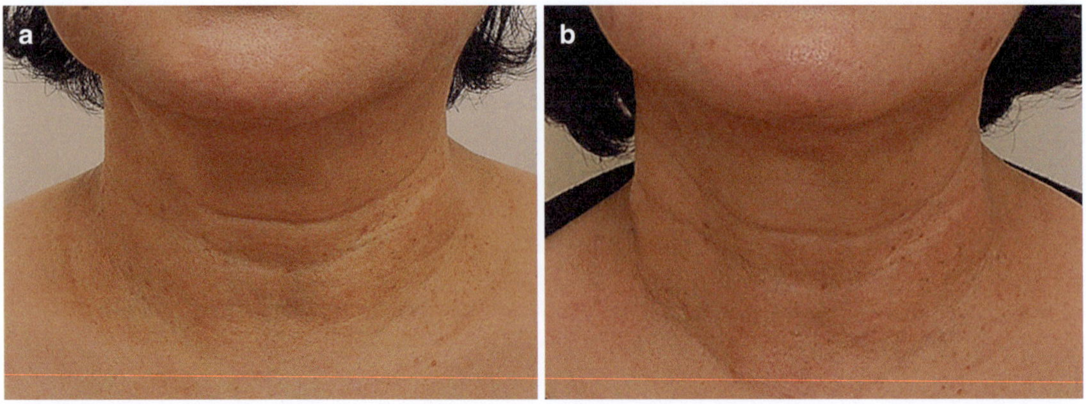

Fig. 4.131 (**a**) Before and (**b**) after treatment of horizontal necklines with HA fillers

Table 4.18 Summary of horizontal neck line injection technique

Item	Contents
Needle vs. Cannula	30-G, 33-G needle 27-G cannula where bruising must be avoided
HA filler	Monophasic HA filler with light Viscoelasticity for thin skin
Amount of HA filler	less than 1 mL per session
Depth of injection	Deep dermis and subdermal layer
Target area	deep horizontal crease
Anesthetics	Topical anesthetics for more than 40 mins
Nondominant hand	Hold the skin to maintain skin tension

a higher risk of bruising. The target plane of injection is the deep dermis/subdermal plane. Where bruising must be avoided as a priority, it is advisable to use a 27-G cannula to fill the etched-in horizontal creases in the subdermal layer using the retrograde linear threading technique. Where the patient is willing to tolerate some degree of bruising, it is preferable to use a 30-G needle both in the deep dermis and the subdermal layer to fill the grooves based on the retrograde linear threading technique. While the needle is more effective for filling in the etched-in creases, care must be taken as utilizing a needle entails a higher risk of bruising and bumpiness.

Meanwhile, the best strategy for treating the vertical platysmal bands is to relax the platysma m. with BoNT-A. It is recommended that 20–30 U of BoNT-A is injected per side to a total of 50–60 U per session [45]. While a touch-up may be administered 2 weeks following the initial treatment, caution is advised as an overdose of BoNT-A in the platysma band may cause complications such as hoarseness, dysphagia, or exacerbation of cervical disc herniation due to the weakening of the cervical neck muscles. In addition, considering that the primary indication of BoNT-A injections is for the treatment of dynamic lines and wrinkles appearing upon facial animation, patients with excess fat (i.e., double chin) or loose skin or under the chin cannot be treated satisfactorily with the use of BoNT-A injections in the platysma bands alone. In such case, BoNT-A should preferably be combined with fat reducing injections or liposuction to address the excess submental fat, while combination with HIFU, thread-lifting, or facelift surgery is advised for tightening or repositioning the loose excess skin hanging under the chin,

Finally, crépey fine wrinkles of the neck can be effectively treated with hydrolifting treatment with HA to restore skin elasticity and firmness in the neck (see Sect. 4.20). For a more even distribution of HA filler, the use of injector devices or Mirajet® system is advised over manual injection. It is recommended to inject 1–2 mL of a soft monophasic HA filler with good cohesivity such as Belotero® Soft evenly across the entire neck [47]. A top-up procedure may be repeated 1 month later, if necessary. For better results, hydrolifting can be combined with skin booster injections or Fraxel® laser or Thermage® radio frequency devices to help build skin elasticity and make the neck look more refreshed.

4.20 Hydrolifting (Multiple Intradermal Injections of HA Filler)

Difficulty Level: B, Effectiveness: A, Complications: B

Summary 1: Use monophasic HA with light-to-moderate viscoelasticity or biphasic HA with fine-sized particles. The suggested volume of injection is 2–4 mL per session for whole face. Administer HA evenly in more than 100 points across the deep dermis using the retrograde linear technique. Inject using a 30-G or 33-G needle bent at a 30° angle.

Summary 2: Hydrolifting helps boost skin elasticity and hydration and is particularly useful for improving the appearance of dynamic lines in the malar, nasolabial folds, cheeks, and perioral regions that are not readily treatable with boutlinum toxin (BoNT-A) due to the risk of altering the facial expression.

Summary 3: Epidermal sliding sign, can be used as an indicator for determing the efficacy of treatment.

Summary 4: Hydrolifting is also effective for treating the wrinkles of the neck, elbow, and knees.

The effects of HA filler injection can be considered as three-fold: It serves to replace lost volume ("space-filling effect"), restore skin elasticity ("structure stabilizing effect"), and stimulate cell regeneration ("cell-stimulating effect"). Space-filling effect refers to the volumizing effect of HA filler to lift etched-in grooves and plump facial depressions by literally "filling out" the areas of volume depletion. Structure stabilizing effect describes how HA filler restores skin elasticity and firmness by reintroducing HA, a naturally occurring substance responsible for skin elasticity, directly into the dermis to replenish the age-related decrease in HA. Cell-stimulating effect describes how the injection of HA in the dermis can boost collagen and elastin production via fibroblast activation [48, 49]. Not only does this help improve skin elasticity but it also allows the rejuvenation effect to persist beyond the longevity of the underlying HA filler. Among these, hydrolifting leverages the structure stabilizing and cell-stimulating effects of HA filler to restore skin elasticity. At the same time, it harnesses the hydrophilic nature of HA to draw water up to1000 times its molecular weight to rehydrate the skin. According to Kerscher et al. [50], marked improvements were reported in skin elasticity and skin surface roughness 24 weeks after administration of hydrolifting, while Distante et al. [45] reported a 20% improvement in skin hydration following three sessions of hydrolifting treatments. As such, hydrolifting captures both the lifting effect (i.e., skin elasticity) and improved hydration HA filler delivers to the skin (Fig. 4.132). Incidentally, as skin retains more moisture it helps improve fine wrinkles and diffuse light reflection, giving the skin a bright, radiant sheen. For this reason, the treatment is colloquially referred to as the "water glow" injection. To the extent hydrolifting is effective for improving skin elasticity, it is ideal not only for improving low elasticity underlying preauricular lines, photoaged skin and crépey neck wrinkles, but also for treating dynamic lines in the malar, nasolabial folds, cheeks, and perioral regions, not readily treatable with BoNT-A due to the risk of altering the facial expression in these areas (Fig. 4.82). Hydrolifting is also well suited for patients who regularly recruit the frontalis m. to open their eyes as a compensatory mechanism against eyelid ptosis or dermatochalasis, as the treatment serves to soften not only static but also severe dynamic wrinkles in the forehead which cannot be fixed entirely with BoNT-A injections alone. Meanwhile, horizontal creases formed

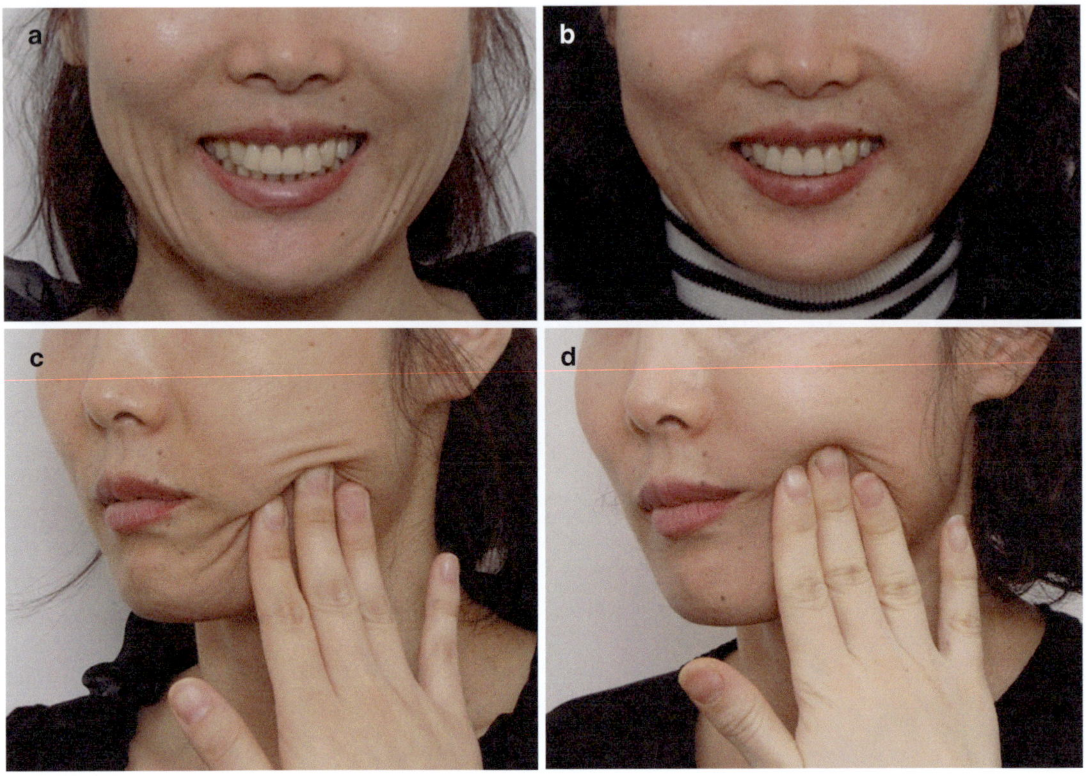

Fig. 4.132 (**a**) Before and (**b**) after hydrolifting. (**c**) Before and (**d**) afer hydrolifting, epidermal sliding signs are improved

above the knees in a standing position or above the elbows when the arm is stretched straight are also good indications for hydrolifting injections, as they also result from decreased skin elasticity (Fig. 4.134).

4.20.1 Pretreatment Assessment

Assess the severity and location of dynamic wrinkles by having the patient animate the facial expression that gives rise to the appearance of wrinkles, and document results in the pretreatment photos (Fig. 4.133). Epidermal sliding signs, or the pleated lines appearing on the skin when cheek is pushed with a finger, attributable to age-related loss of skin elasticity, can be used to determine improvements in skin elasticity before and after the treatment (Fig. 4.132). The choice of HA filler to be used and the desired depth of injection is decided based on a rough estimate of skin thickness in each treatment case. As a general rule, the skin is thicker in men compared with females and in sebaceous skin compared with dry skin. Skin thickness decreases with advancing age and in severely photoaged skin. By facial regions, the skin is thinnest in the periorbital region, while the neck also displays fine skin. By comparison, skin overlying the cheeks, malar, perioral, and forehead areas tends to be relatively thicker. Finally, checks should also be made for the presence of any static deep grooves or facial volume deflation for which concurrent volumization with HA filler may be considered for optimum results.

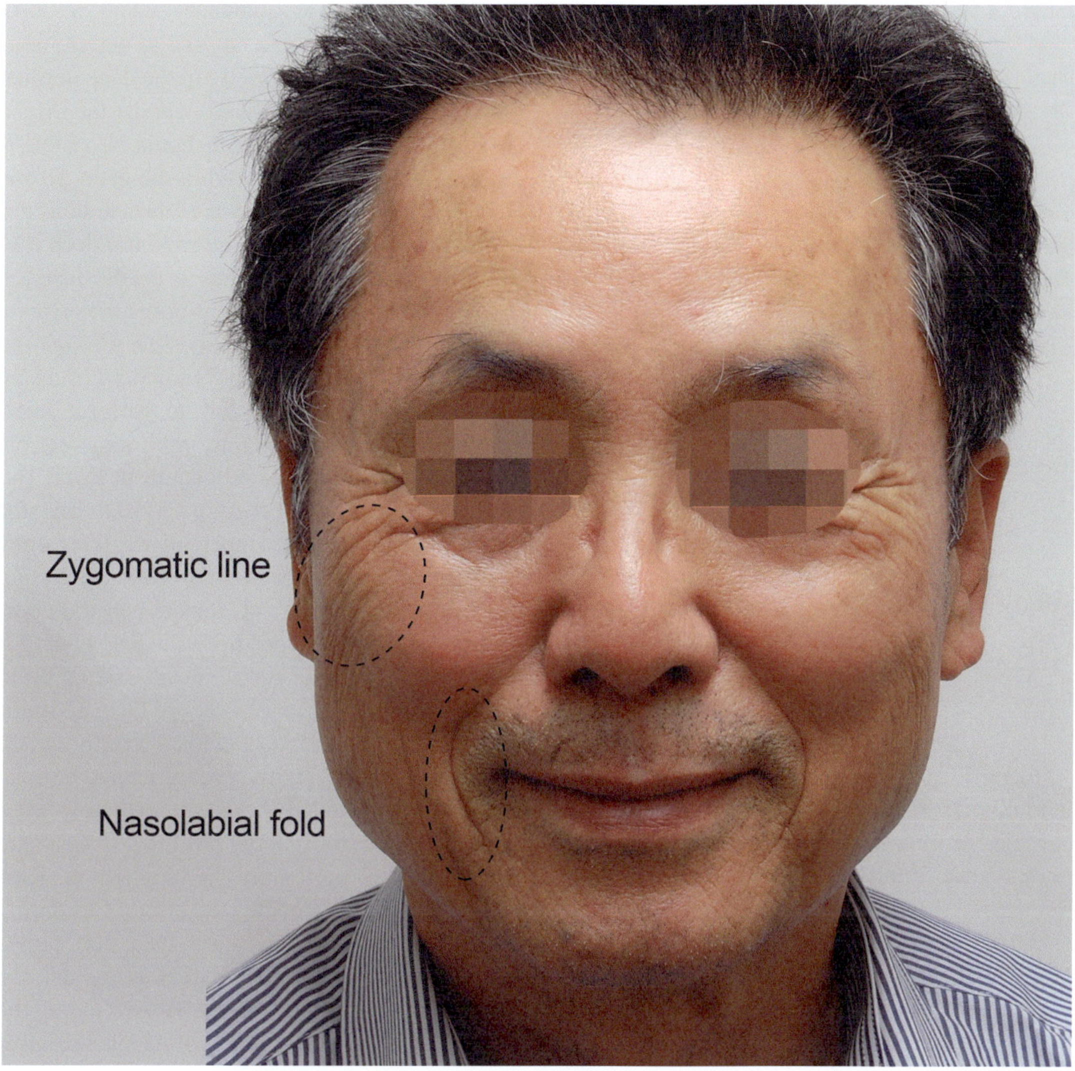

Fig. 4.133 Dynamic expression wrinkles such as zygomatic lines, nasolabial fold and marionette line are good candidates for the hydrolifting treatment

4.20.2 Injection Technique

One of the most commonly practiced techniques for reducing the appearance of dynamic nasolabial folds is the fern technique, which delivers HA filler in the dermis to enhance the skin's integrity and resilience. It involves making multiple intradermal injections of HA filler perpendicular to the direction of the fold from both sides. The name "fern technique" is derived from the rows of HA filler placed on each side of the fold resembling the shape of fern leaves, with the fold itself representing the stem. The hydrolifting technique replicates the same strategy across the entire face, as opposed to treating a single fold or wrinkle, to address the loss of skin elasticity in the face. Accordingly, where applicable, hydrolifting injections should also be made perpendicular to the direction of the relaxed skin tension lines or wrinkles of the face to be treated (Table 4.19) (Fig. 4.134).

Table 4.19 Summary of hydrolifting injection technique

Item	Contents
Needle vs. Cannula	30-G, 33-G needle 27-G cannula where bruising must be avoided Multi-needle injector Laser-assisted needless injector
HA filler	Monophasic HA filler with light viscoelasticity for thin skin Fine biphasic HA filer or monophasic HA filler with moderate viscoelasticity for thick skin
Amount of HA filler	1–4 mL per session
Depth of injection	Deep dermis
Target area	skin with low elasticity and dynamic rhytids in the cheek, the nasolabial folds, perioral area, and malar area
Anesthetics	Topical anesthetics for more than 40 min
Nondominant hand	Hold the skin to maintain skin tension

Regarding the choice of HA filler, injection is to be performed using biphasic HA with fine particles or monophasic HA with light to moderate viscoelasticity, depending on the dermal thickness. Monophasic HA with moderate viscoelasticity (e.g. Belotero® Balance) or biphasic HA with fine particles (e.g. Restylane® Vital) may be acceptable for use in the cheeks and malar where the skin is relatively thick. On the other hand, monophasic HA with low viscosity and greater spreadability (e.g. Belotero® Soft) is more suitable for injecting areas such as the neck and the infraorbital areas demonstrating reduced skin thickness. Note, however, that while monophasic HA fillers offer the advantage of increased spreadability and reduced irregularity, their duration of effect is apparently shorter than that of a biphasic HA filler. In the author's clinical experience, Restylane® Vital was found to last longer than Belotero® Soft. About 50% improvement in dynamic wrinkles can be achieved in a single session where cross-linked HA fillers are used. Where results are deemed insufficient, a follow-up treatment can be undertaken 1 month later.

Meanwhile, the desired depth of injection is at the deep dermis to minimize surface irregularities. When injecting manually using a 30-G needle, a simple test can be used to determine if the needle is located properly in the deep dermis. Lifting the needle upwards from under the skin, a clear silhouette of the needle should be visible if the needle is properly placed in the deep dermis (Fig. 3.12). A clear silhouette of the needle is not visible when the needle is inserted too deep into the subcutaneous layer, while a needle inserted too superficially in the upper dermis generates a gray bluish hue of the needle visible through the skin (Fig. 3.12). To prevent bumpiness in thinly skinned areas, it is advisable to perform small volume injections targeting the deep dermis almost as if injecting the subcutaneous layer. The amount of HA filler required is 0.5 mL for the nasolabial folds or upper lip wrinkles only, 1 mL for partial treatment of the cheeks including the nasolabial folds, 1 mL for the perioral complex including the upper lip wrinkles, 1 mL for each cheek, 1 mL for the forehead, adding up to approximately 4 mL for the entire face. To minimize bruising, it is advisable to constantly switch treatment areas during the procedure and have an assistant compress the area immediately after each injection to reduce bleeding. Anesthetic cream should preferably be applied at least 40 mins in advance to alleviate discomfort during the needle puncture in more than 100 points across the tightly bounded matrix of the dermis. The nondominant hand should be used to pull the skin opposite to the direction of needle advancement to apply tension on the skin surface.

4.20.2.1 Manual Injection Method

Manual injection of HA filler can be time-consuming and prone to surface irregularities when performed with unpracticed hands. Despite such drawbacks, manual injection ensures greater accuracy in treating individual wrinkles, and therefore contributes to maximizing the treatment effect of hydrolifting. For this reason, even where hydrolifting is primarily performed with an injection device, manual injection can be used synergistically to address specific wrinkles such as dynamic nasolabial folds. The use of 30-G or 33-G needle bent at a 30° angle is advised for performing the manual injection technique (Fig. 3.12). The entire length of needle is inserted into the deep dermis, after which HA is delivered via

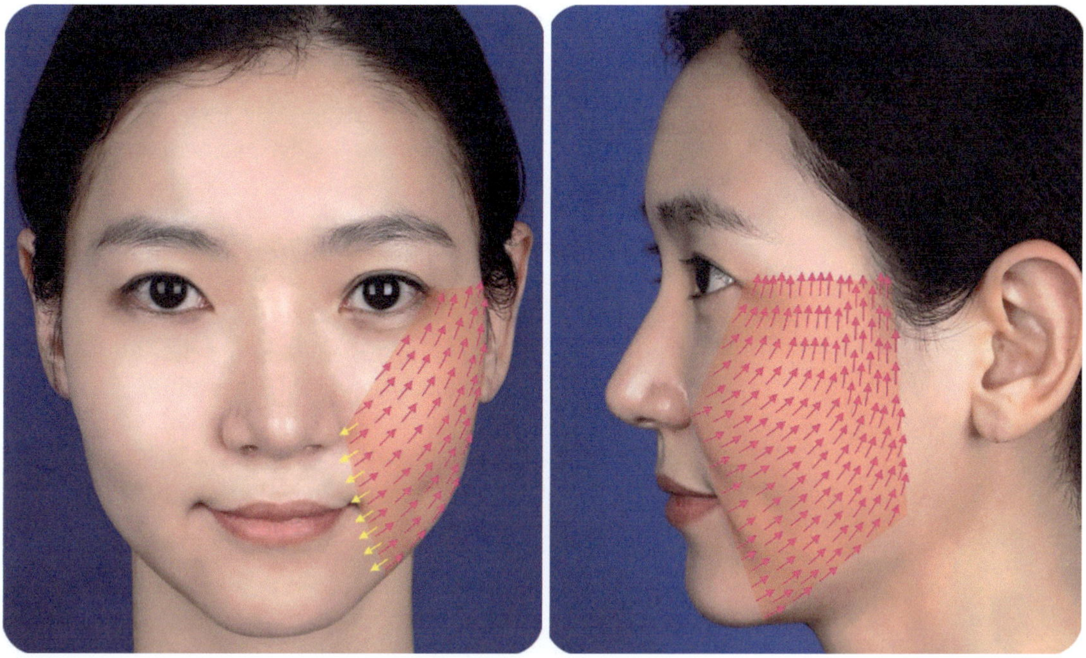

Fig. 4.134 Manual method of hydrolifting technique

retrograde thread technique. The needle should preferably be directed perpendicular to the direction of the relaxed skin tension lines or wrinkles of the face to provide better structural support to the skin and effective treatment of dynamic wrinkles. Note, however, that injections parallel to the fold may also be required to ensure maximum treatment of the deep folds. For ease of injection, injections should preferably be oriented from the medial to lateral and from the inferior to the superior aspects of the face. Regarding the spacing of injection points, HA should be delivered at 3–5 mm intervals from left to right and at 1 cm intervals from the anterior to the posterior when covering wide areas such as the cheek and malar. By comparison, areas such as the upper lip require a more thorough coverage, where HA should be introduced at a tighter interval of 2–3 mm (Fig. 4.134). The amount of HA injected per point is approximately 0.02 mL.

4.20.2.2 Manual Injections Using a Cannula

In case bruising must be avoided as a matter of priority, a cannula may be used instead of a needle for subdermal injection of HA using the same approach as described above. Note, however, that the effects of subdermal HA filler injection for hydrolifting are less pronounced compared with HA injected directly into the dermis. Injection is performed primarily with a 27-G cannula, while the use of a 30-G cannula is advised for injecting delicate fine-skinned areas such as the infraorbital region.

4.20.3 Use of Injectors

Injection devices are capable of delivering HA consistently at the required amount and depth without creating surface irregularities, thus minimizing inter-operator variability. A variety of injectors are currently available on the market, including Vital® injector, Neurajet®, and DermaQueen® (Fig. 4.135). Most of the models are available in the form of a mesogun onto which a disposable 5–9 pin multi-needle tip is mounted. The head of the device uses negative pressure to create a suction between the skin and the needle tip, allowing the needles to penetrate into the skin to deliver the product evenly to the desired amount and depth. The vacuum pressure, needle depth, and injection volume may be adjusted as appropriate according to the indication and injection site. For thin-a

b

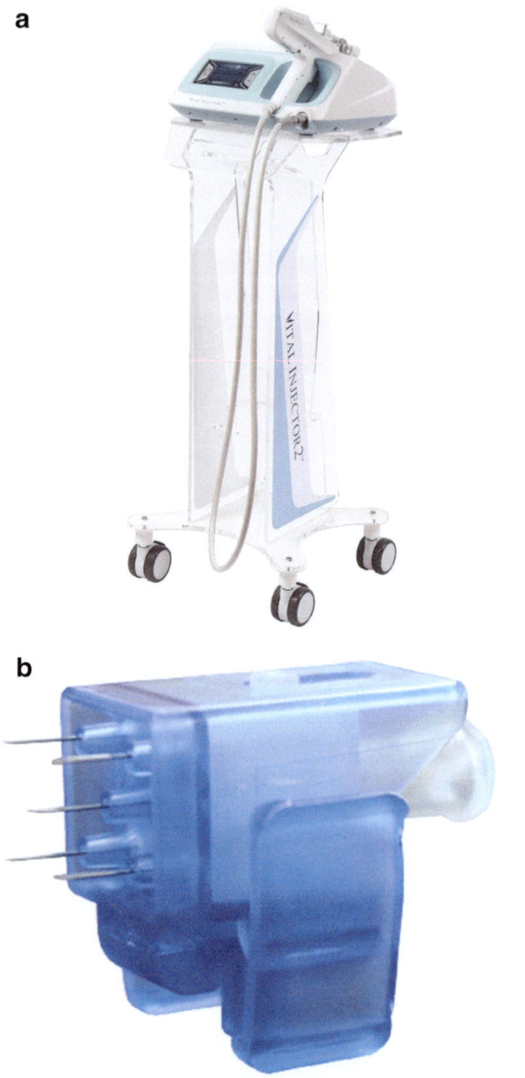

Fig. 4.135 (**a**) Injector for hydrolifting, (**b**) multi-needle injector tip

skinned areas such as the infraorbital region and the neck, a penetration depth of 1.4 mm and injection volume of 1μL per needle is appropriate, while for thicker skinned areas, the relevant penetration depth and injection volume should preferably be adjusted to 1.6 mm and 2μL per needle respectively. It generally takes 10 min to deliver 1 mL of HA filler using a Vital Injector featuring a 5-needle tip, based on an injection volume of 2μL/needle, or 10μL/per shot and an injection speed of 5–6 s per shot.

Consideration must also be given to the product loss that may occur from the leakage of injected HA filler onto the skin surface. Accordingly, the best approach is to use injectors for delivering HA evenly across the entire face in combination with manual injection of HA for treating more severe dynamic wrinkles.

4.20.4 Laser-Assisted Needleless Injector

Laser-assisted needleless injection systems such as Mirajet® also enable hydrolifting treatments with significantly less bruising or irregularity than manual injections (Fig. 4.136). Mirajet® is a novel transdermal drug delivery system capable of delivering drugs into the dermis without the use of needles by leveraging the energy released during the explosion of tissue water into which Erbium YAG laser energy is absorbed. Histologic examination in cadaveric facial skin clearly demonstrates the presence of HA injected into the dermis at the depth of upto 300μm by Mirajet® (Fig. 4.137) (Unpublished data). The system is capable of propelling drugs in a controlled amount and depth at speeds ranging from 10 to 40 Hz, and thus holds a distinct advantage over conventional injector devices in terms of its rapid injection speed. The laser power may be adjusted to 250–450 mW at 10 Hz, 150–300 mW at 20 Hz, and 100–150 mW at 40 Hz, respectively. While increasing the laser power can amplify the amount of drug penetration, care must be taken to tailor the energy level to each patient as appropriate, since an uncontrolled firing of jet injections may inflict severe pain or petechial bleeding (Fig. 4.138). Also, it is advisable to have an assistant apply proper compression on the treatment area immediately after the procedure to minimize the appearance of injection marks. The injected medication used in the author's practice consists basically of HA: placenta extract: PDRN (polydeoxyribonucleotide): epi-lidocaine mixed at a ratio of 2:2:1:1 (i.e., a three-fold dilution of HA filler combining 1 part HA with 2 parts other ingredients). Epi-lidocaine containing 1:100,000 epinephrine effectively helps to prevent severe petechia. The ratio of HA in the formula may be adjusted according to the patient's age and skin elasticity (see Sect. 4.20.5).

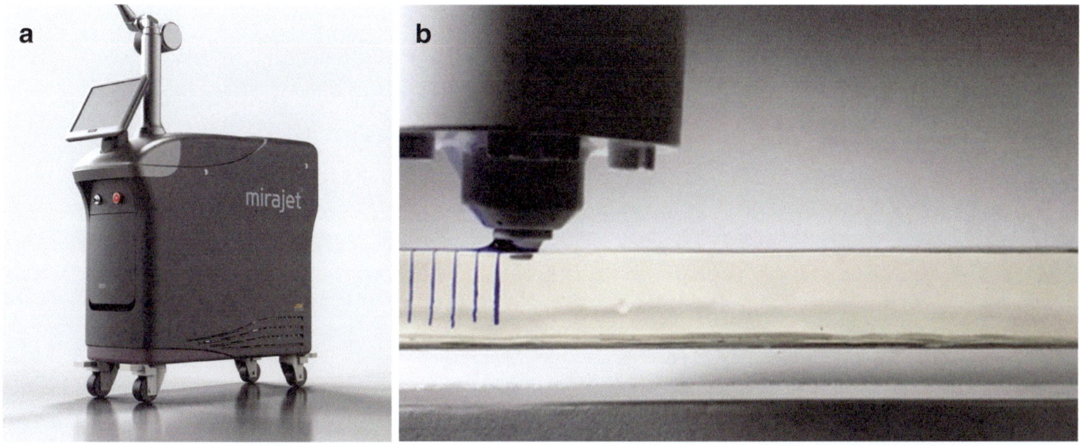

Fig. 4.136 (**a**) Exterior of Mirajet® needle-free injection system, (**b**) transdermal drug delivery system

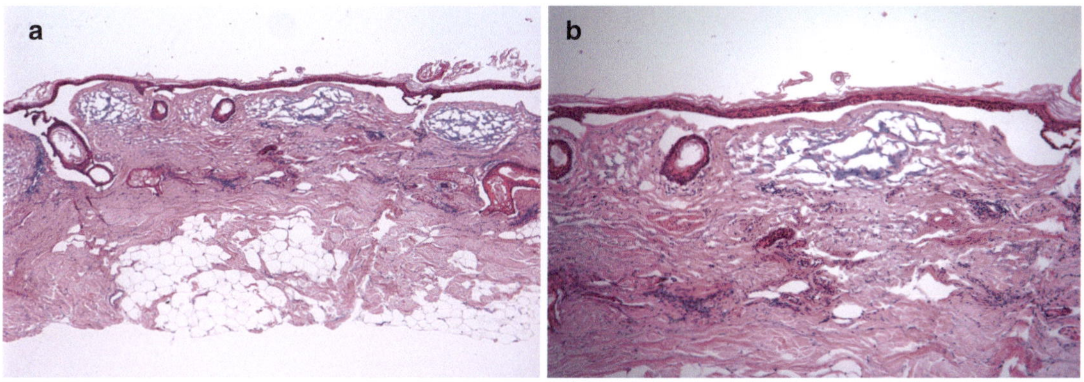

Fig. 4.137 Histologic examination in cadaveric facial skin clearly demonstrates the HA penetrated into the dermis at the depth upto 300μm by Laser-Assisted Needleless Injector, Mirajet® (H&E stain, (**a**) X50, (**b**) X100)

4.20.5 Cocktail Therapy

To further boost the effect of hydrolifting, HA may be synergistically combined with other ingredients such as placenta extracts and PDRN to promote tissue reconstruction and regeneration against cell aging while inducing elastin and collagen remodeling via the HA placement in the dermis. The author's basic formula consists of HA: placenta extract: PDRN blended at a ratio of 2:1:1. The ratio of HA in the mixture can be scaled upwards in patients in their fifth decade and above displaying reduced skin elasticity and downward-adjusted in younger patients in their 30s retaining adequate skin tightness. Some physicians opt to mix HA filler with BoNT-A to further improve the appearance of fine lines and pores. Indeed, multiple intradermal injection of BoNT-A is effective not only for reducing dynamic wrinkles but also for diminishing the appearance of static wrinkles and pore size, which serves to impart a glossy sheen to the skin surface (Fig. 4.139). The improvement of fine wrinkles and tightening of pores is attributable to the mild lymphatic edema in the skin induced by the transient paralysis of underlying musculature from BoNT-A injection, analogous to the swelling of the feet during a long distance flight. The effects of intradermal BoNT-A injections are particularly significant in the forehead, glabella, and periorbital regions, and when combined with hydro lifting, can give further boost to the luminescent, "water glow" effect of hydrolifting injections in these areas. On the other hand, combination with BoNT-A is best avoided in the perioral and cheek regions as inadvertent injection of BoNT-A into

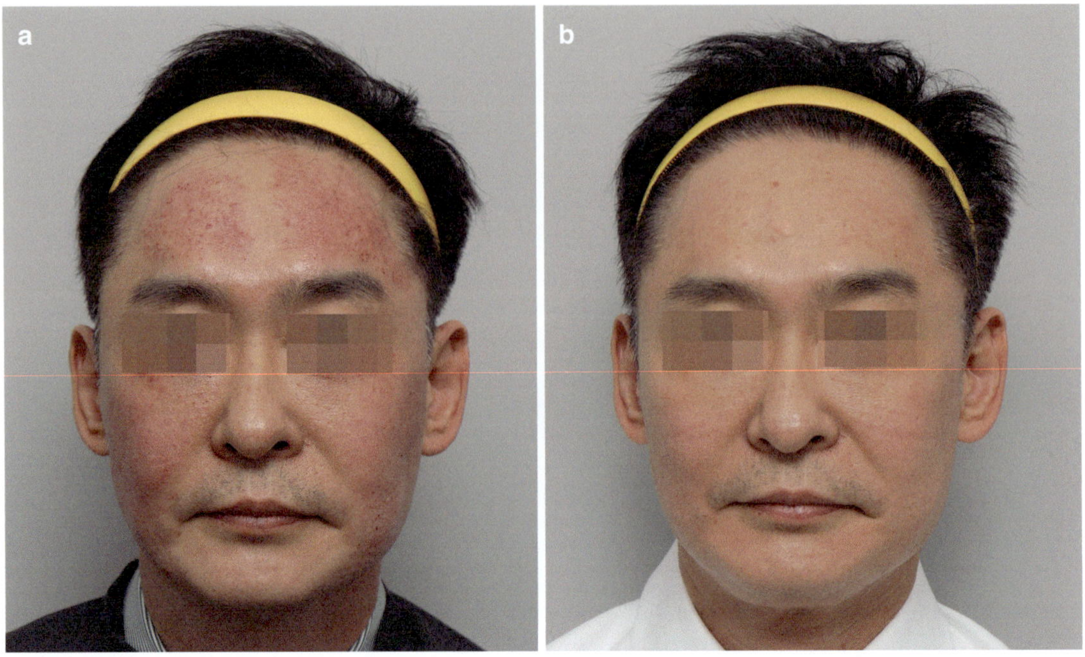

Fig. 4.138 Petechial bleeding (**a**). After treatment of Mirajet® needle-free injection (**b**) Injection marks cleared 5 days after the procedure

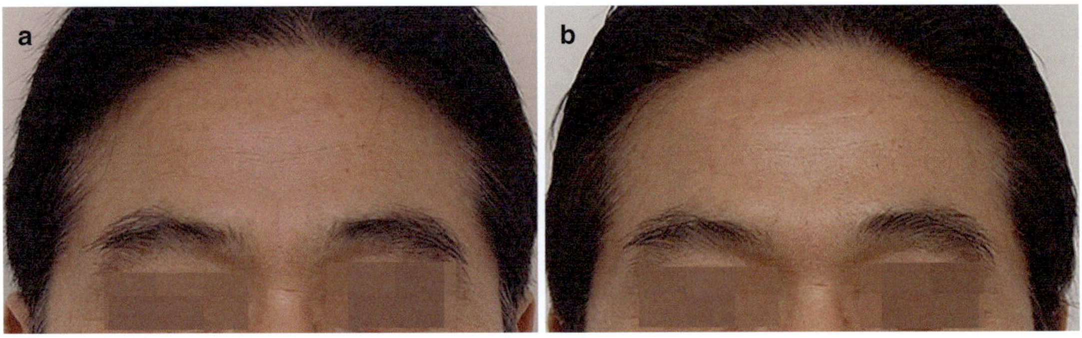

Fig. 4.139 Improvement of pores and static wrinkles in the forehead following intradermal botulinum toxin injection

the underlying mimetic muscles may cause unwanted alterations in facial expression.

4.20.6 Wrinkles Above the Knee

Wrinkling above (i.e., superior to) the knees in a standing position is due to the natural loss of skin elasticity with age and is particularly common in women with reduced body weight. When addressing these wrinkles with hydrolifting, it is important also to concomitantly restore the depletion of soft tissue surrounding the knee itself. At least 4–5 mL of HA is required per side for volumization (replacing lost volume in the knee), and 1–2 mL per side for hydrolifting purposes (Fig. 4.140).

4.20.7 Complications

Irregularity (Fig. 4.141), bruising, and pain are the most significant side effects of hydrolifting. While best efforts should be used to minimize such events, any surface irregularities remaining 2 weeks posttreatment should be dissolved away

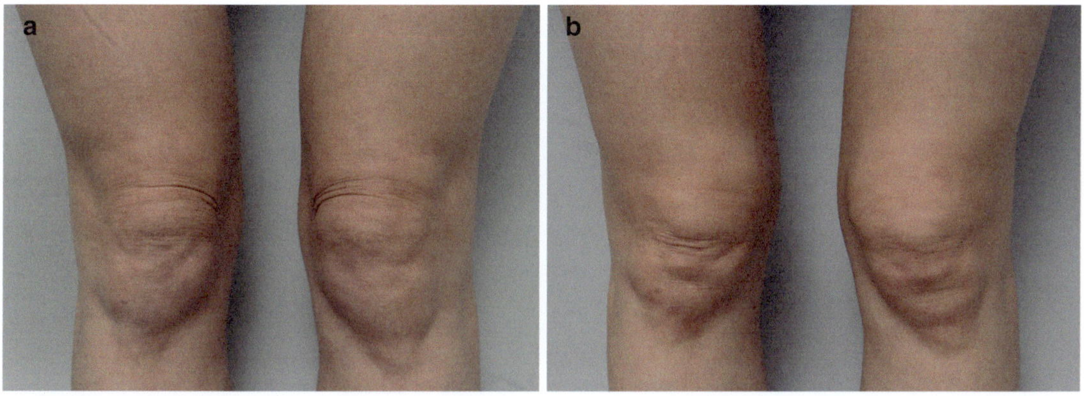

Fig. 4.140 (**a**) Before and (**b**) after, hydrolifting injections, the horizontal creases formed above the knees in a standing position are improved

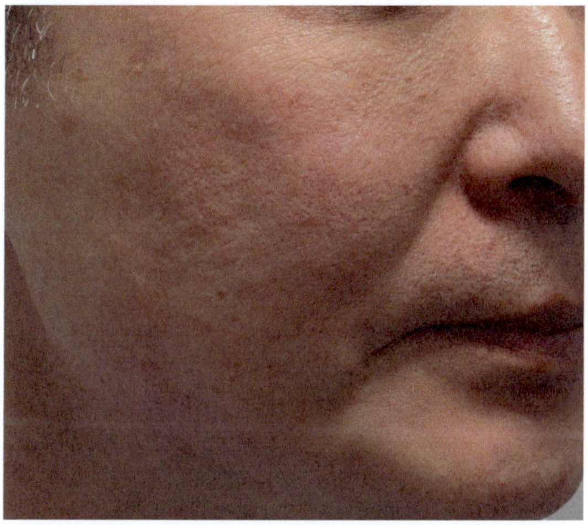

Fig. 4.141 Irregularity is the main complication of hydrolifting performed by manual technique

with hyaluronidase injections. For severe bruising, 2–3 sessions of vascular lasers such as V beam® can be used from the day following treatment to expedite a quick recovery.

References

1. Kim HJ, Seo KK, Lee HK, Kim JS. Clinical anatomy of face for botulinum toxin and filler injection. Berlin: Springer; 2016. p. 93–102.
2. Mariwalla K, Germain M. Forehead refalation. In: Carruthers J, Carruthers A, editors. Soft tissue augmentation. Philadelphia: Elsevier; 2018. p. 85–9.
3. Buso M, Howell DJ. Forehead contouring with calcium hydroxyapatite. Dermatol Surg. 2010;36(s3):1910–3.
4. Yu Chao YY, Chhabra C, Corduff N, Fabi SG, Hornfeldt CS, Kerscher M, Lam S, Pavicic T, Peng PHL, Pooth R, Rzany B, Seo K, Suwanchinda A, Tseng FW, Geister TL. Validation of a photonumeric assessment scale for grading the slope of the Asian forehead. Dermatol Surg. 2019;45(S1):S38–45.
5. Kim HJ, Seo KI, Lee HK, Kim JS. Clinical anatomy of face for botulinum toxin and filler injection. Berlin: Springer; 2016. p. 45–8.
6. Seo KK. Botulinum toxin for Asians. Singapore: Springer Nature Ltd.; 2017. p. 72–81.
7. Kim HJ, Seo KK, Lee HK, Kim JS. Clinical anatomy of face for botulinum toxin and filler injection. Berlin: Springer; 2016. p. 94–103.
8. Carruthers JDA, Carruthers JA. Volumizing the glabella and forehead. Dermatol Surg. 2010;36:1905–9.
9. Beleznay K, JDA C, Humphrey S, Jones D. Avoiding and treating blindness from fillers: a review of the world literature. Dermatol Surg. 2015;41:1097–117.
10. Flynn TC, Carruthers JDA, Carruthers JA. Botulinum toxin treatment of the lower eyelid improves infraorbital rhytides and widens the eye. Dermatol Surg. 2001;27(8):703–8.
11. Cong LY, Lee SH, Tansatit T, Hu KS, Kim HJ. Topographic anatomy of the inferior medial palpebral artery and its relevance to the pretarsal roll augmentation. Plast Reconstr Surg. 2016;138(3):430e–6e.
12. Humphrey S, Fagien S. Infraorbital hollow and nasojugal fold. In: Carruthers J, Carruthers A, editors. Soft tissue augmentation. Philadelphia: Elsevier; 2018. p. 107–13.
13. Kim HJ, Seo KK, Lee HK, Kim JS. Clinical anatomy of face for botulinum toxin and filler injection. Berlin: Springer; 2016. p. 120–4.
14. Kim HJ, Seo KK, Lee HK, Kim JS. Clinical anatomy of face for botulinum toxin and filler injection. Berlin: Springer; 2016. p. 124–8.
15. Kim HJ, Seo KI, Lee HK, Kim JS. Clinical anatomy of face for botulinum toxin and filler injection. Berlin: Springer; 2016. p. P37–41.

16. Almeida ART, Vieira Braz AV. Midfac. In: Carruthers J, Carruthers A, editors. Soft tissue augmentation. Philadelphia: Elsevier; 2018. p. 115–22.
17. Goodman GJ. Facial attractiveness and the central role of volume. In: Carruthers J, Carruthers A, editors. Soft tissue augmentation. Philadelphia: Elsevier. p; 2018. p. 7–15.
18. Sundaram H, Huang PH, Hsu NJ, Huh CH, Wu W, Wu Y, Cassuto D, Kerscher MJ, Seo KI, Pan-Asian Aesthetics Toxin Consensus Group. Aesthetic applications of botulinum toxin A in Asians: an international, multidisciplinary, pan-asian consensus. Plast Reconstr Surg Glob Open. 2016;4(12):e872.
19. Seo KK. Nose. In: Carruthers J, Carruthers A, editors. Soft tissue augmentation. Philadelphia: Elsevier; 2018. p. 123–33.
20. Youn SH, Seo KI. Filler rhinoplasty evaluated by anthropometric analysis. Dermatol Surg. 2016;42:1071–81.
21. Kim HJ, Seo KK, Lee HK, Kim JS. Nose. In: Clinical anatomy of face for botulinum toxin and filler injection. Berlin: Springer; 2016. p. 139–52.
22. Casabona G. Blood aspiration test for cosmetic fillers to prevent accidental intravascular injection in the face. Dermatol Surg. 2015;41(7):841–7.
23. DeLorenzi C. Complications of injectable fillers, part 2: vascular complications. Aesthet Surg J. 2014;34(4):584–600.
24. Kim HJ, Seo KK, Lee HK, Kim JS. Hollow cheek. In: Clinical anatomy of face for botulinum toxin and filler injection. Berlin: Springer; 2016. p. 135–8.
25. Kim HJ, Seo KK, Lee HK, Kim JS. Subzygoma depression. In: Clinical anatomy of face for botulinum toxin and filler injection. Berlin: Springer; 2016. p. 138–9.
26. Seo KK. Botulinum toxin for Asians. Singapore: Springer Nature Ltd.; 2017. p. 87–91.
27. Kim HJ, Seo KK, Lee HK, Kim JS. Nasolabial fold. In: Clinical anatomy of face for botulinum toxin and filler injection. Berlin: Springer; 2016. p. 128–35.
28. Jones IT, FabiS G, Carruthers J. Lip augmentation. In: Carruthers J, Carruthers A, editors. Soft tissue augmentation. Philadelphia: Elsevier; 2018. p. 141–7.
29. Kim HJ, Seo KK, Lee HK, Kim JS. Lip. In: Clinical anatomy of face for botulinum toxin and filler injection. Berlin: Springer; 2016. p. 154–60.
30. Lee KL, Lee HJ, Youn KH, Kim HJ. Positional relationship of superior and inferior labial artery by ultrasonography image analysis for safe lip augmentation procedures. Clin Anat. 2019;2:45–64.
31. Heidekrueger PI, Szpalski C, Weichman K, Juran S, Ng R, Claussen C, Ninkovic M, Broer PN. Lip attractiveness: a cross-cultural analysis. Aesthet Surg J. 2017;37(7):828–36.
32. Kim HJ, Seo KK, Lee HK, Kim JS. Marionette line and jowl. In: Clinical anatomy of face for botulinum toxin and filler injection. Berlin: Springer; 2016. p. 166–9.
33. Seo KK. Botulinum toxin for Asians. Singapore: Springer Nature Ltd.; 2017. p. 93–7.
34. Yu SK, Lee MH, Kim HS, Park JT, Kim HJ. Histomorphologic approach for the modiolus with reference to reconstructive and aesthetic surgery. J Craniofac Surg. 2013;24(4):1414–7.
35. Kim HJ, Seo KK, Lee HK, Kim JS. Chin. In: Clinical anatomy of face for botulinum toxin and filler injection. Berlin: Springer; 2016. p. 160–5.
36. Koh KS, Han SH, Shin KJ, Kim HJ. Sex determination using nonmetric characteristics of the mandible in Koreans. J Forensic Sci. 2006;51(6):1376–82.
37. Naini FB. The chin. In: Facial aesthetics, concepts and clinical diagnosis. Oxford: Blackwell; 2011. p. 312–34.
38. Geraghty LN. Earlobe rejuvenation. In: Carruthers J, Carruthers A, editors. Soft tissue augmentation. Philadelphia: Elsevier; 2018. p. 169–73.
39. Sivek R, Emer J. Use of a blunt-tipped microcannula for soft tissue filler injection in the treatment of linear scleroderma (en coup de sabre). Dermatol Surg. 2014;40(12):1439–41.
40. Pirrello R, Verro B, Grasso G, Ruscitti P, Cordova A, Giacomelli R, Ciccia F, Guggino G. Hyaluronic acid and platelet-rich plasma, a new therapeutic alternative for scleroderma patients: a prospective open-label study. Arthritis Res Ther. 2019;21(1):286.
41. Mashiko T, Mori H, Kato H, Doi K, Kuno S, Kinoshita K, Kunimatsu A, Ohtomo K, Yoshimura K. Semipermanent volumization by an absorbable filler: onlay injection technique to the bone. Plast Reconstr Surg Glob Open. 2013;1(1):e4–e14.
42. Pluijmers BI, van de Lande LS, Caron CJJM, Wolvius EB, Dunaway DJ, Padwa BL, Koudstaal MJ. Part 2: Is the maxillary canting and its surgical correction in patients with CFM correlated to the mandibular deformity? J Craniomaxillofac Surg. 2018;46(9):1436–40.
43. de la Iglesia F, Lopez A, Mareque J, Gutierrez J, Walter A, Puigdollers A. Correction of mandibular deviation and maxillary occlusal canting with mandibular "early" surgery and microscrews: two case reports. Int Orthod. 2019;17(2):384–94.
44. Chalala C, Ghafari JG. Differentiation between maxillary and malar midface position within the facial profile. PeerJ. 2019;7:e8200.
45. Distante F. Rejuvenation influence of a stabilized hyaluronic acid-based gel of nonanimal origin on facial skin aging. Dermatol Surg. 2008;34:720–6.
46. Bae GY. Rheological properties. Filler Toxin. 2016;2(4):15–9.
47. Wilson MV, Fabi SG, Dayan SH. Neck and chest. In: Carruthers J, Carruthers A, editors. Soft tissue augmentation. Philadelphia: Elsevier; 2018. p. 157–60.
48. Landau M, Fagien S. Science of hyaluronic acid beyond filling: fibroblasts and their response to the extracellular matrix. Plast Reconstr Surg. 2015;136(5 Suppl):188s–95s.
49. Wang F, Garza LA, Kang S, Varani J, Orringer JS, Fisher GJ, Voorhees JJ. In vivo stimulation of de novo collagen production caused by cross-linked hyaluronic acid dermal filler injections in photodamaged human skin. Arch Dermatol. 2007;143(2):155–6.
50. Kerscher M, et al. Rejuvenation influence of a stabilized hyaluronic acid-based gel of nonanimal origin on facial skin aging. Dermatol Surg. 2008;34:720–6.

5 Complications

5.1 Vascular Complication

5.1.1 Symptoms

Vascular compromise is the most serious complication associated with filler injection. The causes of vascular compromise are largely two-fold, that is, vascular embolization from inadvertent injection of product directly into the blood supply (i.e., intravascular injection) and vascular insufficiency resulting from external compression by the injected filler material (i.e., extravascular compression) [1]. Extreme care must be taken to avoid vascular occlusion due to intravascular injection as it may bring about skin necrosis and rare incidences of blindness in the most disastrous case. Vascular occlusion typically presents with ischemic color changes such as immediate postinjection blanching or violaceous or greyish skin discoloration occurring 20–30 min of the HA filler injection, for which timely and adequate treatment must be administered (Fig. 5.1) [2, 3]. If left unaddressed, multiple reticular erythematous patches may develop the following day across the nasal dorsum, glabella, and forehead, accompanied by epidermal sloughing and multiple pustules in severe cases. In the extreme, the pustules may progress to skin necrosis accompanied by scab formation (Fig. 4.73).

Vascular complications following the injection of nose fillers are more likely to occur in patients whose vascular circulation has already been modified or compromised by a previous nose surgery, or whose blood vessels have been adhered to the scar tissue in the operated area [3, 4]. Note that vessels trapped inside scar tissue adhesions become easy targets for penetration during filler volumization and are substantially more vulnerable to the risk of intravascular filler injection. Extra care must therefore be taken when treating a patient with a history of a previous nose surgery or removal of the nasal implant.

5.1.2 Prevention

To minimize the risk of vascular occlusion, it is essential for practitioners to be equipped with the knowledge of the underlying anatomy at the injection site, especially regarding the vascular supply, and to strictly adhere to the relevant preventative strategies. However, even with the best knowledge of the facial anatomy and the anatomical hotspots to avoid, the risk for vascular complications nonetheless persists as the vascular supply beneath the skin surface is largely hidden from view. Moreover, individual variations exist in vascular distribution patterns. As a key prevention strategy against vascular embolization, therefore, it is highly recommended that a cannula be used instead of a needle for facial volumization with fillers. That said, precaution is still required even with the use of cannulas as small-diameter cannulas remain capable of piercing through a vessel. To optimize safety during filler administration, the use of cannulas sized 25 or

K. K. Seo, *Facial Volumization with Fillers*, https://doi.org/10.1007/978-981-33-6212-3_5

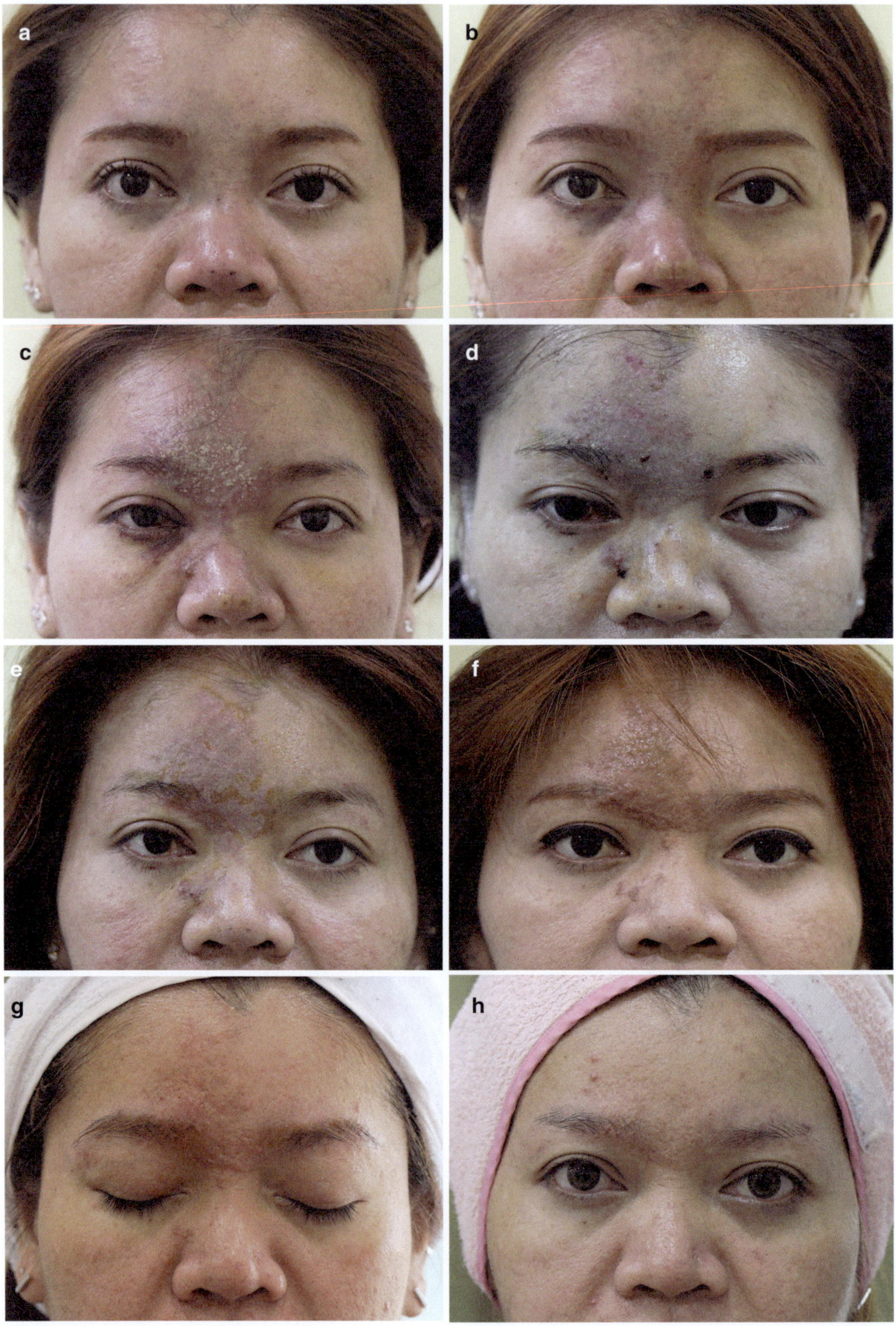
a
b
c
d
e
f
g
h

Fig. 5.1 Case of vascular complication after nose filler which was immediately and successfully treated with hyaluronidase injection. (**a**) Day 1. a 35-year-old woman showed blanching, violaceous or greyish skin discoloration on the dorsum of nose 20–30 minutes after nasal dorsum augmentation using HA filler and a 30G needle. Her nose was immediately injected with hyaluronidase. (**b**) Day 2. Multiple reticular erythematous patches developed across the nasal dorsum, glabella and forehead. Bruising due to injection of hyaluronidase developed in the right lower eyelid and sclera. (**c**) Day 4. Multiple tiny pustules developed in the leseion. (**d**) Day 7. Epidermal sloughing and crust developed in the leseion. (**e**) Day 10. Yellowish crust and erosion still remained. (**f**) 1 Month. The wound healed with surface irregularities and hyperpigmentation on the erythematous base. (**g**) 3 Months. Mild erythematous patches with mild depressed scars still remained. (**h**) 7 Months. The lesions completely resolved without any seqaule. (Photo: Courtesy of Dr. Kim Sang-Yeon)

larger, gentle maneuvering of the instrument, and slow, low pressure injection using the retrograde linear technique are advised wherever feasible to mitigate the risk of intravascular filler injection.

Where the use of a needle is inevitable, it is essential to make sure the injection is made into a relatively avascular plane. For example, when performing reshaping of the nose with a needle, injection should preferably be limited to the nasal radix where deep injection directly onto the periosteum is advised as the vasculature at the upper nasal dorsum runs superficially close to the skin surface (see Sect. 4.9.13). In the case of forehead augmentation, the supraperiosteal layer is a safe avascular zone for the same reason. In addition, aspiration prior to each injection is required when injecting with a needle to ensure the needle tip is not placed in a blood vessel. Note, however, that the results of blood aspiration tests are not necessarily failproof as the test may produce false negatives, especially where the injection was performed using gel-type HA fillers or small diameter needles (see Sect. 4.9.13).

Practitioners should pay close attention to any ischemic color changes occurring during or immediately after filler injection that alert them to a possible vascular occlusion, in which case timely and adequate intervention including injection of hyaluronidase in and around the lesion is required. Of the five cases of vascular occlusions from filler rhinoplasty encountered by the author, the event went unnoticed during the treatment in three cases, and it was not until the next day that mottled erythematic patches began appearing on the patient's face, which took approximately 1 month to fully disappear without severe sequelae. Since then, it has been the author's policy to have the patient remaining in the office for 30 mins after nose filler injections to ensure early detection of any ischemic skin changes. Patients are also advised to immediately revert back to the clinic upon noticing any violaceous changes in the skin occurring within 1–2 h of their departure. Finally, one cannot overstate the value of using reversible HA fillers to guard against unexpected events of vascular occlusion occurring even with the best preventative procedures in place. Specifically, HA should be the preferred choice for treating the high-risk areas for vascular occlusion including the nose, glabella, nasolabial fold, and forehead (Table 5.1).

5.1.3 Treatment

In the event of vascular embolization due to intravascular filler injection or vascular insufficiency from external compression of weak vessels by the surrounding HA filler, the injected HA must be dissolved away immediately with hyaluronidase. While it is next to impossible to inject hyaluronidase into the precise location in the vessel where the occlusion is present, it has been postulated by De Lorenzi et al. that hyaluronidase infused in sufficient amounts generally around the area where the ischemic symptoms are present may effectively traverse and diffuse *across* the arterial wall to reach the hyaluronic acid held

Table 5.1 Prevention and management of vascular complication from filler injection

Prevention	Management
1. Thorough knowledge of the facial anatomy, especially facial vessels 2. Routine use of HA filler 3. Routine use of cannulas 25-gauge or larger 4. Routine aspiration prior to injection when needle is used 5. Injection into the avascular plane such as deep supraperiosteal layer of forehead and nasal radix when needle is used 6. Retrograde injection technique 7. Slower injection speed with lower pressure 8. Smooth progression of the cannula 9. Extra precaution when treating patients with a previous record of surgical procedure in the area	1. Hyaluronidase injection subcutaneously in large amounts (3–6 mL) at a high concentration (750 U/mL) into the lesion and the adjacent area for HA fillers. Immediate retrobulbar administration of hyaluronidase in large volumes (>4500–6000 U) and high concentrations (1500 U/mL) can help counteract the risk of permanent blindness. 2. Application of topical nitroglycerine 3. Sublingual nitroglycerin 4. PO sildenafil or tadalafil 5. PO aspirin (100 mg) 6. PO steroid 7. PO antibiotics 8. Warm massage 9. Hyperbaric oxygen treatment if available.

in the blood vessel [4]. Hence, in order to resolve occlusions of hyaluronic acid fillers it is advised to infiltrate hyaluronidase subcutaneously in copious amounts (3–6 mL) at a high concentration (750 U/mL) around the tissue where ischemic symptoms such as blanching, greyish decolorization, or mottled erythema are suspected (see Sect. 5.4).

The effective timing of hyaluronidase injection for such vascular events is within 24 hours of HA filler injection. This is also backed up by the findings of an animal study in which vascular occlusion was induced in rabbit ears using HA filler, to which hyaluronidase was subsequently injected at different intervals [5]. While hyaluronidase injected within 4 h was beneficial in clearing the occlusion, it had little effect after 24 h. Accordingly, patients demonstrating even the slightest signs of ischemia should be observed for 20–30 min in the office for any further development of symptoms. Progression of symptoms calls for immediate injection of hyaluronidase. Regardless, even after the 24-hour window, there may still be some value to giving hyaluronidase injections as a placebo for the patient and as protection for the practitioner from the legal consequences of denying such intervention. Apart from the administration of hyaluronidase, sublingual nitroglycerin tablets administered twice at 30 min intervals (i.e., two tablets given 30 min apart) together with oral aspirin and sildenafil (or tadaifil) is necessary to facilitate systemic blood circulation. Intramuscular injection of steroids such as dexamethasone is also recommended for reducing inflammatory reaction while antibiotic administration is advised to prevent secondary infection.

In case the patient presents to the clinic after the golden hour of treatment (i.e., the first 24 h) has passed, presenting with severe symptoms including multiple pustules, skin necrosis, and crust formation, all of the aforementioned treatment modalities, including hyaluronidase injection, should be applied in tandem, except for oral nitroglycerin which should be given only during the acute phase. The use of hyperbaric oxygen treatment (HBO) is also advisable, where applicable, for treating peripheral ischemic symptoms [2] (Table 5.1). Concurrent injection of PRP (platelet-rich plasma), stem cell extracts, or placenta extract once daily during the first week, twice weekly during the first month, and once weekly thereafter for 3 months can also be helpful combined with EGF (epidermal growth factor) spray or ointment (Fig. 4.73). Bleaching treatment such as laser toning using Nd:YAG laser is recommended combined with bleaching topical agents such as hydroquinone in the case of postinflammatory hyperpigmentation. Vascular lasers such as V-beam would be helpful for the treatment of erythematous lesions after the crust has been removed, with fractional laser for the scar tissue.

5.1.4 Cause and Treatment of Blindness Following HA Filler Injection

Occlusion of facial arteries due to intra-arterial injection of HA filler can lead to the serious complication of skin necrosis. Inadvertent entry of the product into branches of the ophthalmic a. including the supratrochlear a., supraorbital a., and dorsal nasal a., however, can lead to the instantaneous and catastrophic consequence of visual loss. Blindness secondary to filler injection is caused by the backflow of the filler embolus from the above arterial branches into the ophthalmic a., from which the material is pushed down by the arterial pressure into the central retinal a. and posterior ciliary a. which supply the retina, resulting in retinal embolism [6, 7] (Fig. 5.2). According to the literature review by Beleznay et al. regarding cases of blindness following filler injection, the risk of blindness from filler was the highest at the glabella (38.8%), followed by the nasal region (25.5%), nasolabial folds (13.3%), and forehead (12.2%) [6]. By filler type, autologous fat (47.9%) was the most common cause followed by hyaluronic acid (23.5%) [6]. In 23.5% of the cases, blindness was also accompanied by incidence of central nervous system complications caused by the introduction of the filler material into the cerebral circulation.

As noted, various facial regions commonly injected with fillers can serve as unintended pathways to vision loss if not become targets of localized vascular occlusion. For example, HA filler placed in the glabella and forehead and accidentally entering the supratrochlear a. or supraorbital a. may flow retrograde into the ophthalmic a. and obstruct blood supply to the retina. Likewise, HA filler injected in the nose or nasolabial folds may also be transported up to the ophthalmic a. via the rich anastomoses present between the dorsal nasal a. (as a direct branch of the ophthalmic a.) and the various branches of the facial a. such as the angular a. and lateral nasal a.

Blindness has been found to occur even from HA filler injection in the lips and the chin. The mechanism may best be explained by the reverse flow of the HA filler emboli from either the inferior and/or superior labial a. back into the facial a. after which the material is sent traveling up the branches of the facial a. and into their interconnections with the dorsal nasal a. which joins into the ophthalmic a. Meanwhile, HA filler inadvertently injected into the inferior medial palpebral artery (IMPA) running parallel to the lower eyelash during pretarsal roll augmentation can also cause vision loss since the IMPA constitutes a branch of the ophthalmic a [1]. Rare cases of blindness have also been reported following temple enhancement with HA filler [6]. Presumably, this is caused by the retrograde flow of HA filler from the deep temporal a. into the maxillary a. and its subsequent delivery into the infraorbital branch of the maxillary a. which communicates with the dorsal nasal and inferior palpebral branches of the ophthalmic a.

Arterial occlusion of the retina presents with immediate impairment of vision and acute pain in the eyes. As of yet, no treatment has proven to be entirely successful in restoring patients from filler–related blindness except for retrobulbar hyaluronidase injection [8–11]. According to Zhu et al. [9], even retrobulbar hyaluronidase injection has been shown to lack efficacy as a rescue treatment for patients with HA filler-induced vision loss, despite being the most novel treatment protocol so far. However, one possible counterargument might be that such findings stem from the untimely implementation of the retrobulbar technique, that is, *after* the critical golden hour for the treatment had elapsed. Indeed, in an animal study involving monkeys, the critical window of opportunity for restoring retinal function was found to be within 97 min of clamping of the central retinal a., with irreversible blindness occurring after 4 h of the clamp down and blockage of the blood supply.

On the contrary, Lee et al. [11] have found in their recent animal study that retrobulbar hyaluronidase injection administered in high doses and concentrations within minimum time was effective in dissolving the HA filler emboli from the central retinal a. in rabbit eyes. Specifically, three out of four rabbit eyes with an occluded central retinal a. achieved immediate arterial

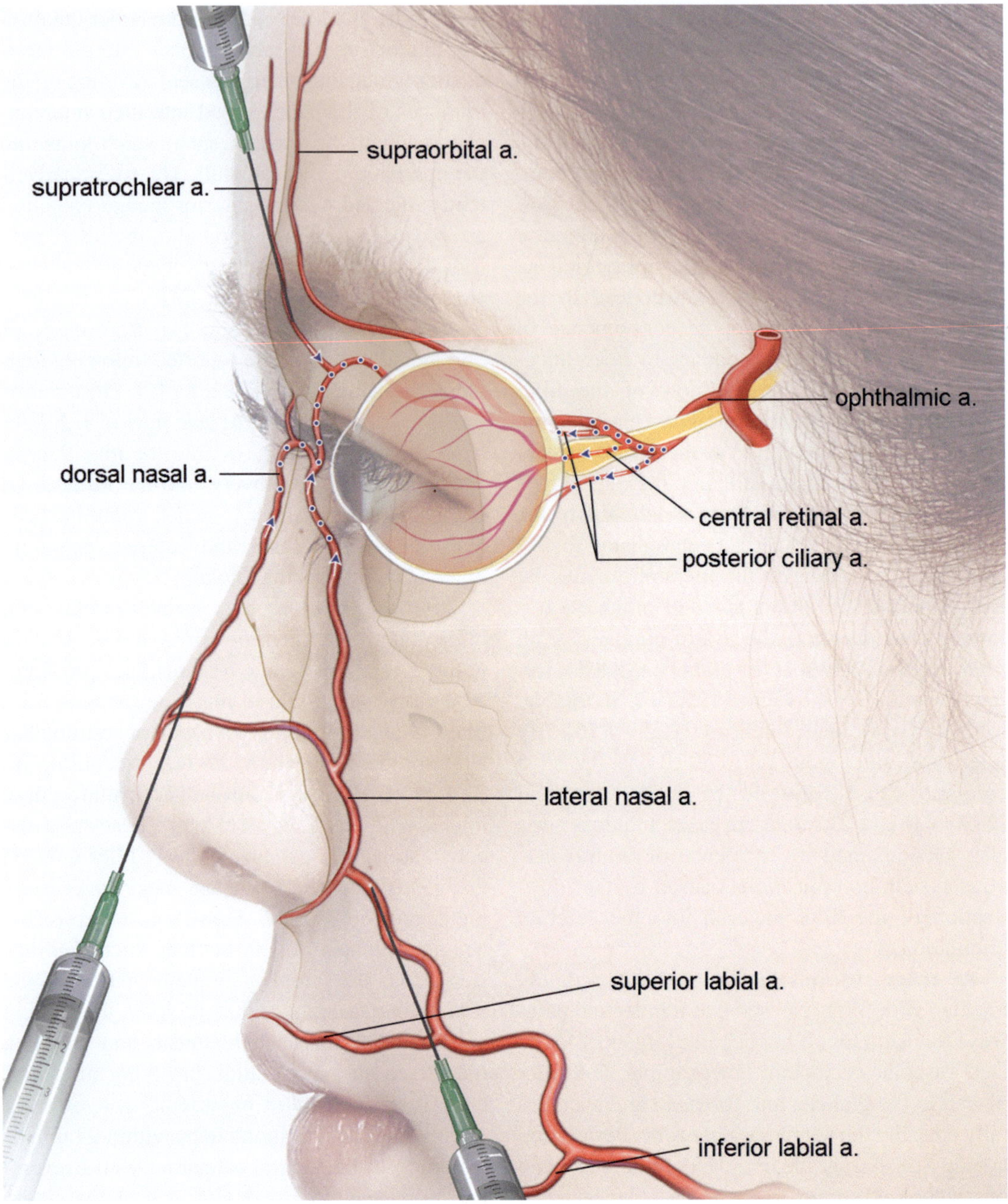

Fig. 5.2 Blindness secondary to filler injection is caused by the backflow of the filler embolus from the supratrochlear a., supraorbital a. and dorsal nasal a. into the ophthalmic a., from which the material is pushed down by the arterial pressure into the central retinal a. and posterior ciliary a. which supply the retina, resulting in retinal embolism

recanalization upon retrobulbar injection of 3000 U (2 mL) of hyaluronidase within 10 min of the onset of the arterial occlusion.

From this, it may be surmised that hyaluronidase infiltrated in high doses and high concentrations may diffuse effectively across the walls of the ophthalmic/central retinal arteries to dissolve the HA filler held in the blood vessels. Such findings suggest that, if vision loss is suspected, immediate retrobulbar administration of hyaluronidase in large volumes (>4500–6000 U) and high concentrations (1500 U/mL) can help counteract the risk of permanent blindness. To prevent injury to the eyeball, a 27G 3 cm cannula or blunt tip needle (Atkinson needle) should be used to perform the retrobulbar injection of hyaluronidase, with the cannula inserted through the inferior eyelid and advanced to the back of the eye parallel to the orbital floor. The cannula entry point is created where a vertical line drawn from the lateral canthus meets the bony orbital rim (Fig. 5.3). To avoid

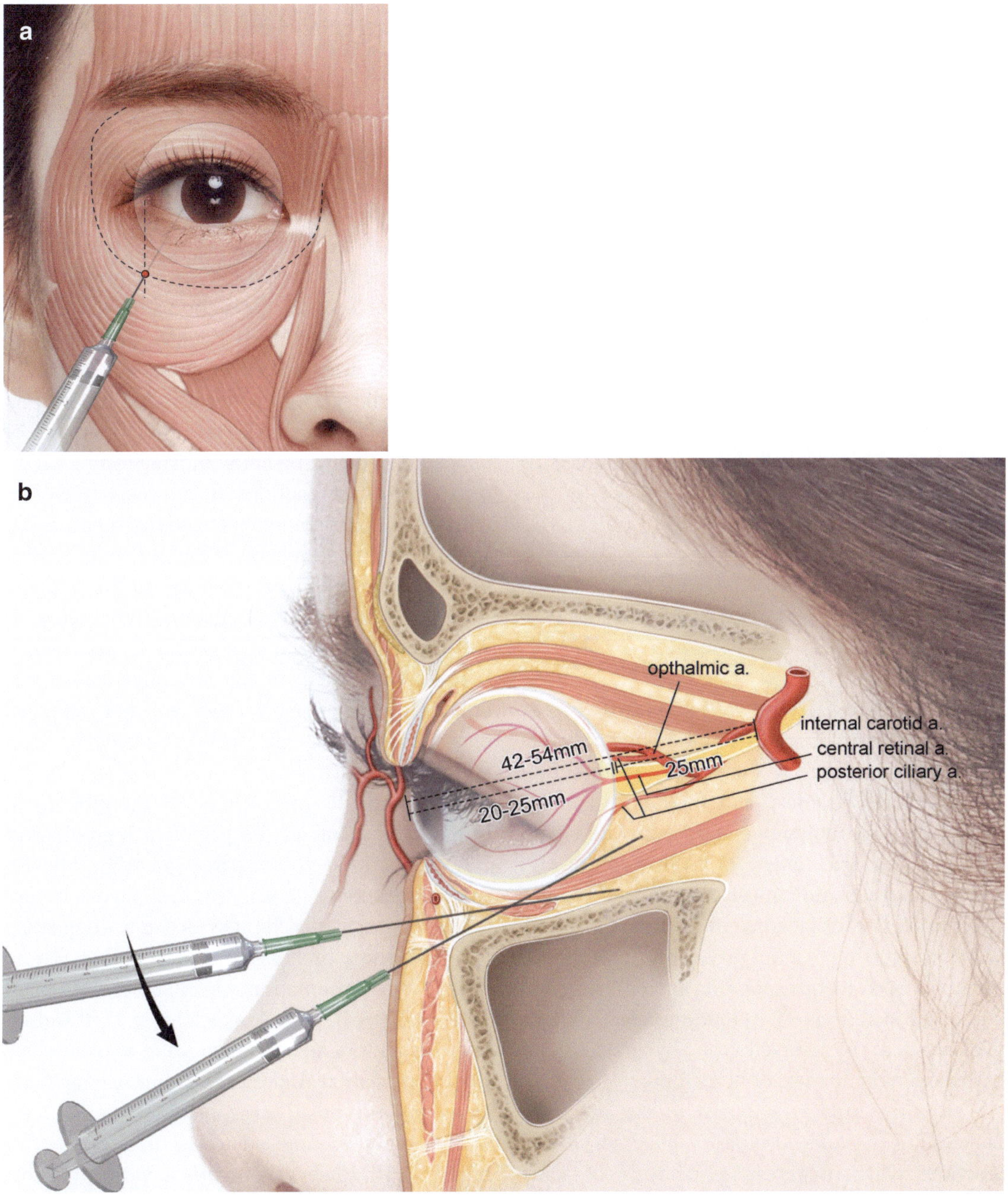

Fig. 5.3 Technique for retrobulbar injection of hyaluronidase. (**a**) The cannula entry point is created where a vertical line drawn from the lateral canthus meets the bony orbital rim. (**b**) To avoid injury to the eyeball, the cannula should be inserted in an inferomedial direction 2 cm into the orbital floor, after which it should be redirected superiorly and advanced for an additional 1 cm before hyaluronidase is injected

injury to the eyeball, the cannula should be inserted in an inferomedial direction 2 cm into the orbital floor, after which it should be redirected superiorly and advanced for an additional 1 cm before hyaluronidase is injected [12]. However, it must be noted that this technique carries the risk of retrobulbar hemorrhage in rare cases. Another option for placement of hyaluronidase into the extraocular muscle cone is performing a Sub-Tenon's block. This technique requires first making a small opening in the conjuctiva and then another opeing in the Tenon's layer using Wescott scissors and toothed forceps. The Wescott scissors are then used to bluntly dissect into the retrobulbar space, or the sub-Tenon's plane. Next hyaluronidase is delivered via a blunt cannula into the muscle cone [13]. Retrobulbar injection of hyaluronidase must be administered immediately upon presentation of symptoms as the critical window of treatment is 7 mins and irreversible blindness begins occurring after 4 h. In case the first injection yields no results, reinjection of hyaluronidase may be attempted 10 mins. later.

5.2 Inflammation from Delayed-Type Hypersensitivity to HA Filler

Hyaluronic acid (HA) is well-suited for use as injectable filler as it consists of the same polysaccharides that constitute our body and therefore has an excellent safety and tolerability profile with minimum immunogenicity compared with protein-based injectables. For this reason, HA represents the world's most widely used type of injectable filler for facial volumization. However, with the surge in HA filler procedures performed, there has been a corresponding increase, though still rare, in reports of immune-related adverse events such as delayed-type hypersensitivity associated with the use of H A fillers.

Currently, little is reported in the literature concerning delayed-type hypersensitivity reactions which manifest in the form of acute inflammation, symptoms of which include swelling, tenderness, or local heating distinct from granuloma formation. Further, due to its apparent overlap in symptoms with inflammation from infection, delayed-type hypersensitivity is often incorrectly diagnosed and treated as an infectious reaction. However, it is important for the injecting physician to be able to identify and distinguish inflammation from delayed-type hypersensitivity from an infection as it can be treated effectively with the use of steroid alone without implicating the use of antibiotics.

5.2.1 Cause of Delayed-Type Hypersensitivity Following HA Injection

According to the Gell and Coombs classification, delayed-type hypersensitivity is categorized as a type IV hypersensitivity reaction which is defined as an antibody-independent cell-mediated immune memory response [14]. It is initiated when a memory T cell previously activated by an antigen releases various cytokines upon repeat exposure to the same antigen, triggering a plethora of late-onset reactions. In contrast to the other antibody-dependent hypersensitivity types (I–III) in which immune reactions kick off within minutes or hours upon presentation to the antigen, type IV hypersensitivity reactions characteristically start after a delay of 48–72 h. Exactly which specific component of the HA filler causes this delayed-type hypersensitivity has not yet been clearly identified, and may conceivably vary from case to case.

According to one school of thought, hyaluronic acid itself, as the principal ingredient of HA fillers, may be capable of triggering an immune response [3, 15, 16]. This theory is supported, in particular, by a prior study suggesting the possibility of low-molecular-weight HA to induce the presentation of inflammatory cytokines such as IL (interleukin)-12 or TNF (tumor necrosis factor)-alpha, which serve to exacerbate the inflammation. Indeed, HA skin testing occasionally yields positive responses, while HA antibodies are sometimes detected in the patient's blood. [16] However, perhaps a more plausible explanation involves the presence of trace impurities not entirely removed during the HA filler manufacturing process [17]. These include residual bacterial protein, DNA or the cell organelle, bacterial endotoxin, or any lingering amounts of the cross-linking agents (BDDE) in the final product. Most of the commercially available HA fillers are manufactured through the process of extraction and purification of HA from bacteria, that is, streptococcus, and may contain trace quantities of bacterial impurities such as protein, DNA, cell organelle, or endotoxin. HA is classified as food grade, cosmetic grade, or medical grade which is further subclassified as those licensed for use as ophthalmic agents or as injectable preparations, depending on the stringency of the purification performed [16]. In each case, market authorization is granted upon the product satisfying the *minimum* regulatory standard, which is also the case for the licensing of medical-grade HA. [17] HA purification is a costly process requiring a hefty investment of time, resources, and CAPEX on the part of the manufacturer. The sheer cost burden, combined with the minuscule incidence of delayed-type hypersensitivity reactions associated with the product, may disincentivize manufacturers from committing additional resources solely for the purpose of minimizing bacterial impurities. This naturally explains the varying incidence of inflammation from delayed hypersensitivity in different HA filler products. Meanwhile, the cross-linking agent BDDE may also play a role in causing inflammation from delayed-type hypersensitivity. In this respect, it bears noting that delayed-type hypersensitivity has also been found to occur in the recently launched longer lasting HA products which incorporate a higher degree of cross-linking or higher BDDE content to boost longevity.

While the exact cause of delayed type hypersensitivity to HA remains largely open to debate, in the author's view, residual bacterial impurities not fully removed during purification appear to be the primary culprit. In my practice, I have found cases where a patient with a history of delayed inflammation to one HA filler brand was treated uneventfully with a different brand of HA filler. I have also anecdotally observed cases where a patient who had been injected with two different types of HA filler respectively in two different facial areas developed hypersensitivity reactions subsequently in only the area injected with a particular HA filler. On top of this, there has been cases, though rare, of continued recurrence of inflammatory reactions even after the full dissolution of the underlying HA filler several months prior. Together, these cases point to the likelihood of residual bacterial impurities being the more likely root cause of delayed type hypersensitivity than the HA itself.

5.2.2 Symptoms

5.2.2.1 Case

A 26-year-old female patient presented complaining of swelling and induration in her left medial malar, which had occurred since the previous day (Fig. 5.4a). She had previously received 2 cc of HA injection in each medial malar 8 weeks prior. There had been no subsequent history of trauma or the use of injectables or surgery in the relevant site, except for the patient returning from a trip 1 week prior, after which she reportedly experienced some degree of fatigue. Upon physical examination, the presence of erythematous swelling, induration, and mid tenderness were noted in the area. An intramuscular injection of 5 mg of Dexamethasone was administered together with oral prednisolone 20 mg/day for 2 days. Rapid recovery was achieved with no relapse thereafter.

Illustrated above is a classic case of an inflammatory reaction from delayed-type hypersensitivity following HA injection. Clinical symptoms generally include swelling, induration, erythema, localized heat, and pain or tenderness in the treated area, though in mild cases, only swelling and induration may be present. Occasionally, eczema seborrheicum, lupus erythematosus or other forms of dermatitis of the face unrelated to HA injection may be confused as inflammation from delayed-type hypersensitivity since the former symptomatically displays erythema and localized heat as well. However, delayed-type hypersensitivity cannot be diagnosed simply based on the presence of erythema and localized warmth alone. Instead, swelling and induration must be identified as they are present even in mild cases of delayed-type hypersensitivity hence serving as more reliable indicators.

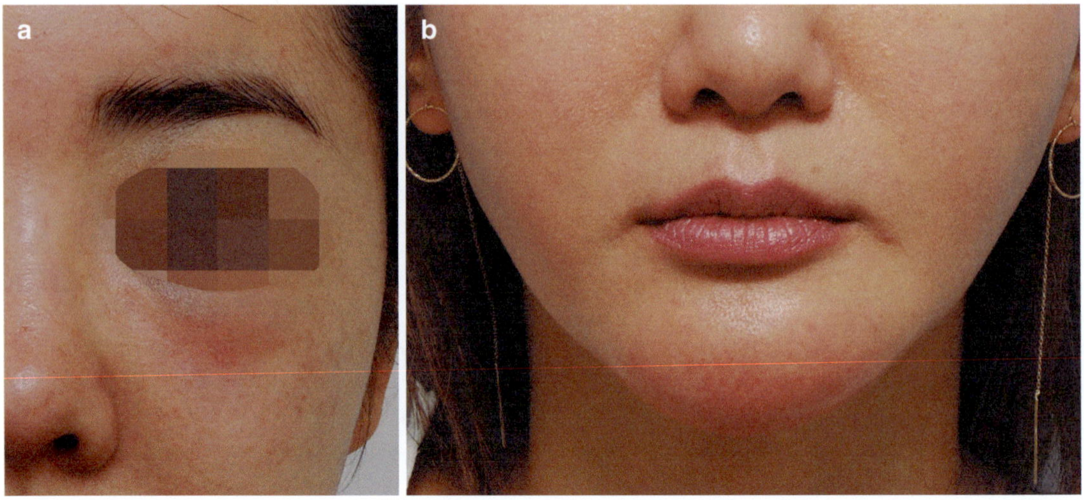

Fig. 5.4 Cases of inflammation from a delayed-type hypersensitivity reaction to HA filler. (**a**) The tender erythematous swelling with induration developed in the right cheek 8 weeks post-injection in a 26-year-old female patient injected with Restylane® SubQ to address hollowness in the bilateral infraorbital and anterior medial malar regions. (**b**) A 36-year-old female patient injected with Neuramis® Volume for the chin augmentation developed tender erythematous swelling in the chin 16 month post-injection

Concerning the timing of onset, a wide variation exists among published reports, ranging from 1 month postinjection to as long as 3 years postinjection [17]. Contrary to acute inflammatory reactions due to infection which typically occur within 2–3 days of HA filler injection, inflammation from delayed-type hypersensitivity starts 2–4 weeks postprocedure at the earliest and may occur even as late as 16 months postprocedure based on the author's clinical experience.

Incidence of inflammation from delayed-type hypersensitivity varies by product. Based on the literature review, the prevalence of immune-mediated reactions following HA injections was found to vary, from 0.8% in one study, of which 0.3% represented delayed hypersensitivity to 0.04–0.7% in a European study [16]. However, these numbers do not pertain squarely to the prevalence of delayed inflammation from delayed-type hypersensitivity to HA filler as they also cover cases of delayed granuloma due to delayed-type hypersensitivity.

The incidence of inflammation from delayed-type hypersensitivity in the HA products used in the author's own practice at Modelo Clinic is less than 0.3%. On a related note, a local HA product is known to have been voluntarily withdrawn from the market shortly following its release due to the high incidence (>10%) of delayed-type hypersensitivity inflammatory reactions. While less than 0.3% may seem negligible numbers-wise, understanding that it can be deeply distressing for the individual patient going through the symptoms, it may be worthwhile to alert them to this risk during consultation as the patient may assume the reaction to be the result of faulty filler placement. Personally, my preferred product to use in patients visiting from abroad or outside of Seoul is Belotero® (Merz), given its minimal incidence of delayed-type hypersensitivity reactions. That being said, I have observed cases of inflammatory reactions from delayed-type hypersensitivity even with the use of Belotero® Volume, while Restylane® SubQ in the same patient had proven to be uneventful. In other cases, the patient responded unfavorably to both products.

While the exact etiology of inflammation from delayed hypersensitivity to HA remains unclear, more than half of the patients who eventually developed hypersensitivity reactions in my practice reported of having undergone a certain stressful event such as a flu, long-distance trip abroad, or working late hours prior to the outbreak, which may possibly have primed their body's immune response. Indeed, according to one study, approximately 40% of delayed-onset granuloma following Juvederm® Voluma injection was found to have been accompanied by a trigger, such as a cold or a dental procedure, which may have disrupted the patients' immune system. While together these cases suggest a higher likelihood of inflammatory reaction from delayed-type hypersensitivity during a state of reduced immunity, they fall short of establishing a clear causation given that delayed-type hypersensitivity also occurred in the absence of a trigger.

In 2/3 of cases based on the author's experience, inflammation from delayed hypersensitivity is a one-off event with no recurrence of symptoms thereafter. However, in the remaining 1/3 of the affected patients, a relapse has been found to occur 1–4 weeks after the initial resolution of symptoms. In extremely rare cases, however, the patient may experience similar symptoms even after the HA filler had been fully dissolved with hyaluronidase.

5.2.3 Differential Diagnosis

An important distinction should be drawn between inflammation arising from delayed-type hypersensitivity and inflammation with an infectious origin since a striking similarity exists in their symptoms, namely tenderness, erythematous swelling, induration, and local heating.

On diagnostic tests, inflammation from delayed-type hypersensitivity can show elevated levels of nonspecific acute phase proteins such as fibrinogen or CRP, which also happen to appear in testing for infection-induced acute inflammation. While ideally, culture identification should provide conclusive evidence of any bacterial infection, it often produces negative results due to its failure to isolate the causative bacteria [18]. Infection from HA filler injection is caused primarily by the introduction of the staphylococcus residing on the skin surface into the tissue, where it forms a biofilm around the injected filler. The staphylococcus then tends to maintain a low level of virulence to evade host immune response or the effect of antibiotics.

HA filler-related infection may also be caused by the activity of a nontuberculous mycobacterium. Based on the speed of growth, mycobacteria consist of the rapidly growing nontuberculous mycobacterium and the slow-growing nontuberculous mycobacterium. Of these, the rapid growers, specifically, M. fortuitum and M. abscessus are mainly responsible for the lesions caused during an invasive procedure. As a matter of fact, there is one case of M. abscessus infection following HA injection reported overseas, where the procedure had been performed by a nonlicensed injector [19]. Lesions of nontuberculous mycobacterial infection manifest as nodules, patches, or abscess.

Given the remarkable similarity in symptoms between inflammation arising from delayed-type hypersensitivity and infection-induced inflammation, both of which manifest as acute inflammatory reactions, the key distinguishing factor is the timing of their onset. An inflammatory reaction occurring within 2–3 days of treatment suggests infection, while inflammation developing at least 2–4 weeks after the HA injection most likely indicates delayed-type hypersensitivity. In the author's clinical experience, the longest duration from HA injection until the outbreak of inflammatory reactions around the site of filler injection was 16 months. Also, inflammation occurring sporadically in multiple sites is more likely to be a delayed-type hypersensitivity reaction. More specifically, inflammation spreading simultaneously or consecutively in multiple areas in and around the injection site indicates a delayed-type hypersensitivity reaction whereas infections tend to be confined mainly to one localized area. Of course, this does not represent the absolute criteria as delayed-type hypersensitivity reactions can also start initially from one localized area before developing in other facial regions with time. Infection may also involve the formation of an abscess, in which case a throbbing fluctuation may be felt in the infected area. The final point of differentiation is whether the symptoms respond to standalone treatments using steroid without the combined use of antibiotics, since infections do not respond to such monotherapy without antibiotics.

5.2.4 Treatment

Steroids alone provide effective treatment for inflammation from delayed-type hypersensitivity. A single intramuscular injection of 5 mg dexamethasone where practicable combined with oral administration of prednisolone 10 mg twice daily for 3–5 days results in complete resolution [16, 19]. The combined use of analgesics and anti-inflammatory drugs may be considered to relieve any accompanying pain. Significantly, antibiotics are not necessary for treating inflammations from delayed-type hypersensitivity as symptoms do not arise from an infection. While I had also previously relied on the combined use of antibiotics for treating delayed-type hypersensitivity due to fears of possible infection, since some 6 years ago I converted to the use of steroids alone, based on which 100% recovery is achieved. As previously noted, roughly 2/3 of hypersensitivity cases are cleared as a single isolated episode with no recurrent attacks. However, a relapse may occur in the remaining 1/3 of the cases 1–4 weeks following a successful resolution, in which case it is preferable to dissolve the problematic HA filler with hyaluronidase. Reversal of HA filler may be considered even upon initial presentation of the inflammation where symptoms are particularly severe or where a speedier 1-day recovery is desired. While no published guidelines are available regarding the appropriate dose of hyaluronidase, in my clinical experience, 30 U of hyaluronidase per each 0.1 mL of HA filler provides quick resolution as the HA filler softens within hours and completely dissolves away within a day.

5.2.5 Summary

To recap, HA represents the world's most widely used injectable filler for facial volumization owing to its biocompatibility and minimal immunogenicity. While rare, however, immune responses may occur following HA filler injections, and in ths respect, understanding the characteristics of delayed-type hypersensitivity reactions is critically important. Inflammations from delayed-type hypersensitivity share many clinical symptoms with infection but must be distinguished as the pertinent treatment is different.

In contrast to infection, delayed-type hypersensitivity characteristically develops with a time lag of at least 2–4 weeks if not several months from the HA injection, and responds favorably to steroid monotherapy without the combined use of antibiotics. While the exact cause of inflammation from delayed-type hypersensitivity remains unclear, I theorize that it is most likely caused by the delayed release of trace bacterial impurities or BDDE not properly removed during the purification of HA filler.

In my experience, I have anecdotally found that a patient treated using two different HA fillers in two different facial areas may present inflammatory reactions from delayed-type hypersensitivity only in the site injected with a particular HA product.

Also, I had patients who had previously developed an inflammatory reaction from delayed-type hypersensitivity to one brand of HA filler but were treated without event when switched on to a different HA fillerbrand. Finally, while rare, there have been cases where inflammatory reactions were found to reoccur months after the complete dissolution of the underlying HA filler.

While inflammation from delayed-type hypersensitivity arises primarily due to product/patient factors, patients may mistakenly assume it to be a technique issue on the part of the pratictitioner, and should therefore be alerted to such risks before treatment. In case a delayed-type hypersensitivity reaction occurs, steroids alone provide excellent treatment. However, in approximately 1/3 of the cases, a relapse may occur 1–4 weeks following successful treatment, in which case it is best to have the HA filler dissolved with hyaluronidase. The dissolved HA filler can be replaced with a different HA product if the patient so desires. Note, however, that hypersensitivity reactions may recur even after switching to a different HA filler. In this case, the use of HA filler should be contraindicated in the patient as recurrence suggests the patient has an inherent hypersensitivity to either the HA itself and/or the crosslinker.

5.3 Posttreatment Contour Irregularity

Contour irregularity represents the most common complication associated with the use of volumizing HA fillers. Depending on the underlying cause, they range from transient lumpiness from immediate postinjection swelling which resolves spontaneously within a week, or an uneven contour caused by inadequate placement technique or insufficient injection volume, to those occurring weeks or months following an otherwise successful procedure due to variations in individual physiological factors. Fortunately, such undesirable outcomes can readily be reversed by the administration of hyaluronidase to the extent HA filler had been used for the treatment.

Contour irregularity following a HA filler procedure falls largely into those stemming from the inadequate placement of HA filler and those developing gradually long after the initial HA filler procedure. Inadequate placement, in turn, is attributable to the practitioner's lack of skill or insufficient injection volume. Alternatively, it can also occur when only one localized area of the face is treated without regard to the balance and harmony with the rest of the face.

Meanwhile, there are cases where the irregularities may not be apparent in the first instance but appear over time due to the following factors: subsequent aggregation of HA filler caused by surrounding muscle contraction, gradual swelling of HA filler due to its hydrophilicity, or variations in the longevity of HA fillers at different facial regions [20]. This chapter elucidates the various underlying causes of posttreatment contour irregularities and provides the relevant strategies for their correction and management.

5.3.1 Inadequate Placement

5.3.1.1 Inadequate Positioning

Overfilling the lower pretarsal area during a pretarsal roll augmentation may cause the injected volume to spill over into the adjacent infraorbital fat region exacerbating the puffiness of any undereye bags. Likewise, overcorrection of the canine fossa during a nasolabial fold correction may cause the excess volume to migrate upward, creating a doughy, pillowy appearance in the nasolabial fat pads (Fig. 5.5).

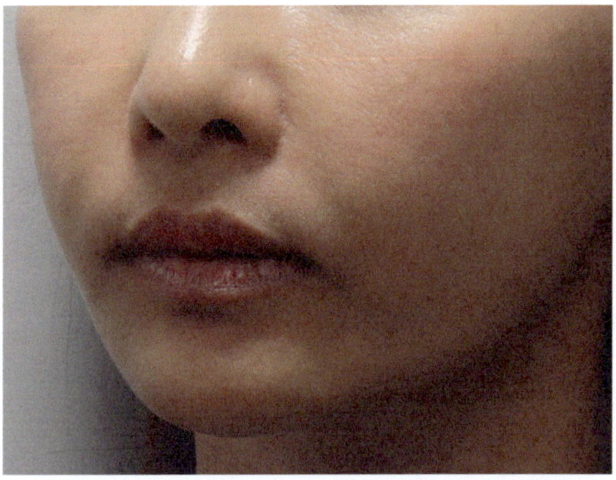

Fig. 5.5 A case of inadequate placement. Overcorrection of the canine fossa during a nasolabial fold correction may cause the excess volume to migrate upward, creating a doughy, pillowy appearance in the nasolabial fat pads

5.3.1.2 Inadequate Technique

While no facial region is immune to the risk of contour irregularity where suboptimal techniques have been employed, certain areas are particularly at risk, namely, the periorbital area where the skin is exceptionally thin and the nasal and frontal regions where only limited space is available for HA filler placement.

Irregularity is a common complication of forehead augmentation. Unevenness in forehead contour may occur immediately after HA injection or develop with a time lag of 3–6 months posttreatment due to the contraction of the surrounding muscles. The former is most likely the result of a suboptimal placement technique, that is, failure on the part of the practitioner to distribute filler evenly across the forehead. Such failures are more apt to occur with the use of a needle as opposed to a cannula. When I was first in practice, it was common practice to use a 1.25 cm sharp needle to perform forehead augmentation as cannulas had yet to be introduced at the time. The exercise was not only time-consuming but was also fraught with the risk of irregularities. In contrast, a cannula is ideal for creating a smooth, even forehead contour as its longer length allows better reach into multiple different areas across the forehead into which volume can be distributed evenly from a given entry point.

Meanwhile, the periorbital area, with its reduced dermal thickness, is also vulnerable to contour irregularities. For example, overcorrection of the tear trough can often lead to the development of the Tyndall effect or the appearance of disfiguring lumps. Unevenness can occur particularly where the HA filler is added in the tear trough only without considering the lack of volume in the malar region below to support it (Fig. 5.6). Treatment of sunken eyes with filler is also prone to developing unevenness in contour, which may become more noticeable when the eyes are closed (Fig. 4.23). Therefore, a moderate undercorrection is advised when treating the sunken eyes, preferably aiming for only 60–70% correction with the eyes open. Pretarsal roll augmentation is also susceptible to lumpiness where the injection lacks smooth consistency, or too little volume is injected into loose saggy lower pretarsal skin. Also, in patients with a history of lower eyelid blepharoplasty or trichiasis surgery, postsurgical scar tissue adhesions in the area tend to prevent adequate filler placement along the lash line and are likely to cause lumpiness even when the filler is placed inferior to the lash line (Fig. 4.28).

5.3.1.3 Insufficient Injection Volume

Occasionally, treatment may appear perfect in the first instance owing to the additional volume created by postinjection edema, only to reveal subtle irregularities 1–2 weeks later as the swelling subsides. It is necessary to inform the patient of this possibility in advance since he/she might otherwise misunderstand it as a technique issue. The patient should be further advised that the purpose of scheduling a follow-up visit 1–2 weeks post-treatment is so that any such opportunities for adjustments may be identified.

It also bears noting that the primary purpose of volumizing fillers is to literally *fill out* areas of volume deficit or depletion. As such, achieving an aesthetically desirable outcome can be elusive when working with an insufficient amount of HA filler. To draw an analogy, imagine filling a balloon with water. To inflate the balloon to capacity, a certain threshold volume of water is required. If not filled enough, the balloon would remain loose and saggy rather than becoming taut and tight. The amount of water required to fill the balloon in this case depends on the size of the balloon, that is, the larger the balloon, the more water that is needed. Likewise, the more severe the volume deflation, the larger the amount of filler that is required. Otherwise, contour irregularity would continue to persist (Fig. 3.15).

Significantly, however, it is a customary practice of many aesthetic clinics to charge patients by the number of syringes used, which creates an incentive for patients to demand minimum doses in order to lower their costs. Injecting too little,

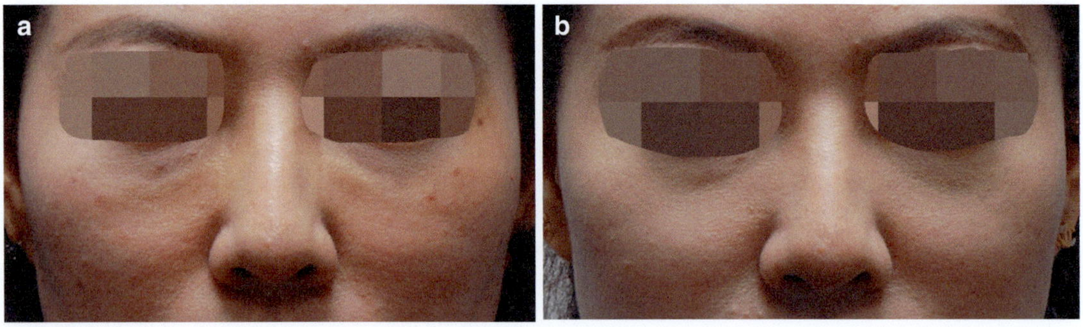

Fig. 5.6 (**a**) Unevenness after HA fller injection in the tear trough only without considering the lack of volume in the anterior malar region below to support it. (**b**) After hyaluronidase injection

however, often leads to suboptimal outcomes which the patient may attribute instead to faulty placement. Patients should therefore be counseled on the drawbacks of underfilling and be further advised that when it comes to facial volumization treatments the volume of injection also matters. The bottom line should be *to get more, they may need more*.

5.3.2 Inadequate Balance

Enumerated below are the key regions of the face where the overcorrection can take its toll, though the same cardinal principle holds true for practically any facial area treated with volumizing fillers; that is, there *can* be too much of a good thing.

1. Overfilling the nasal dorsum can widen the nose, creating the appearance of the *Avatar nose* or a *lion nose*. Unlike nasal implants carved and inserted to fit precisely onto the patient's nose, filler rhinoplasty consists of a fluid gel-type material injected in the dorsum to lift the overlying soft tissue from within. However, given that the tight skin envelope of the nose exerts as much downward pressure on the liquid filler as the filler pushing upward, excess volume placed with the intention of elevating the nasal dorsum may end up spreading sideways, broadening the nose as a consequence. For reference, the ratio between the width of dorsum to the nasal base should be 0.6 or less in men, and even smaller in a female nose.
2. The canine fossa located lateral to the nasal ala is a quintessential structure constituting a natural curvature of the face. Regardless, in all too many cases, overtreatment of the canine fossa during nasolabial fold correction tends to be a common occurrence (Fig. 5.5). Note that volume should be restored only up to a contour that looks natural. Completely effacing the subtle concavity naturally created by the canine fossa removes three-dimensionality from the face, blows the malar cheeks out of proportion, and in the extreme, gives a monkey-like appearance to the face. The *absence* of this vital structure on the face of a monkey bears noting in this respect.
3. Overtreating the central forehead during forehead augmentation without addressing the lateral forehead regions lying above the brows can lead to an odd localized protrusion in the middle of the forehead. Meanwhile, placing too much volume across the entire expanse of the forehead can produce a disproportionately bulbous forehead resembling that of a dolphin.
4. In patients with pronounced bilateral zygoma, volume added only in the medial malar to address infraorbital hollowness may cause lateral expansion of the cheeks as the injected volume blends with the fullness already present in the lateral zygomatic region. In such a case, concurrently filling the submalar depression and/or subzygomatic depressions (the posterior cheek) can help to subdue the cheekbone prominence due to optic illlusion.
5. Overfilling the pretarsal roll should be avoided as it may disrupt the balance and harmony of the eyes. Notably, an overly thick pretarsal roll in patients with horizontally short eye apertures can create a particularly odd, worm-like appearance (Fig. 4.31). Note that the ideal thickness of the pretarsal roll is within 30% of the length of the eye aperture (see Sect. 4.5.2).
6. To prevent the appearance of overdone, duck-like lips following lip augmentation, no more than 3 cc of filler should be injected in a single session. In patients with a naturally protruded upper lip, the practitioner may consider not injecting the upper lip at all or injecting conservative amounts only in its lateral aspects (Fig. 4.98).

5.3.3 Delayed Irregularity

As previously noted, the gradual appearance of irregularity in the injected area over time is generally attributable to the subsequent clumping of HA filler due to the surrounding muscle activity or to the hydrophilic tendency of HA to attract water and gain volume.

5.3.3.1 Aggregation of Filler Due to Muscle Contraction

HA is known for its excellent safety profile involving minimum adverse reactions in the body. Nonetheless, when placed in regions of heavy facial animation, corresponding muscle contractions may cause the filler to shift and migrate from the implanted site, resulting in aesthetically displeasing bulges and irregularities. Classic examples include HA filler placed in the forehead, glabella, and the infraorbital regions. The hyperactivity of frontalis or corrugator muscles following forehead augmentation may create subsequent dimples or indentations in the forehead, glabella, or above-brow areas. In severe cases, a large visible V-shaped indentation may develop across the glabella and the central forehead region, evoking the image of the classic animation character super robot *Mazinger Z.*

This occurs most commonly in patients who rely heavily on the frontalis m. to lift the upper eyelid due to a preexisting blepharoptosis, aging-related eyelid hooding, or other genetic factors. In such patients, BoNT-A injection is required in the forehead/and glabella regions both before and regularly after forehead augmentation to relax and minimize relevant muscle movement. The same applies when undertaking glabella volumization in patients with a hypertrophic corrugator m; adjunctive BoNT injection to the corrugator m. is required to prevent the migration and collection of HA filler.

The infraorbital region is also significantly impacted by surrounding muscle contractions. Protrusion of the hypertrophic medial muscular band of the orbicularis oculi m. during smiling is a normal and common occurrence in Koreans, found in as many as 50–60% of the population (Fig. 4.37). In people presenting such traits, however, HA filler or fat graft injected in the anteromedial malar may accentuate the appearance of this bulge upon smiling. With repeated muscle contraction, the filler may clump up and protrude even when the face is at rest. In such a case, adjunctive BoNT-A injection into the medial band of the orbicularis oculi m. before and after filler injection can help to avoid such occurrences.

5.3.3.2 Postinjection Swelling of HA Filler

Due to its hydrophilic nature, HA filler is known to expand compared to its original volume within 2–4 weeks of placement [20] (Fig. 2.14). On the upside, the propensity of HA filler to attract water from surrounding tissues and become voluminous contributes to increased longevity. However, undesired swelling when placed in areas of reduced dermal thickness such as the delicate periorbital region is a countervailing drawback.

The tear trough represents a key risk area in this respect as well as the lower pretarsal region where the thickening of pretarsal rolls due to the swelling of HA may appear *worm-like* and unnatural. The nasal bridge is also an area where the skin is thin and where the water retention property of HA can cause lateral expansion of HA filler, resulting in an unnaturally thick bulky nasal dorsum resembling a *lion nose*. In this respect, I made a serendipitous discovery many years ago in which I found that patients who routinely drank more than two liters of water per day were more susceptible to this phenomenon. I had a patient some 10 years ago who was treated in her tear trough with HA, but had to have the filler dissolved 2 weeks later due to excessive swelling. It took three iterations of reversing and reinjecting the HA filler to finally reach the desired outcome, and it was at some later point the patient conveyed to me that she made it a rule to regularly drink at least two liters of water per day.

Different types of HA fillers have different water absorption capacity. Monophasic HA fillers tend to demonstrate a higher water retention capacity compared with biphasic HA fillers. According to one study, monophasic HA fillers (Belotero®, Juvederm®) absorbed more water than biphasic HA fillers (Restylane®, Yvoir®) and demonstrated a greater incremental increase in volume 2–4 weeks postinjection vis-a-vis the initial injection volume (Fig. 2.14). Accordingly, biphasic HA filler is better suited for treating delicate areas such as the tear trough and the lower pretarsal region, as undesired bulging or expansion of HA filler is minimized.

5.3.3.3 Different Durations of Effect by Facial Region

The rate at which HA filler is metabolized by our body's enzyme depends on the amount of HA filler injected. Assuming the HA filler was injected in the form of a bolus, the injected volume would be the greatest at the center of the bolus while displaying a gradual tapering toward the peripheral aspects. Correspondingly, the thicker, more robust volume concentrated at the center is better able to withstand enzymatic biodegradation compared with the thinner peripheral volume which dissipates more quickly with time. A classic example is the HA filler placed in the anteriormedial malar region. Here, most of the peripheral volume would wear off within a space of 1–2 years, leaving only the central portion, reduced to the size of a button by this time, to become visible in patients with thin skin and little subcutaneous fat to cover it.

Likewise, HA filler injected superficially at the dermal or subdermal level tends to last considerably longer than the HA filler placed more deeply in the subcutaneous fat or muscular layers where it tends to break down more rapidly. For example, the superficially placed filler in the tear trough is generally well maintained for more than a year while the HA filler concurrently placed at the deep subcutaneous fat of the anterior malar tends to degrade more substantially during the same period. This may create an unnatural "ledge" in the lid–cheek junction as the superficial filler in the tear trough sits by itself with no structure to support it from below. To smoothen the transition in this case, a more feasible approach is to restore the lost volume in the anterior malar rather than dissolve the filler in the tear trough.

5.3.4 Solution: Administration of Hyaluronidase

Temporary lumpiness from postinjection reactive swelling is normal and to be expected during the first week of treatment. However, lumps and bumps continuing beyond the first 1–2 weeks deserve prompt resolution as they would persist for months if not years if left attended. While the ideal approach would be to strategically fill in areas of relative volume deficiency to even out the surface contour, in some cases the height of bump is such that this becomes impracticable. In such situations, reversing the HA filler with hyaluronidase is the only remaining alternative.

For complete dissolution of HA filler, hyaluronidase diluted to 150 U/mL should be administered at double the dose of the injected HA filler. For partial dissolution of a localized bump hyaluronidase should be injected at a diluted concentration of 30–50 U/mL [20] and a dose equal to the volume of the injected filler. Given the fluid nature of hyaluronidase injection, it should be noted that the actual pattern of HA dissolution cannot be predicted with precision and that the risk of over-dissolving or under-dissolving exists in any case.

The use of a cannula is generally preferred also for administering hyaluronidase to prevent tissue trauma and bruising. However, a 30G needle may become the preferred option where the body has formed a hard nodule or encapsulation around the HA filler due to collagen stimulation.

Precaution must be taken when injecting hyaluronidase, given its animal origin as allergic reactions to hyaluronidase, including erythema and edema, may continue for several days. Prior allergy skin test on the patient's forearm is therefore strongly advised. Positive testing requires intravenous injection of steroids and antihistamine prior to the hyaluronidase injection.

Hyaluronidase takes immediate effect and completely dissolves the filler within hours of injection [8]. Any reapplication of HA following its reversal should preferably be undertaken after 1 day has elapsed. Considering that hyaluronidase has a short half-life of several minutes, HA filler may theoretically be injected back after 8 h of administering hyaluronidase. That said, in my clinical experience where I had HA filler dissolved in the morning and reapplied in the evening of the same day, I perceived that a certain amount of the freshly applied filler was partially affected by the lingering hyaluronidase (See the Sect. 5.4).

5.4 The Adequate Use of Hyaluronidase

HA dominates the world market for injectable fillers driven significantly by its excellent safety profile as a natural constituent of the human soft tissue that is well-tolerated by the body. That aside, it can be said that the true beauty of HA filler lies in its reversibility, the assurance that results could be dissolved instantaneously if so desired using hyaluronidase as the reversal agent. In my earlier practice, I had once worked with semi-permanent synthetic fillers such as polyacrylamide gel (PAAG)-based Aquamid® or polymethylmethacrylate (PMMA)-based Artecoll® or collagen stimulators such as Radiesse® which provided prolonged longevity. However, after experiencing a few cases where I was unable to assist patients who, due to fluctuations in their facial dimensions from subsequent weight gains, wished to have the filler removed 1–2 years posttreatment, I converted entirely to using only HA fillers in my practice. Contingencies may occur even in the most experienced hands, and for the sake of ensuring peace of mind as well as my own longevity (!), I opted to use only fully reversible HA fillers.

In volumizing HA filler treatments, hyaluronidase is commonly used to treat overcorrection or unevenness from HA filler placement. Temporary lumpiness from immediate postinjection swelling is normal and to be expected during the first week of treatment. However, lumps and bumps persisting beyond the initial 1–2 weeks deserve prompt resolution since they would persist for months if not years if left addressed. The use of hyaluronidase is also a critical step in responding to vascular complications arising from embolization by the HA filler, in which case hyaluronidase should be injected to flush the occluded blood vessel of the filler embolus. This chapter provides specific details concerning the use of hyaluronidase as the dissolving agent of HA, including the pharmacological mechanism of action, the clinical use of hyaluronidase for correcting HA filler misplacement, the clinical use of hyaluronidase for managing vascular complications, and potential adverse events associated with its administration.

5.4.1 Pharmacological Characteristics

Hyaluronic acid, as a constituent of the body's extracellular matrix, plays a pivotal role in providing the tissue with the necessary structural support, in modulating cellular migration and proliferation, and in regulating inflammation and wound repair/regeneration. In the human body, 50% of the native hyaluronic acid exists in the skin, while the rest is present in various other parts of the body such as the joints and the eyes. Hyaluronic acid absorbs moisture in the tissues to keep the tissue lubricated and hydrated while providing it with structural support. Meanwhile, as an enzyme, hyaluronidase is responsible for breaking down the glucosaminidic bond between C1 of the *N*-acetylglucosamine and C4 of the D-glucuronic acid in the hyaluronic acid [22]. By catalyzing the hydrolysis of the HA and effectively breaking up the cellular linkages in the interstitial tissue, hyaluronidase spurs the dispersion and absorption of injected drugs into the interstitial tissue while promoting the resorption of extravasated fluids back into the tissue.

Consequently, it is used clinically for hastening the absorption of postsurgical hematoma or edema in plastic surgery; for enhancing the diffusion and permeation of drugs such as local anesthetics; and also for hypodermoclysis, i.e., the subcutaneous administration of fluid in conjunction with other drugs in infants and elderly patients who are not amenable to receiving an intravenous injection. 1 U of hyaluronidase is defined as the enzyme dosage discharged for degrading 1 μmole of *N*-acetylglucosamine at 37 °C pH 4 for 1 min [23]. The relevant dose/strength of commercial hyaluronidases varies depending on manufacturers from 150 to 2000 U (2000 U/vial) per vial, though variations may exist between different products and formulations. Six types of human hyaluronidase have been reported in humans, including HYAL-1, -2, -3, -4, HYALP1, and PH20.

5.4.2 **Products** (Fig. 5.7)

In the United States, bovine testicular hyaluronidase Hydase™ (PrimaPharm, Inc.), bovine tes-

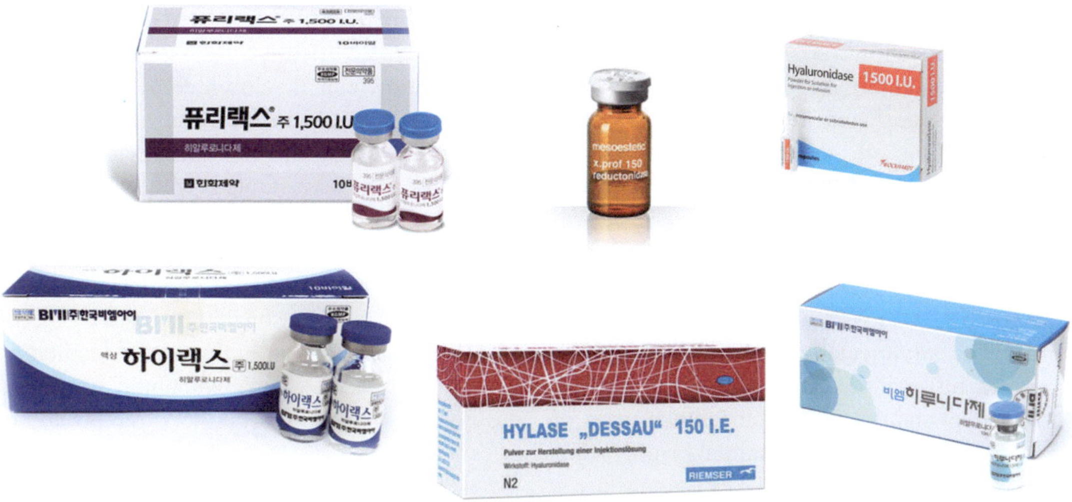

Fig. 5.7 Commercial hyaluronidase products

Table 5.2 Hyaluronidase products (available in the market)

Country	Brand name	Manufacturer	Type	Dose	Source
Korea	Hirax Injection 0.15%	BMIkorea	Solution	750IU/0.5 ml 2000IU/1.3 ml 1500IU/1 ml 5000IU/3.4 ml	Bovine
Korea	Purirax Inj	Hanwha Pharma Co, Ltd.	Solution	1500IU/1 ml	Bovine
Korea	Liporase Inj.	DaehanNew Pharm Co, Ltd.	Powder	1500 IU	Bovine
Korea	BM Hylunidase Inj.	BMIkorea	Powder	1500 IU	Bovine
Korea	Hyalase Inj.	Huons. Co, Ltd.	Powder	1500 IU	Bovine
USA	Vitrase	Bausch&Lomb incorporated	Solution	200 IU	Ovine (sheep)
USA	Hylenex recombinant	Halozyme Therapeutics, Inc.	Solution	150 IU	rHuPH20 (recombinant human hyaluronidase)
Germany	Hyalase Dessau	Riemser Pharma GmbH	Powder	150 IU 300 IU	Bovine
Ireland	Hyalase	Wockhardt UK Limited	Powder	1500 IU	Ovine
Spain	Reductonidasa	Mesoestetic Pharma	Solution	1500 IU	Bovine
Brazil	Hyaluronidase 2000	Biometil Swiss	Powder	2000 IU	Bovine

ticular hyaluronidase Amphadase® (Amphastar Pharmaceutical Inc.), ovine testicular hyaluronidase Vitrase® (ISTA Pharmaceutical), and human recombinant DNA-derived hyaluronidase (r-HuPH20) Hylenex® (Halozyme Therapeutics) have been approved for use. In Korea, there are more than 27 brands of hyaluronidase currently available on the market including Hyalase® (Huons), BM Hylunidase® (SH-Pharm), H-Lase® (Kuhnil Pharm), and Hirax® (BMI Korea) with an identical product marketed under the tradename PURIRAX® by HanWha Pharma, all of which are derived from bovine sources (Fig. 5.7) (Table 5.2). Incidence of allergic reaction varies by formulation. Among Korean products, notably, Hirax® (BMI Korea) is a hyaluronidase preparation in injectable form which reportedly has achieved more than 95% purity and hence a dramatic reduction in allergic reactions arising from extraneous impurities remaining in the product. Except for Vitrase®, Hylenex® and Hirax® supplied as a liquid formulation, all others are available in the form of powder for injection which require reconstitution with normal saline. Upon reconstitution, the product must be stored at refrigeration and used preferably within 10 hours considering its loss of potency over time. Hirax®, as an injectable solution, should be stored at refrigeration while the other powder formulatons should be kept at temperatures of 25 °C or below.Due to their animal origin, products derived either from bovine or ovine sources may contain remnants of protein impurities remaining in the product, which may trigger undesired immunogenic responses. Incidence of allergic reaction varies by product. Notably, Hirax® (BMI Korea) as an injectable solution has reportedly achieved more than 95% purity and hence a dramatic reduction in allergic reactions arising from any extraneous impurities remaining in the product.

5.4.3 Use of Hyaluronidase in the Correction of HA Filler Placement (Table 5.3)

5.4.3.1 Dilution and Concentration of Hyaluronidase

Most commercial hyaluronidase products in Korea are available in the form of powder for solution contained in 1500 U/mL vials. Hence, they must be reconstituted with an adequate amount of saline solution. The pertinent concentration of hyaluronidase to be used for dissolving HA filler is open to debate. At the very least, however, it should reasonably be higher than the 15 U/mL concentration indicated for facilitating retrobulbar anesthesia in ophthalmic surgery to ensure minimum impact on the vitreous body of the eyeball.

While a hyaluronidase concentration of 20 U/mL is described as sufficient for reversing HA according to a prospective controlled study of dissolution of HA placed in the human dorsum, my preferred concentration for completely dissolving the HA filler is 150 U/mL [24]. The concentration of 20–30 U/mL described in the study may be entirely valid for making partial corrections as a higher dose of 50 U/mL, in my experience, tends to degrade not only the excess amount of HA but also HA placed in adjacent areas (Fig. 5.8). That said, a higher concentration of 150 U/mL is clinically preferable for the complete removal of HA, as it delivers full resolution in a single session. For

Table 5.3 Recommended use of hyaluronidase for filler procedure

Indication		Concentration of hyaluronidase	Volume of hyaluronidase	Needle vs Cannula
Partial dissolution	Tiny bumps in upper eyelid, and tear trough	20–50 U/mL	0.1–0.3 mL	Cannula
	Overcorrection or irregularity in the cheeks	20–50 U/mL	0.5–1 mL depending on the size of correction	Cannula
Complete dissolution	Overcorrection	150 U/mL	Hyaluronidase corresponding to at least 2–3 times the volume of the injected filler is required	Cannula
	Round, palpable encapsulations	150 U/mL	0.5–1 mL	Needle
	Where previous attempts at dissolution have proved unsatisfactory	1500 U/mL	1–2 mL	Needle
Inflammation		150 U/mL	2–4 mL per site	Cannula
Vascular complications	Intravascular embolization	750 U/mL	3–6 mL	Needle
	Blindness	1500 U/mL	3–6 mL	Cannula

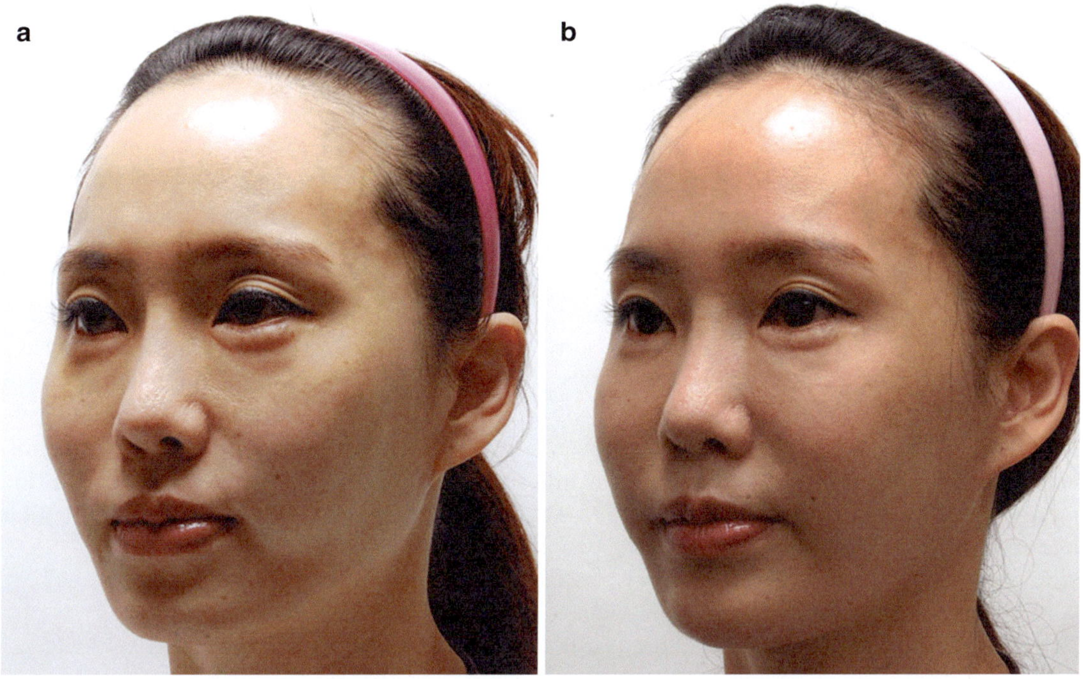

Fig. 5.8 Disfiguring irregularities caused by inappropriate HA filler injection, thread lifting and liposuction was improved using the combined treatment involving hyalurodiase for addressing the lumpiness in the pretarsal roll and tear trough, and filler for restoring the depressed area

partial removal of HA filler, I inject small doses of hyaluronidase at a reduced concentration of 20–50 U/mL to minimize the impact on the adjacent volume. On the other hand, where the HA filler had proven to be resistant to dissolution with hyaluronidase, I use a ten times higher concentration 1500 U/mL by reconstituting hyaluronidase into a 1 mL solution.

5.4.3.2 Injection Dosage of Hyaluronidase

The dosing of hyaluronidase for HA dissolution varies according to the specific indication. To completely dissolve the filler, hyaluronidase (150 U/mL) corresponding to at least 2–3 times the volume of the injected filler is administered. Where the exact volume of the injected filler cannot be determined, 2–4 mL (300–600 U) of hyaluronidase per site is advised as a general rule of thumb. For partial dissolution, hyaluronidase should be injected at both reduced doses and lower concentrations. Hyaluronidase dosage is also adjusted according to the size of the area and the overcorrection to be treated. For example, for fine corrections of tiny bumps in small areas such as the pretarsal roll, upper eyelid, and tear trough, 0.1–0.3 mL of hyaluronidase diluted to 20–50 U/mL is advised according to the size of the bump. On the other hand, when addressing overcorrection or irregularities in larger areas such as the cheeks, a higher dose of 0.5–1 mL is advisable depending on the size of excess volume injected. Gentle massage with fingers on the injected site helps to dissolve the HA and immediate dissolution of HA can be felt by palpation.

5.4.3.3 Cannula vs. Needle

The use of a cannula is preferred to prevent the risk of bruising while delivering hyaluronidase. That notwithstanding, the use of a 30G needle is advised for piercing and dissolving round, palpable encapsulations, or where previous attempts at dissolution have proved unsatisfactory, or otherwise where granuloma or scar-like hardness is present.

5.4.3.4 Timing of HA Filler Reinjection

Most patients wish to have their HA filler redone following the dissolution of the problematic HA with hyaluronidase. In this respect, the optimal timing of HA filler reinjection becomes an issue, given concerns over the lingering impact of hyaluronidase. Views are divided on this point, with some suggesting an interval of 2–3 days before HA reinjection and others describing a much longer timeframe of 2–4 weeks to avoid the action of residual hyaluronidase. However, given the short half-life of hyaluronidase, HA filler may safely be injected back 1 day after the injection of hyaluronidase. This is corroborated by the findings of a rat study, which shows HA filler reinjected in rats 6 hrs after dissolution with hyaluronidase managed to substantially regain most of the previous shape and volume [25].

Certainly, in my own clinical experience where I regularly dissolve and reinject HA filler in more than 3–4 patients per day, I have never encountered any issues when HA filler was replaced the day after its dissolution with hyaluronidase. Even in the one isolated case where the filler was dissolved in the morning and reapplied 8 h later in the evening due to the patient's scheduled departure the following day, I merely perceived a smaller-than-expected volume augmentation at follow-up. Conceivably, this suggests HA filler may be reinjected as early as 6 h following its reversal in certain inexplicable circumstances.

5.4.3.5 Reinjection of Hyaluronidase

Given the short half life of hyaluronidase which lasts for only a few minutes in blood, the injection may be repeated 5 minutes after the first injection if residual amounts of HA filler is palpated. Occasionally, the patient may request reinjection of hyaluronidase following the initial administration, stating that the underlying HA filler had not been fully dissolved. Indeed, in some cases, residual amounts of HA filler may be palpated upon physical examination. In other cases, the problematic HA may no longer be palpable contrary to the patient's belief. Reinjection of hyaluronidase generally follows the same approach as the initial injection, except where any soft encapsulations or hard nodules can be felt, in which case a needle should be used for performing the injection, with the relevant dose upscaled to 750 U/mL. Occasionally, even after the reinjection of hyaluronidase and despite the absence of palpable lumps, the patient may remain unconvinced that the filler had been effectively removed, requesting repeat treatment for the third or fourth round. In other cases, what may initially have been perceived as a hard nodule from the HA injection may turn out to have been a previous fat graft or Sculptra. To avoid further doubt and to spare the need for unnecessary intervention, it may be helpful to use ultrasonic devices to conclusively establish the presence or absence of any lingering HA filler in the tissue (see Sect. 5.4.8).

5.4.4 Use of Hyaluronidase for Managing Inflammation from Delayed-type Hypersensitivity to HA or Bacterial Infection

Though rare, acute inflammation may occur from bacterial infection during HA filler treatment, calling for the immediate removal of the product. Also, in the rare case where the patient develops delayed-type hypersensitivity to the cross-linking agent BDDE or trace impurities such as the residual bacterial protein, DNA, or the intracellular organelle not fully removed during the HA filler manufacturing process, the underlying filler may need to be removed (see Sect. 5.3). Here, sufficient dosing of hyaluronidase 150 U/mL injected at doses of 2–4 mL per site (i.e., 300–600 U in total) is advised to achieve complete degradation of the HA filler.

5.4.5 Use of Hyaluronidase in the Treatment of Vascular Complications from HA Filler Injection

In the event of a vascular embolization due to intravascular filler injection or vascular insufficiency from the compression of weak vessels by the surrounding HA filler, the HA filler at issue must immediately be dissolved away with hyaluronidase. While it is next to impossible to inject hyaluronidase into the precise location in the vessel where the occlusion is present, it has been postulated by Di Lorenzi et al. that hyaluronidase infused in sufficient amounts generally around the area where ischemic symptoms are present may effectively traverse and diffuse *across* the arterial wall to reach the hyaluronic acid held in the blood vessel. Hence, in order to dissolve occlusions of hyaluronic acid fillers, it is advised to infiltrate hyaluronidase subcutaneously in copious amounts (3–6 mL) at a high concentration (750 U/mL) around the tissue where ischemic symptoms such as blanching, greyish decolorization, or mottled erythema are present. The effective timing of hyaluronidase injection for such vascular events is within 24 hrs of HA filler injection. This is also backed up by the findings of an animal study in which vascular occlusion was induced in rabbit ears using HA filler, to which hyaluronidase was subsequently injected at different intervals. While hyaluronidase injected within 4 hrs was beneficial in clearing the occlusion, it had little effect after 24 hours. Accordingly, patients demonstrating even the slightest signs of ischemia should be observed for 20–30 mins in the office for any further development of symptoms. Progression of symptoms calls for immediate injection of hyaluronidase for an effective resolution. Regardless, there may still be some value to giving hyaluronidase injections even after the 24-hour window as a placebo for the patient, while protecting the practitioner from the legal consequences of denying such intervention.

5.4.6 Allergic Reaction to Hyaluronidase and Allergy Testing

Allergic reaction to hyaluronidase injection may be caused either by the enzyme itself or by other extraneous protein impurities in the product as most commercial hyaluronidase products consist of protein derived from bovine or ovine testicular tissue. The reported incidence of allergic reactions to hyaluronidase varies widely, ranging from 0.1% to 7%, depending on the product. The vast majority of these reactions are antibody-mediated Type 1 hypersensitivity reactions with typical symptoms being angioedema with severe erythema and edema, or, in more serious situations, anaphylaxis. Though rare, the onset of symptoms may start hours from the exposure to hyaluronidase or even on the next day. While occurring primarily in patients who have previously been treated with hyaluronidase for dissolving HA filler, allergic reactions to hyaluronidase may occur even upon the first exposure independent of such treatment history. In those without a prior history of hyaluronidase injection, allergic reactions may occur instead as a result of an allergy to bovine protein or even from a previous bee venom therapy, given that hyaluronidase is also found in fire ants, bees, and arthropods such as scorpions.

Alternatively, the patient may have been unknowingly sensitized to hyaluronidase by receiving fat dissolving injections or facial contouring injections from aesthetic clinics whose proprietary formulations not disclosed to the patient happened to contain hyaluronidase. Simply put, allergies may develop irrespective of previous hyaluronidase injections. As such, a preliminary skin test must be performed as a matter of course, to determine the presence of allergies in patients wishing to undergo hyaluronidase treatment. The skin test is undertaken by an intradermal injection of 0.1 mL of 150 Unit/mL hyaluronidase in the forearm. The development of erythema or a red raised wheal with pseudopods appearing within 15 min accompanied by localized itching indicates a positive reaction (Fig. 5.9).

Note once again that, although rare, allergic reactions may not appear until several hours later, if not until the day following hyaluronidase injection. Where the patient tests positive, intravenous injection of *dexamethasone* (1 ampoule) combined with antihistamine Avil (1 ampoule) administered 10 min prior to hyaluronidase injection provides effective cover against allergic reactions, if not reducing the symptoms to a mild edema. Oral prednisolone 10 mg bid 8 mg for 2 days is also prescribed following treatment.

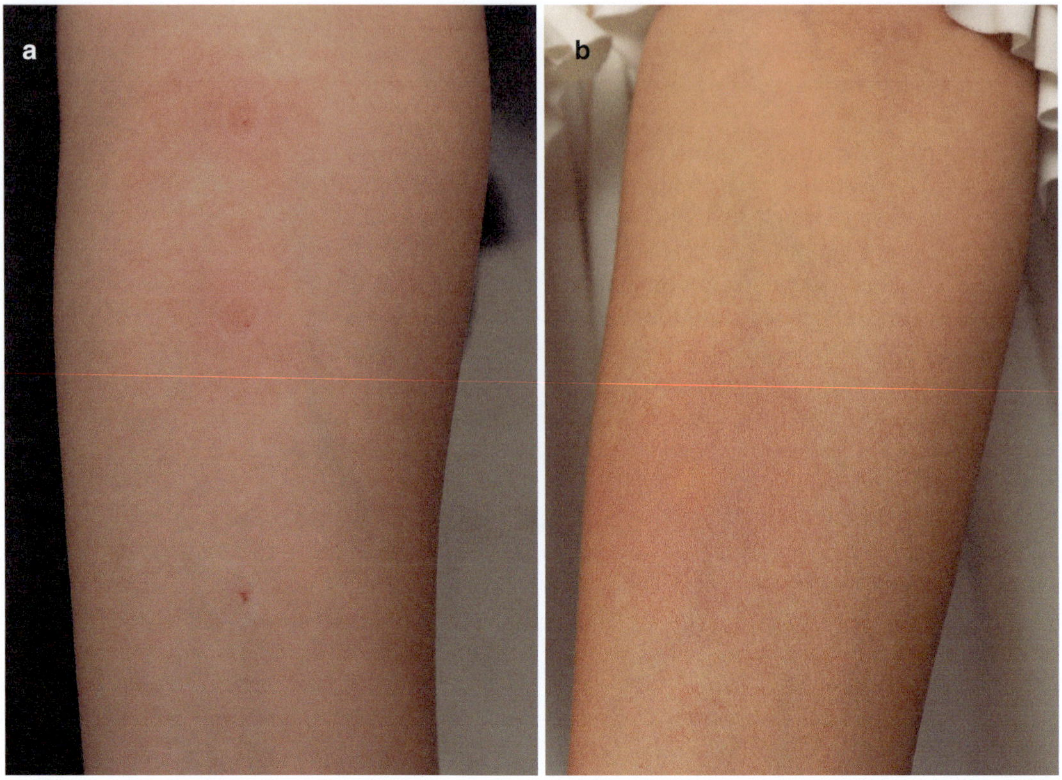

Fig. 5.9 The skin test for the hyaluronidase. (**a**) Liporase®; positive, hylunidase®; positive, Hirax®; negative. (from the top to bottom). (**b**) The development of erythema or a red raised wheal with pseudopods appearing within 15 minutes accompanied by localized itching, indicates a positive reaction

The incidence of allergic reaction varies by product. Among Korean products, Hirax® (BMI Korea), with identical product marketed under the trade name PURIRAX® by HanWha Pharma Co., Ltd., has shown a relatively lower incidence of allergic reactions. Notably, Hirax® (BMI Korea) is a hyaluronidase preparation in injectable form, which reportedly demonstrates more than 95% purity and results in a dramatic reduction in allergic reactions arising from impurities.

5.4.7 Skin Atrophy

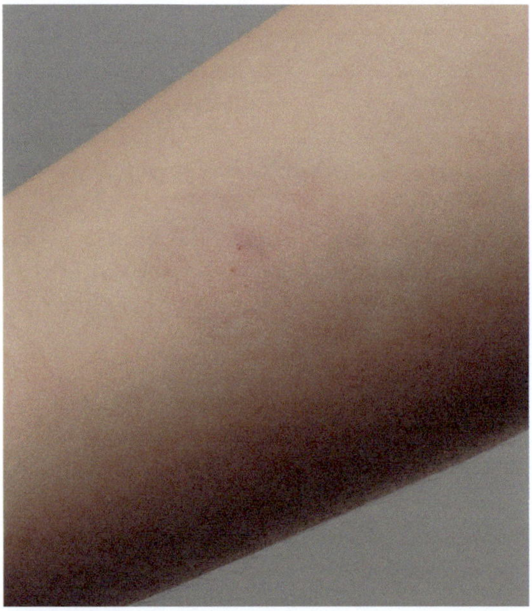

Fig. 5.10 Skin atrophy deveoped on the forearm after allergy testing for hyaluronidase

Granted, hyaluronidase may dissolve the body's own native hyaluronic acid in the skin or tissue (Fig. 5.10). Significantly, hyaluronidase injection made directly into the dermis is highly likely to induce skin atrophy, given that more than 50%

of the body's naturally occurring hyaluronic acid is present in the skin (Fig. 5.11). By contrast, hyaluronidase injected in the subcutaneous fat will not cause any visible deformities or atrophic indentations on the skin surface since the level of hyaluronic acid contained in the subcutaneous fatty layer is much lower by default. In my practice, I regularly inject hyaluronidase subcutaneously to dissolve HA filler at doses as high as 300–600 U. Yet, I have never encountered any noticeable skin atrophy or tissue deformation in my patients, even though I typically handle more than 3–4 such cases on any given day. Even when hyaluronidase is injected in the dermis, it will not cause long-term detriment to the skin, as the body substantially replenishes the native hyaluronic acid within 2 weeks, allowing the skin to naturally regains its normal integrity within 1 month.

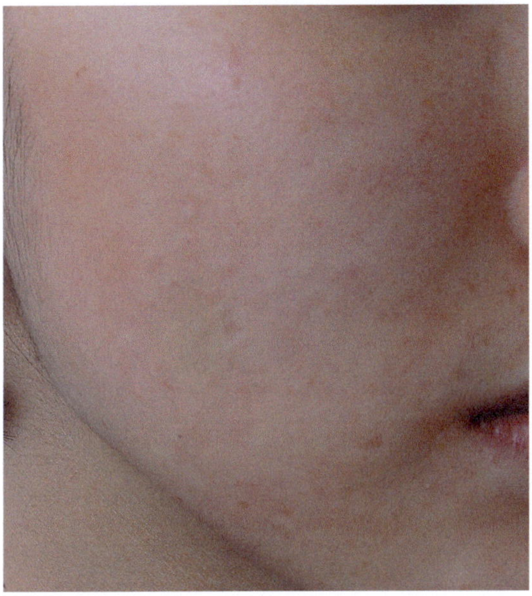

Fig. 5.11 Multiple atrophied depressions in face developed after intradermal injection of hyaluronidase with the concentration of 500 U/ml

5.4.8 Use of Ultrasonic Imaging to Establish the Presence of HA in the Tissue

In ultrasonic scans, HA is easily distinguished from other tissues since it consists of 99% water and appears anechoic (black) on ultrasound image (Fig. 5.12). Therefore, the use of ultrasound can be instrumental in locating the HA filler before its dissolution or establishing the specific nature of the material in question, that is, whether it consists of dissolvable HA filler or any other substance (Fig. 5.13).

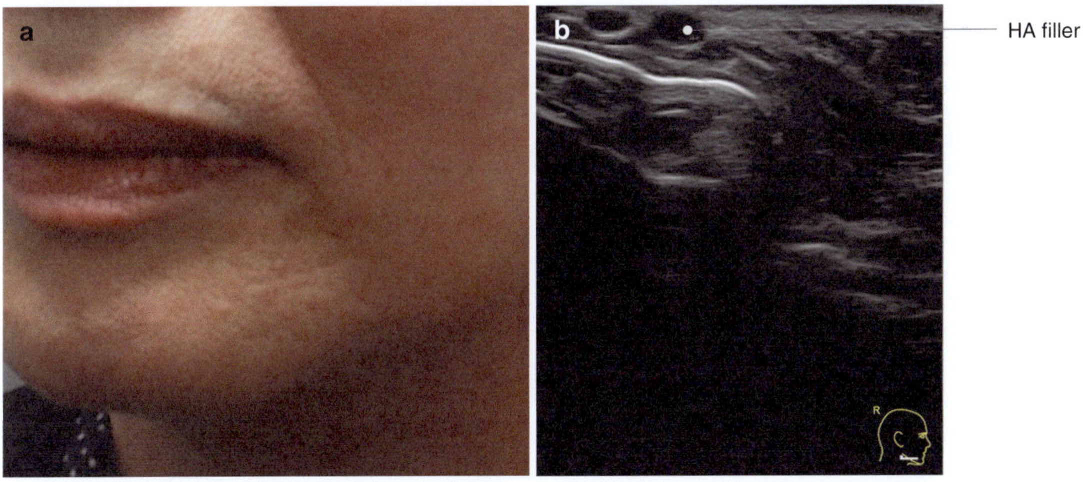

Fig. 5.12 (**a**) Small nodules are observed 1 year after HA filler injection for the treatment of marrionett lines. (**b**) Two round anechoi nodules are observed by ultrasound evaluation

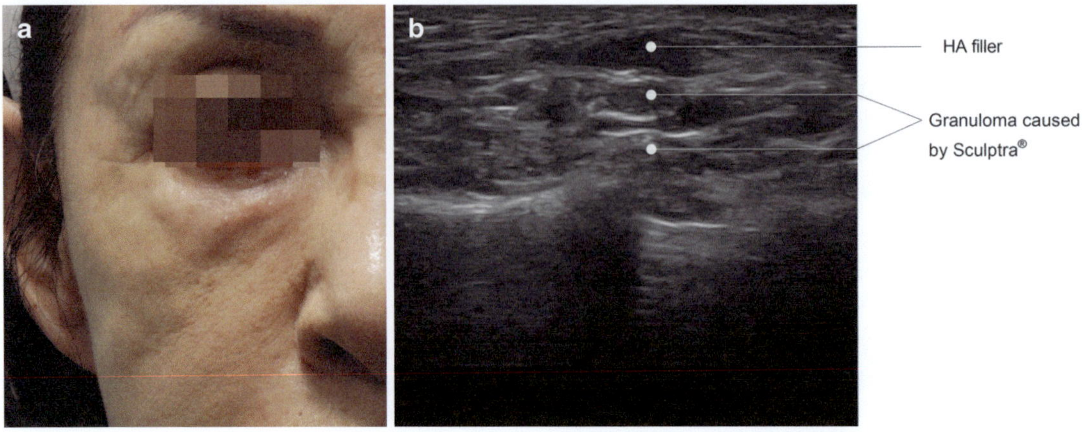

Fig. 5.13 (**a**) Irregularity cuased by Sculptra® injection into the infraorbital depression. (**b**) Hyperechoic masses are observed by ultrasound evaluation

References

1. Kim HJ, Kyle Seo HK, Lee JS. Kim. In: Clinical anatomy for botulinum toxin and filler injection. Berlin: Springer; 2016.
2. Beleznay K, Jones D. Vascular compromise. In: Carruthers J, Carruthers A, editors. Soft tissue augmentation. Philadelphia: Elsevier; 2018. p. 185–9.
3. Bolton JG, Fabi SG. Complications of Temporary Fillers. In: Carruthers J, Carruthers A, editors. Soft tissue augmentation. Philadelphia: Elsevier; 2018. p. 191–201.
4. DeLorenzi C. Complications of injectable fillers, part 2: vascular complications. Aesthet Surg J. 2014;34(4):584–600.
5. Kim DW, Yoon ES, Ji YH, Park SH, Lee BI, Dhong ES. Vascular complications of hyaluronic acid fillers and the role of hyaluronidase in management. J Plast Reconstr Aesthet Surg. 2011;64:1590–5.
6. Beleznay K, JDA C, Humphrey S, Jones D. Avoiding and treating blindness from fillers: a review of the world literature. Dermatol Surg. 2015;41:1097–117.
7. Park KH, Kim YK, Woo SJ, Kang SW, Lee WK, Choi KS, Kwak HW, Yoon H, Huh K, Kim JW. Iatrogenic occlusion of the ophthalmic artery after cosmetic facial filler injections a national survey by the Korean retina society. JAMA Ophthalmol. 2014;132(6):714–23.
8. Casabona G, Montes JR, Marchese P. Reversers. In: Carruthers J, Carruthers A, editors. Soft tissue augmentation. Philadelphia: Elsevier; 2018. p. 215–26.
9. Zhu GZ, Sun ZS, Liao WX, Cai B, Chen CL, Zheng HH, Zeng L, Luo SK. Efficacy of retrobulbar hyaluronidase injection for vision loss resulting from hyaluronic acid filler embolization. Aesthet Surg J. 2017;38(1):12–22.
10. Surek CC, Said SA, Perry JD, Zins JE. Retrobulbar injection for hyaluronic acid gel filler-induced blindness: a review of efficacy and technique. Aesthet Plast Surg. 2019;43(4):1034–40.
11. Lee W, Oh W, Ko HS, Lee SY, Kim KW, Yang EJ. Effectiveness of retrobulbar hyaluronidase injection in an iatrogenic blindness rabbit model using hyaluronic acid filler injection. Plast Reconstr Surg. 2019;144(1):137–43.
12. Parness G, Underhill S. Regional anesthesia for intraocular surgery. Contin Educ Anaesth Crit Care Pain. 2005;5(3):93–7.
13. Kumar CM, Eid H, Dodds C. Sub-Tenon's anaesthesia: complications and their prevention. Eye (Lond). 2011;25(6):694–703.
14. Gell PGH, Coombs RRA, editors. Clinical aspects of immunology. 1st ed. Oxford, England: Blackwell; 1963.
15. Ahn JS. J Korean Soc Dermatol Surg. 2017;4:41–7.
16. Alijotas-Reig J, Garcia-Gimenez V. Delayed immune-mediated complications related to hyaluronic acid and acrylic hydrogel dermal fillers: clinical findings, long-term follow-up, and review of the literature. J Eur Acad Dermatol Venereol. 2008;22(2):150–61.
17. Roh NK. The things filler manufacturers won't let you know. Filler Toxin. 2018;2018:31–4.
18. Friedman PM, Mafong EA, Kauvar AN, Geronemus RG. Safety data of injectable nonanimal stabilized hyaluronic acid gel for soft tissue augmentation. Dermatol Surg. 2002;28:491–4.
19. Beleznay K, Carruthers JD, Carruthers A, et al. Delayed-onset nodules secondary to a smooth, cohesive 20mg/ml hyaluronic acid filler: cause and management. Dermatol Surg. 2015;41(8):929–39.
20. Park KY, Kim JM, Seok J, Seo SJ, Kim MN, Youn CS. Comparative split-face study of durational

changes in hyaluronic acid fillers for mid-face volume augmentation. Dermatol Ther. 2019;32(4):e12950. https://doi.org/10.1111/dth.12950.

21. Juhász MLW, Levin MK, Marmur ES. The kinetics of reversible hyaluronic acid filler injection treated with hyaluronidase. Dermatol Surg. 2017;43(6):841–7.
22. Ferraz RM, Sandkvist U, Lundgren B. Degradation of hylauronic acid fillers using hyaluronidase in an in vivo model. J Drugs Dermatol. 2018;17(5):548–53.
23. Dunn AL, et al. Hyaluronidase: a review of approved formulations, indications and off-label use in chronic pain management. Expert Opin Biol Ther. 2010;10(1):127–31.
24. Margit LW Juhász, Melissa K Levin, Ellen S Marmur. The Kinetics of Reversible Hyaluronic Acid Filler Injection Treated With Hyaluronidase Dermatol Surg. 2017;43(6):841–7.
25. Kim HJ, Kwon SB, Whang KU, Lee JS, Park YL, Lee SY. The duration of hyaluronidase and optimal timing of hyaluronic acid (HA) filler reinjection after hyaluronidase injection. J Cosmet Laser Ther. 2018;20(1):52–7.

MIX
Papier aus verantwortungsvollen Quellen
Paper from responsible sources
FSC® C105338

If you have any concerns about our products,
you can contact us on
ProductSafety@springernature.com

In case Publisher is established outside the EU,
the EU authorized representative is:
Springer Nature Customer Service Center GmbH
Europaplatz 3, 69115 Heidelberg, Germany

Printed by Libri Plureos GmbH
in Hamburg, Germany